THE WASHINGTON MANUAL™

Rheumatology   Subspecialty Consult

Second Edition

Editors

Leslie E. Kahl, MD
Professor of Medicine
Department of Internal Medicine
Division of Rheumatology
Washington University School of Medicine
St. Louis, Missouri

Series Editors

Thomas M. De Fer, MD
Professor of Internal Medicine
Washington University School of Medicine
St. Louis, Missouri

Katherine E. Henderson, MD
Assistant Professor of Clinical Medicine
Department of Medicine
Division of Medical Education
Washington University School of Medicine
Barnes-Jewish Hospital
St. Louis, Missouri

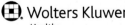 Wolters Kluwer | Lippincott Williams & Wilkins
Health
Philadelphia • Baltimore • New York • London
Buenos Aires • Hong Kong • Sydney • Tokyo

Senior Acquisitions Editor: Sonya Seigafuse
Senior Product Manager: Kerry Barrett
Vendor Manager: Bridgett Dougherty
Senior Marketing Manager: Kimberly Schonberger
Manufacturing Manager: Ben Rivera
Design Coordinator: Stephen Druding
Editorial Coordinator: Katie Sharp
Production Service: Aptara, Inc.

**WE
39
W319
2012**

© **2012 by Department of Medicine, Washington University School of Medicine**

Printed in China

Library of Congress Cataloging-in-Publication Data
The Washington manual rheumatology subspecialty consult. — 2nd ed. /editor, Leslie E. Kahl.
    p. ; cm.
    Rheumatology subspecialty consult
    Includes bibliographical references and index.
    ISBN 978-1-4511-1412-6 (alk. paper) — ISBN 1-4511-1412-5 (alk. paper)
    I. Kahl, Leslie E.   II. Title: Rheumatology subspecialty consult.
    [DNLM: 1. Rheumatic Diseases—diagnosis—Handbooks.   2. Rheumatic Diseases—
therapy—Handbooks. WE 39]
616.7′23—dc23

                                                                2012004717

The Washington Manual™ is an intent-to-use mark belonging to Washington University in St. Louis to which international legal protection applies. The mark is used in this publication by LWW under license from Washington University.

Care has been taken to confirm the accuracy of the information presented and to describe generally accepted practices. However, the authors, editors, and publisher are not responsible for errors or omissions or for any consequences from application of the information in this book and make no warranty, expressed or implied, with respect to the currency, completeness, or accuracy of the contents of the publication. Application of the information in a particular situation remains the professional responsibility of the practitioner.

The authors, editors, and publisher have exerted every effort to ensure that drug selection and dosage set forth in this text are in accordance with current recommendations and practice at the time of publication. However, in view of ongoing research, changes in government regulations, and the constant flow of information relating to drug therapy and drug reactions, the reader is urged to check the package insert for each drug for any change in indications and dosage and for added warnings and precautions. This is particularly important when the recommended agent is a new or infrequently employed drug.

Some drugs and medical devices presented in the publication have Food and Drug Administration (FDA) clearance for limited use in restricted research settings. It is the responsibility of the health care provider to ascertain the FDA status of each drug or device planned for use in their clinical practice.

To purchase additional copies of this book, call our customer service department at (800) 638-3030 or fax orders to (301) 223-2320. International customers should call (301) 223-2300.

Visit Lippincott Williams & Wilkins on the Internet: at LWW.com. Lippincott Williams & Wilkins customer service representatives are available from 8:30 am to 6 pm, EST.

10 9 8 7 6 5 4 3 2 1

Contributing Authors

Zarmeena Ali, MD
Fellow
Department of Internal Medicine
Division of Rheumatology
Washington University School of Medicine
St. Louis, Missouri

Amy Archer, MD
Resident
Department of Internal Medicine
Division of Rheumatology
Washington University School of Medicine
St. Louis, Missouri

John P. Atkinson, MD
Samuel Grant Professor of Medicine
Department of Internal Medicine
Division of Rheumatology
Washington University School of Medicine
St. Louis, Missouri

Rebecca Brinker, MD
Fellow
Department of Internal Medicine
Division of Rheumatology
Washington University School of Medicine
St. Louis, Missouri

Lesley Davila, MD
Fellow
Department of Internal Medicine
Division of Rheumatology
Washington University School of Medicine
St. Louis, Missouri

Maria C. Gonzalez-Mayda, MD
Fellow
Department of Internal Medicine
Division of Rheumatology
Washington University School of Medicine
St. Louis, Missouri

Richa Gupta, MD
Fellow
Department of Internal Medicine
Division of Rheumatology
Washington University School of Medicine
St. Louis, Missouri

Amy Joseph, MD
Associate Professor of Medicine
Department of Internal Medicine
Division of Rheumatology
Washington University School of Medicine
St. Louis VA Medical Center
St. Louis, Missouri

Reeti Joshi, MD
Fellow
Department of Internal Medicine
Division of Rheumatology
Washington University School of Medicine
St. Louis, Missouri

Leslie E. Kahl, MD
Professor of Medicine
Department of Internal Medicine
Division of Rheumatology
Washington University School of Medicine
St. Louis, Missouri

Alfred H. J. Kim, MD, PhD
Instructor in Medicine
Department of Internal Medicine
Division of Rheumatology
Washington University School of Medicine
St. Louis, Missouri

Ashwini Komarla, MD
Resident
Department of Internal Medicine
Division of Rheumatology
Washington University School of Medicine
St. Louis, Missouri

Kristine A. Kuhn, MD, PhD
Fellow
Department of Internal Medicine
Division of Rheumatology
Washington University School of Medicine
St. Louis, Missouri

Hyon Ju Park, MD
Fellow
Department of Internal Medicine
Division of Rheumatology
Washington University School of Medicine
St. Louis, Missouri

Prabha Ranganathan, MD
Associate Professor of Medicine
Department of Internal Medicine
Division of Rheumatology
Washington University School of Medicine
St. Louis, Missouri

Michael L. Sams, MD
Fellow
Department of Internal Medicine
Division of Rheumatology
Washington University School of Medicine
St. Louis, Missouri

Jeffrey Sparks, MD
Resident
Department of Internal Medicine
Division of Rheumatology
Washington University School of Medicine
St. Louis, Missouri

Wayne M. Yokoyama, MD
*Sam and Audrey Loew Levin Professor of
 Medicine*
Department of Internal Medicine
Division of Rheumatology
Washington University School of Medicine
St. Louis, Missouri

Chairman's Note

I t is a pleasure to present the new edition of *The Washington Manual*® Subspecialty Consult Series: *Rheumatology Subspecialty Consult*. This pocket-size book continues to be a primary reference for medical students, interns, residents, and other practitioners who need ready access to practical clinical information to diagnose and treat patients with a wide variety of disorders. Medical knowledge continues to increase at an astounding rate, which creates a challenge for physicians to keep up with the biomedical discoveries, genetic and genomic information, and novel therapeutics that can positively impact patient outcomes. The *Washington Manual* Subspecialty Series addresses this challenge by concisely and practically providing current scientific information for clinicians to aid them in the diagnosis, investigation, and treatment of common medical conditions.

I want to personally thank the authors, which include house officers, fellows, and attendings at Washington University School of Medicine and Barnes-Jewish Hospital. Their commitment to patient care and education is unsurpassed, and their efforts and skill in compiling this manual are evident in the quality of the final product. In particular, I would like to acknowledge our editor, Dr. Leslie Kahl, and the series editors, Drs. Tom De Fer and Katherine Henderson, who have worked tirelessly to produce another outstanding edition of this manual. I would also like to thank Dr. Melvin Blanchard, Chief of the Division of Medical Education in the Department of Medicine at Washington University School of Medicine, for his advice and guidance. I believe this Subspecialty Manual will meet its desired goal of providing practical knowledge that can be directly applied at the bedside and in outpatient settings to improve patient care.

Victoria J. Fraser, MD
Dr. J. William Campbell Professor
Interim Chairman of Medicine
Co-Director of the Infectious Disease Division
Washington University School of Medicine

Preface

We have written this manual as a guide to inpatient and outpatient rheumatology consultations. The target audience includes medical students, residents, and other medical professionals who care for patients with rheumatologic problems. In addition, this manual could also serve as a pocket reference for medical professionals specializing in rheumatology. It is not intended as a compendium of rheumatology but, rather, focuses on how to approach rheumatologic problems. As such, it provides guidance on how to perform the musculoskeletal examination and arthrocentesis, what laboratory testing may prove useful, and which medications are appropriate (including dosages and recommended monitoring), all framed within a brief overview of the major rheumatologic diseases.

The editor would like to thank the contributing authors for their participation in this project. A special thanks goes to Dr. Tom De Fer for his ongoing support and oversight, and to the authors and editors of the first edition of the manual for leading the way.

L.E.K.

Contents

PART II. COMMON RHEUMATIC DISEASES

PART III. CRYSTALLINE ARTHRITIS

PART IV. SPONDYLOARTHROPATHIES

PART V. VASCULITIS

PART VI. INFECTION AND RELATED DISORDERS

PART VII. OTHER RHEUMATIC DISORDERS

Approach to the Rheumatology Patient

Maria C. Gonzalez-Mayda and
Leslie E. Kahl

GENERAL PRINCIPLES

- Musculoskeletal conditions may be classified according to their symptom presentation, that is, inflammatory versus noninflammatory and articular versus nonarticular.
- A thorough history and physical examination is necessary in order to help narrow your diagnosis.
- Use specific ancillary tests such as radiographs, labs, and arthrocentesis to help confirm your initial diagnosis.
- Rheumatic diseases mainly involve the musculoskeletal system.
  - Inflammatory disorders are often accompanied by systemic features (fever and weight loss) and other organ involvement (kidney, skin, lung, eye, blood).
  - Since these diseases affect multiple organ systems, they are therefore challenging to diagnose, complicated to treat, and often humbling to study.
- Musculoskeletal complaints account for a majority of outpatient visits in the community.
  - Many are self-limited or localized problems that improve with symptomatic treatment.
  - Other conditions (e.g., septic arthritis, crystal-induced arthritis, fractures) require urgent diagnosis and treatment.
- Musculoskeletal problems may also be the initial presentation of diseases such as cancer and endocrinopathies.
- Inpatient consultations usually involve patients with known diagnoses (a patient with lupus admitted with a flare) or with multiple organ system involvement and the suspicion of a systemic rheumatic disease (a patient with respiratory and kidney failure with positive antineutrophil cytoplasmic antibody [ANCA]).

Classification

The following is an approach to patients with musculoskeletal complaints and to common inpatient consults. Regional problems (i.e., nonsystemic musculoskeletal disorders) are discussed in Chapter 8, Regional Pain Syndromes.

Inflammatory versus Noninflammatory

The characteristics of inflammatory and noninflammatory disorders are presented in Table 1-1.

- **Inflammatory disorders**
  - Characterized by **systemic symptoms** (fever, stiffness, weight loss, fatigue).
  - Signs of joint inflammation on physical examination (**erythema, warmth, swelling, pain**).

TABLE 1-1	NONINFLAMMATORY VERSUS INFLAMMATORY DISORDERS	
Symptoms	Noninflammatory Disorders (e.g., OA)	Inflammatory Disorders (e.g., RA, lupus)
Morning stiffness	Focal, brief	Significant, prolonged, >1 hour
Constitutional symptoms	Absent	Present
Peak period of discomfort	After prolonged use	After prolonged inactivity
Locking or instability	Implies loose body, internal derangement, or weakness	Uncommon
Symmetry (bilateral)	Occasional	Common

OA, osteoarthritis; RA, rheumatoid arthritis.

- ○ Lab evidence of inflammation (elevated erythrocyte sedimentation rate [ESR], elevated C-reactive protein [CRP], hypoalbuminemia, normochromic normocytic anemia, thrombocytosis).
- ○ **Joint stiffness** is common after prolonged rest (morning stiffness) and improves with activity.
  - ■ Duration of >1 hour suggests an inflammatory condition.
  - ■ Noninflammatory conditions may cause stiffness usually lasting <1 hour and the joint symptoms increase with use and weight bearing.
- ○ These distinctions are useful but not absolute.
- ○ Inflammatory disorders may be **immune-mediated** (systemic lupus erythematosus [SLE], rheumatoid arthritis [RA]), **reactive** (reactive arthritis [ReA]), **infectious** (gonococcal [GC] arthritis), or **crystal induced** (gout, pseudogout).
- • **Noninflammatory disorders**
  - ○ Characterized by absence of systemic symptoms, **pain without erythema or warmth,** normal lab tests.
  - ○ Osteoarthritis (OA), fibromyalgia, and traumatic conditions are common noninflammatory disorders.

Articular versus Nonarticular
- • Pain may originate from:
  - ○ **Articular structures** (synovial membrane, cartilage, intra-articular ligaments, capsule, or juxtaarticular bone surfaces).
  - ○ **Periarticular structures** (bursae, tendons, muscle, bone, nerve, skin).
  - ○ **Nonarticular structures** (i.e., cardiac pain referred to the shoulder).
- • **Articular disorders**
  - ○ Cause deep or diffuse pain that worsens with active and passive movement.

○ Physical examination may show deformity, warmth, swelling, effusion, or crepitus.

  ▪ **Synovitis** (inflammation of the synovial membrane that covers the joint) is a boggy, tender swelling around the joint. The joint loses its sharp edges on examination. Synovitis is easy to detect in finger and wrist joints.

○ **Arthralgia** refers to joint pain without abnormalities on joint examination.

○ **Arthritis** indicates the presence of abnormality in the joint (warmth, swelling, erythema, tenderness).

• **Nonarticular disorders**

○ Usually have point tenderness and increased pain with active, but not passive, movement.

○ Physical examination does not usually show joint deformity or swelling.

DIAGNOSIS

Clinical Presentation

• The evaluation of musculoskeletal complaints should determine whether the disorder is inflammatory or noninflammatory, whether the joints or the periarticular structures are involved, and the number and pattern of joints involved.

• Number and pattern of joints involved:

○ The number and pattern of joints involved are important in the diagnosis.

○ **Acute monoarthritis** suggests infection but gout and trauma are possible.

○ **Asymmetric, oligoarticular** (<5 joints) involvement, particularly of the lower extremities, is typical of OA and ReA.

○ **Symmetric, polyarticular** (≥5 joints) involvement is typical of RA and SLE.

○ Involvement of the **spine, sacroiliac (SI) joints, and sternoclavicular** joints is characteristic of ankylosing spondylitis (AS).

○ In the hands, **distal interphalangeal (DIP) joints** are involved in OA (Heberden's nodes) and in psoriatic arthritis (PsA) but are spared by RA.

○ **Proximal interphalangeal (PIP) joint** involvement is seen in OA (Bouchard's nodes) and RA.

○ **Metacarpophalangeal (MCP) joints** are involved in RA but not in OA.

○ **Acute first metatarsophalangeal (MTP) joint** arthritis is classic for gout (podagra) but is also seen in OA and ReA.

○ Vasculitis and SLE may present with **multiple organ system involvement,** often without major joint complaints.

○ Fibromyalgia presents with **diffuse pain** but without arthritis.

○ Myositis presents with **muscle weakness** and rashes and occasionally peripheral arthritis.

History

• A comprehensive history and physical examination are often enough to make a diagnosis.

• Ask about **pain,** swelling, weakness, tenderness, limitation of motion, stiffness, as well as constitutional symptoms when presented with a musculoskeletal complaint since these clues will help you narrow your diagnosis.

○ For example, joint pain that occurs at rest and which worsens with movement suggests an inflammatory process versus pain elicited with activity and relieved by rest usually indicates a mechanical disorder such as a degenerative arthritis.

- Inquire about what **medications** they are taking since many have side effects and patients on immunosuppressive drugs are predisposed to developing infections.
  - Some medications may cause a **lupus-like syndrome** (e.g., hydralazine, procainamide), **myopathies** (e.g., statins, colchicine, zidovudine), or **osteoporosis** (e.g., corticosteroids, phenytoin).
  - **Alcohol** commonly precipitates gout and may rarely cause myopathies and avascular necrosis (AVN).
  - Vasculitis, arthralgias, and rhabdomyolysis may also be seen with **substance abuse** (e.g., cocaine, heroin).
- Certain areas of the United States and Europe have an increased incidence of **Lyme disease;** therefore, it is important to inquire about recent trips to these areas.
- A **family history** may be important in AS, gout, and OA.
- The **review of systems** may identify other organ involvement and support the diagnosis.
  - The **nervous system** may be involved in SLE, vasculitis, and Lyme disease.
  - **Eye involvement** may be severe and occurs in Sjögren's syndrome (SS), RA, seronegative spondyloarthropathies, giant cell arthritis, Behçet's disease, and Wegener's granulomatosis (WG).
  - **Oral mucosal ulcers** are common in SLE, enteropathic arthritis, and Behçet's disease.
  - **Rashes** are seen in SLE, vasculitis, PsA, dermatomyositis (DM), adult-onset Still's disease, and Lyme disease.
  - **Raynaud's phenomenon** is a reversible, paroxysmal constriction of small arteries that occurs most commonly in fingers and toes and is precipitated by cold. The classic sequence is initial blanching followed by cyanosis and finally erythema due to vasodilation and is accompanied by numbness or tingling. It may be idiopathic or associated with scleroderma, SLE, RA, and mixed connective tissue disease (MCTD).
  - **Pleuritis and pericarditis** may be seen in RA, SLE, MCTD, and adult-onset Still's disease.
  - **Gastrointestinal (GI) involvement** is seen in enteropathic arthritis; **polymyositis** (PM), and scleroderma. The latter may be associated with dysphagia.
- Certain diseases are more frequent in specific **age groups and genders.**
  - SLE, juvenile RA, and GC arthritis are more common in the young.
  - Gout, OA, and RA are more common in middle-aged persons.
  - Polymyalgia rheumatica (PMR) and giant cell arthritis occur in the elderly.
  - Gout and AS are more common in men; gout is rare in premenopausal women.
  - SLE, RA, and OA are more common in women.

Physical Examination
- Tailor the physical examination based on the presenting complaint.
- If the main complaint is arthritis or arthralgia, look for signs of inflammation such as swelling, warmth, erythema over the joint and surrounding structures, tenderness, deformity, limitation of motion, instability of the joint, and crepitus.
- If the pain appears to be nonarticular in origin, examine the surrounding bursae, tendons, ligaments and bones for tenderness and inflammation.

- If there is suspicion of systemic involvement, make sure to perform a thorough examination from head to toe so as not to miss any important findings that could help you determine the etiology of their symptoms.
  - Examine the hair for signs of alopecia and or rashes.
  - The skin for any type of discoloration, rash, ulceration, blistering as well as the nails for pitting.
  - The nose and mouth for signs of ulceration.
  - The heart and lungs for signs of pericardial and or pleural rubs, and/or decreased breath sounds from underlying pulmonary fibrosis.
  - The abdomen for signs of serositis, pain related to ischemic bowel, etc.
  - A thorough examination of all the joints to look for the signs mentioned above.
  - Examine the back thoroughly at the spinous processes, paraspinal and surrounding muscles. Do not forget to examine the SI joints as well.
  - If there is clinical suspicion for Behçet's disease and/or inflammatory bowel disease, a genital examination would be indicated since ulcerations can be seen.

Differential Diagnosis

Approach to Monoarthritis

- Common causes of monoarthritis are **infection, crystal-induced arthritis, and trauma** (Table 1-2).
- Acute pain or swelling of a single joint requires immediate evaluation for septic arthritis that can rapidly destroy the joint if left untreated (Fig. 1-1).
- It is also important to distinguish pain arising from periarticular structures (tendons, bursa), which usually requires only symptomatic treatment, and cases of referred pain (shoulder pain due to peritonitis or heart disease).
- The history should exclude trauma and can provide clues such as:
  - History of tick bite (Lyme disease).
  - Sexual risk factors (GC arthritis).
  - Colitis, uveitis, and urethritis (ReA).
- Physical examination usually distinguishes between articular and nonarticular disorders.
- **Perform arthrocentesis in patients with acute monoarthritis** (see Chapter 4, Synovial Fluid Analysis). Send synovial fluid for:
  - Leukocyte count with differential (>2000/mm^3 suggest an inflammatory process).
  - Gram stain and culture.
  - Crystal analysis. A wet mount of the fluid examined under polarizing microscopy may identify crystals, but **the presence of crystals does not exclude infection.**
- **Culture other potential sources** of infection (throat, cervix, rectum, wounds, blood).
- Synovial biopsy and arthroscopy are sometimes used to diagnose chronic monoarthritis.
- Radiographs are useful in cases of trauma and may show OA or chondrocalcinosis in calcium pyrophosphate deposition disease.
- **A patient with synovial fluid that is highly inflammatory requires empiric antibiotic therapy until the evaluation, including cultures, is completed.**

TABLE 1-2	FEATURES AND CAUSES OF MONOARTHRITIS	
Type	Features	Causes
Infectious arthritis	Common; acute; may or may not have fever or leukocytosis; synovial fluid culture usually confirmatory in nongonococcal arthritis	Bacteria (gonococci and *Staphylococcus aureus*) most common. Also viruses (HIV, hepatitis B), fungi, mycobacteria, Lyme disease
Crystal-induced arthritis	Common; very acute onset; extremely painful; crystals on microscopic examination of synovial fluid	Monosodium urate crystals (gout), calcium pyrophosphate dihydrate crystals, and others
OA	Common; usually in lower extremities; synovial fluid is noninflammatory	May be primary or secondary to trauma, hemochromatosis
Trauma	Common; history is diagnostic; occurs rarely in inpatients	Fracture, hemarthrosis, internal derangement
AVN of bone	Uncommon; more common in hip, knee, shoulder	Risk factors include trauma, corticosteroid use, alcohol
Tumors	Uncommon	Benign or malignant, primary or metastatic
Systemic diseases with monoarticular onset	Uncommon (follow-up may be needed for diagnosis)	Psoriatic arthritis, SLE, ReA, RA

OA, osteoarthritis; AVN, avascular necrosis; SLE, systemic lupus erythematosus; ReA, reactive arthritis; RA, rheumatoid arthritis.

Approach to Polyarthritis
- Polyarthritis is one of the most common problems in rheumatology (Fig. 1-2).
- The number and pattern of joint involvement suggest the diagnosis (Table 1-3).
- There are many nonarticular causes of generalized joint pain.
  - Disorders of periarticular structures (tendons, bursae) cause joint pain but usually involve a single joint.
  - Myopathies occasionally cause widespread pain, but muscle weakness is the primary symptom.
  - PMR causes shoulder and pelvic girdle pain with morning stiffness, but there is usually no arthritis on examination; weakness is not a feature of this disease.
  - Neuropathies, primary bone diseases (Paget's disease), and fibromyalgia can also cause widespread pain but are distinguished by history and physical examination.

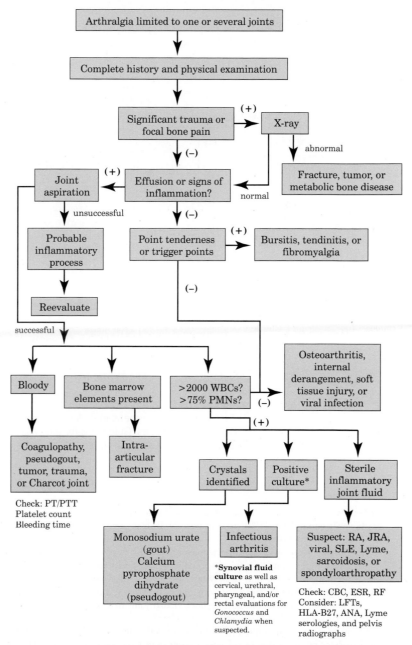

FIGURE 1-1. Approach to monoarthritis. JRA, juvenile rheumatoid arthritis; PMNs, polymorphonuclear cells. (Adapted from American College of Rheumatology ad hoc Committee on Clinical Guidelines. Guidelines for the initial evaluation of the adult patient with acute musculoskeletal symptoms. *Arthritis Rheum.* 1996;39:1.)

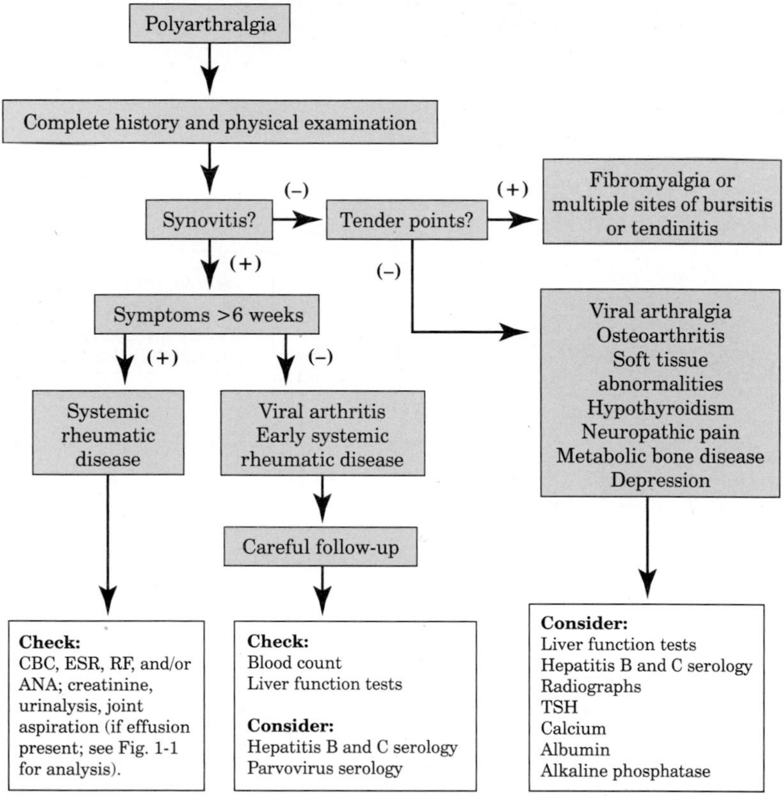

FIGURE 1-2. Approach to polyarthritis. (Adapted from American College of Rheumatology ad hoc Committee on Clinical Guidelines. Guidelines for the initial evaluation of the adult patient with acute musculoskeletal symptoms. *Arthritis Rheum.* 1996;39:1.)

- **Rheumatoid arthritis** is the prototypical polyarticular arthritis.
  - Given its frequency (1%), it is important to recognize and distinguish RA from other types of arthritis.
  - RA usually begins with **symmetric peripheral arthritis** of multiple small joints of hands, wrists, and feet which progresses over weeks to months. Morning stiffness is prominent and usually lasts >1 hour. Other joints (knees, ankles, shoulders, elbows) are sequentially involved. Involvement of the cervical spine, temporomandibular joint, and sternoclavicular joint may also be seen.
  - Lumbar spine and SI involvement is very rare.
- **SLE** may present with polyarthritis similar to RA that may be intermittent. Fever, rashes, serositis, and other organ involvement may accompany arthritis in SLE.
- **Viral arthritis** (due to parvovirus B19, hepatitis B, rubella, HIV) may have an acute onset with fever and rashes and persist for months.

TABLE 1-3   CAUSES OF POLYARTHRITIS

Inflammatory
  Polyarticular peripheral (usually symmetric)
    RA (usually presents insidiously, additive)
    Viral arthritis (usually acute onset)
    SLE
    PsA (occasionally)
    Palindromic rheumatism (recurrent attacks)
  Oligoarticular with axial involvement (usually asymmetric, lower extremity
      joints)
    Seronegative spondyloarthropathies (AS, ReA, PsA, and enteropathic
      arthritis)
  Oligoarticular without axial involvement (usually asymmetric)
    PsA
    ReA
    Enteropathic arthritis
    Lyme disease
    Polyarticular gout (more commonly monoarticular)
    CPDD
    Bacterial endocarditis
    Septic arthritis (particularly in patients with RA)
    Sarcoidosis
    Behçet's disease and relapsing polychondritis (rare)
    Rheumatic fever (usually migratory)
Noninflammatory
  OA
    OA of the hands
    Generalized OA
    Posttraumatic OA
    OA secondary to metabolic diseases (hemochromatosis, ochronosis,
      acromegaly)
  Sickle cell disease
  Hypertrophic osteoarthropathy
  Others (rare)
    Leukemia
    Hemophilia
    Amyloidosis

RA, rheumatoid arthritis; SLE, systemic lupus erythematosus; PsA, psoriatic arthritis; AS, ankylosing spondylitis; ReA, reactive arthritis; CPDD, calcium pyrophosphate deposition disease;
  OA, osteoarthritis.

- **Palindromic rheumatism** causes recurrent attacks of symmetric arthritis that affect hands, wrists, and knees and are self-limited over several days.
- The **seronegative spondyloarthropathies** are characterized by spine and SI joint involvement, enthesopathy (pain at sites of tendon insertion to bone) and varying degrees of peripheral joint, eye, skin, and GI involvement.
  - Peripheral joint involvement is usually **asymmetric, oligoarticular,** and of the lower extremities (knee, ankle).

- ○ **Dactylitis,** a diffuse swelling of a digit ("sausage digit"), may be seen in fingers and toes and is characteristic of ReA and PsA.
  - ○ A symmetric, polyarticular form of PsA exists that is similar to RA.
- Oligoarticular disease may also be seen with Behçet's disease, sarcoidosis, and relapsing polychondritis.
- **Bacterial arthritis** may be polyarticular in patients with preexisting joint damage (RA).
- **GC arthritis** may be migratory and is accompanied by fever, pustular skin lesions, and tenosynovitis.
- Fever and migratory arthralgias or mild arthritis may be seen in early **Lyme disease,** and a persistent oligoarticular arthritis occurs months later.
- **Bacterial endocarditis** often presents with fever, low back pain, and arthralgias and may have a positive RF.
- **Gout** is usually monoarticular, but polyarthritis is sometimes seen, particularly later in disease.
- Pseudogout may present as "pseudo-RA" with bilateral hand and wrist involvement.
- Rheumatic fever occurs after streptococcal infection and is characterized by migratory arthritis of large joints, fever, and extra-articular involvement (carditis, chorea, rash).
- OA is the most common form of noninflammatory polyarthritis.
  - ○ DIP, PIP, **first carpometacarpal (CMC), knees, hips, and first MTP joints** are typically involved.
  - ○ Hemochromatosis predisposes to OA in unusual joints (second and third MCP).

Approach to Patients with Positive Antinuclear Antibodies

- **Antinuclear antibodies (ANAs)** are autoantibodies that target nucleic acid and nucleoprotein antigens, and are usually detected by indirect immunofluorescence (see Chapter 5, Laboratory Evaluation of Rheumatic Diseases) (Figure 1-3).
- ANAs are **very sensitive** (their absence by current assays practically rules out SLE) but not too specific for SLE.
- ANAs are present in other rheumatic diseases (e.g., scleroderma, MCTD, PM, SS), in drug-induced lupus (DIL), in some infectious diseases (e.g., HIV), and in up to 5% of healthy individuals (in low titers).
- They are also present in many patients with chronic liver or lung disorders, and in those with nonarticular autoimmune diseases such as thyroiditis.
- **An ANA test should be ordered only when you suspect a patient has an underlying autoimmune condition such as SLE.**
- A positive ANA should be followed by a complete history and physical examination to identify those conditions.
  - ○ A history of hydralazine or procainamide use suggests DIL.
  - ○ Myositis, skin changes, and Raynaud's phenomenon suggest MCTD, myositis, or scleroderma.
  - ○ Sicca symptoms (dry eyes and dry mouth) suggest SS.
- **SLE** is a multisystem disease that is diagnosed clinically.
  - ○ Criteria developed for the classification of lupus (see Chapter 12, Systemic Lupus Erythematosus) can be used as a framework for assessing whether a patient has SLE.
  - ○ Certain other diseases (acute HIV infection, endocarditis, autoimmune hepatitis) may fulfill criteria for SLE.

○ High-titer ANAs (>1:640) should be followed by assays for antibodies to certain antigens (double-stranded DNA, SSA/Ro, SSB/La, ribonucleoprotein [RNP], Smith [Sm]) that may be more specific for SLE and other rheumatic diseases.
○ If no certain diagnosis is made, follow-up may be indicated.
○ Up to 40% of patients referred to a rheumatologist for evaluation of positive ANAs who do not fulfill criteria on presentation do fulfill criteria for SLE after months to years of follow-up.

Approach to Patients with Possible Systemic Vasculitis

- The vasculitides are a heterogeneous group of disorders characterized by inflammation of blood vessels.
- Vasculitis is often suspected in patients with multiple organ involvement. Vessels in the respiratory tract, kidneys, GI tract, peripheral nerves, and skin may be involved in varying degrees depending on the category of vasculitis and the size of the blood vessel involved.
- Perform a complete history and physical examination on these patients.
  ○ Patients with suspected vasculitis should be questioned about fever, rashes, arthralgias or arthritis, abdominal pain, weight loss, and any underlying rheumatic diseases (SLE, RA).
  ○ The physical examination should identify other organ system involvement (purpura, peripheral neuropathy, joint abnormalities) that may not be obvious on initial presentation
- **ANCA** should be ordered if suspecting some types of vasculitis.
  ○ ANCA is sensitive and specific for some vasculitides but may be seen in infections (such as HIV).
  ○ Positive ANCA tends to require confirmation with more specific assays for antibodies against myeloperoxidase (MPO) and proteinase-3 (PR3) (see Chapter 5, Lab Evaluation of Rheumatic Diseases).
- Other lab tests (ANA, complement levels, hepatitis panels, cryoglobulins, urinalysis) may be useful to establish etiology.
- Chest and sinus radiographs may reveal occult respiratory tract involvement.
- Diagnosis may require pathologic examination of skin, nerve, kidney, or lung tissue.
- Infection should be ruled out before treatment with corticosteroids or immunosuppressives is considered.
- Bacterial endocarditis, embolic disease and cocaine use may mimic vasculitis and therefore should also be considered.

SPECIAL CONSIDERATIONS

Perioperative Considerations

- There are special considerations for patients with rheumatic diseases who undergo elective surgical procedures, related to joint deformities that limit mobility, medications the patient is taking, and existing end-organ damage.
- **Joint deformities** in patients with RA, juvenile RA, and AS may include limited jaw opening and cervical spine fusion or laxity, which can contribute to difficult intubation.
  ○ Patients with RA should have preoperative cervical spine radiographs (lateral in flexion and extension) to detect severe instability.
  ○ Fiberoptic or awake intubation may be needed.

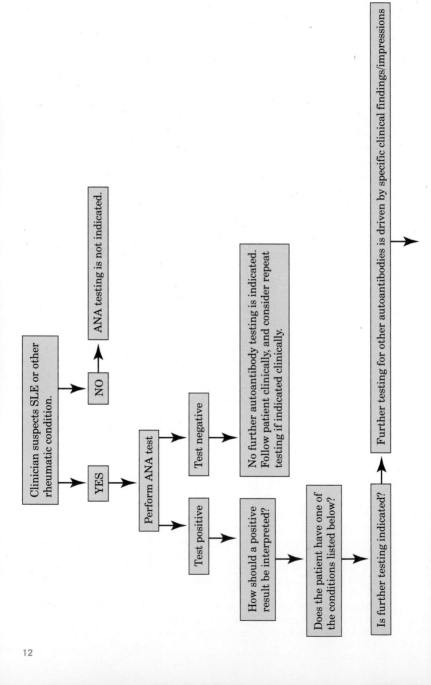

Clinician suspects SLE or other rheumatic condition.

NO → ANA testing is not indicated.

YES → Perform ANA test

Test negative → No further autoantibody testing is indicated. Follow patient clinically, and consider repeat testing if indicated clinically.

Test positive → How should a positive result be interpreted? → Does the patient have one of the conditions listed below? → Is further testing indicated? → Further testing for other autoantibodies is driven by specific clinical findings/impressions →

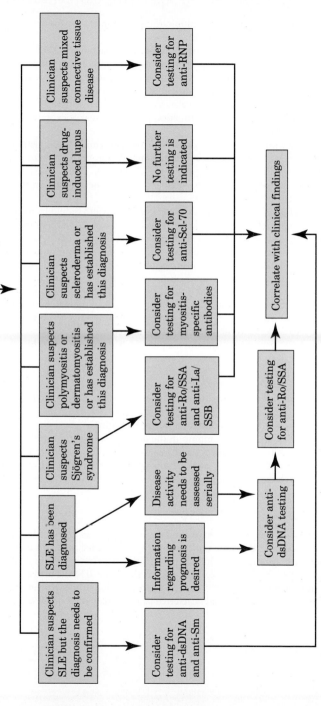

FIGURE 1-3. Approach to a positive ANA. dsDNA, double-stranded DNA; Sm, Smith. (From Kavanaugh A, Tomar R, Reveille J, et al. Guidelines for clinical use of the antinuclear antibody test and test for specific autoantibodies to nuclear antigens. *Arch Pathol Lab Med.* 2000;124:71–81.)

○ Patients with AS may also have limitations in thoracic expansion that may complicate mechanical ventilation.

- Cystitis, skin infections, and possible sources of bacteremia such as caries should be treated before joint replacement to prevent seeding of the prosthesis.
- Patients with SS are at risk for corneal abrasions in surgical settings and need to receive ocular lubricants before and after surgery.
  ○ NPO orders may be made more tolerable with artificial saliva.
  ○ Particular care is needed with intubation given the usual poor state of dentition in these patients.
- Many patients with rheumatologic diseases are on nonsteroidal anti-inflammatory drugs (NSAIDs), corticosteroids, disease-modifying anti-rheumatic drugs (DMARDs), and/or biologic agents (see Chapter 9, Drugs Used for the Treatment of Rheumatic Diseases). Below are recommendations on when to hold specific medications perioperatively.
  ○ Aspirin and other NSAIDs affect platelet aggregation and should be discontinued 5 to 7 days before surgery. Selective cyclooxygenase-2 (COX-2) inhibitors do not affect platelet aggregation and may be used until the day of surgery.
  ○ Patients who are on or have received corticosteroids in the previous year may be at risk for adrenal insufficiency during the stress of surgery. Hydrocortisone, 100 mg IV q8h, is the traditional "stress dose," but lower doses may be sufficient. Taper the corticosteroid dose to the daily dose (or to zero in patients not previously on corticosteroids) within a few days if the patient is stable.
  ○ Methotrexate should be withheld 48 hours before surgery and restarted within 1 to 2 weeks to prevent a flare of arthritis.
  ○ Nephrotoxic agents such as cyclophosphamide should also be withheld preoperatively.
  ○ Biological agents including etanercept, infliximab, adalimumab, and anakinra may be withheld for 1 week before and after surgery.
- Prophylaxis against deep vein thrombosis is mandatory in joint replacement patients.
- Aggressive physical therapy is essential for rehabilitation.
- Acute crystalline arthritis is common in the postoperative period, and management may be difficult in patients with renal dysfunction or who cannot have oral intake. In these patients, narcotic analgesics or intra-articular corticosteroids (after excluding infection) may be an option (see Chapter 13, Gout).

FOLLOW-UP

- Many rheumatologic diseases have similar clinical pictures at onset but evolve into distinct patterns over time and close follow-up is needed to make a diagnosis.
- A patient with symmetric, peripheral polyarthritis may have a self-limited viral arthritis, but persistence for >12 weeks suggests that RA will be the final diagnosis.
- Urgent treatment is required in cases with active infection. Other patients may be treated with NSAIDs and should be referred to a rheumatologist if disease persists.

Rheumatologic Joint Examination

Michael L. Sams and Leslie E. Kahl

2

GENERAL PRINCIPLES

- The full joint examination is often excluded from the general complete physical examination because it is considered too time-consuming for minimal diagnostic gain. The joints are usually addressed only if the patient has a specific complaint.
- Musculoskeletal disorders, however, are common in patients who present to physicians and are the most common reason for disability in the population.
- The joint examination, if done consistently, can be performed with increasing efficiency and brevity.
- A brief screening examination is presented in Table 2-1.

DIAGNOSIS

Clinical Presentation

History

- History should focus on the following points: The onset of the symptoms, insidious versus abrupt, the length of time symptoms have been present, the specific location of the symptoms within or around the joint, aggravating and relieving factors, the presence of stiffness, and if stiffness is present how long it takes for it to resolve with activity.
- It is also important to ascertain functional impairment, including how well the patient can perform activities of daily living (e.g., dressing, grooming, cooking) and how the musculoskeletal disorder interferes with occupation or hobbies.

Physical Examination

- In general, the examination should begin with a **visual inspection** noting asymmetry, alignment, swelling, deformities, and changes in color.
- The examination continues with **palpation** for warmth, tenderness, and crepitus.
  - ○ Any specific structures of the joint that are tender should be noted, as patients with rheumatologic disease can also have common musculoskeletal complaints, such as meniscal tear.
  - ○ Hard swelling around joints may be due to bony deformities, whereas tender, "boggy" swelling may be due to synovial inflammation (synovitis).
- Simultaneously notice the **bulk, tone, and strength** of the associated muscle groups.
- Assess **active and passive ranges of motion**, making note of any pattern of joint involvement.

TABLE 2-1	BRIEF JOINT SCREENING EXAMINATION

Upper extremities
  Squeeze across MCP joints collectively and ask patient if it is painful
  "Make a fist"
  "Touch your fingers to the tip of your thumb"
  "Turn your hands over"
  "Place your hands behind your head"
  "Place your hands behind your back"

Neck and back
  "Touch your chin to your chest"
  "Look up at the ceiling"
  "Turn your head to the left and to the right"
  "Bend over and touch your toes"

Lower extremities
  Squeeze across MTP joints collectively and ask patient if it is painful
  Perform the FABER maneuver (of hip)
  "Straighten your knee"
  "Step on the gas" (plantar flexion)
  "Pull your foot up" (dorsiflexion)

———

Note: Examination may be performed in a few minutes. It may be easier to ask the patient to follow the examiner's lead and copy the movements. Any abnormality should be followed by a complete examination.

MCP, metacarpophalangeal; MTP, metatarsophalangeal; FABER, flexion, abduction, and external rotation.

Adapted from: Doherty M, Dacre J, Dieppe P, Snaith M. The "GALS" locomotor screen. *Ann Rheum Dis.* 1992;51:1165–1169.

- Finally, perform **specific provocative tests** for each joint to help identify a source of pain. A good example is Phalen's test for carpal tunnel syndrome.
- Note the patient's gait as he or she walks into the room. Is the patient using any adaptations to protect a particular joint? How does the patient sit in a chair? Is the patient able to get up to the examination table unassisted? Note the use of canes or other assistive devices. Look for uneven wear on shoes.
- **Perform a general physical examination**, paying close attention to the skin, eyes, oropharynx, and nervous system.

Examining Individual Joints

Hands
- Begin with **visual inspection** by instructing the patient to stretch out all fingers with the palms down. Then, palms up, have the patient make a fist and oppose the thumb to the base of the fifth finger. Note any finger lag. Inspect for visible swelling or erythema. Observe for deformity. For example, sublimations of the metacarpophalangeal (MCP) joints with ulnar deviation of the digits are seen with rheumatoid arthritis (RA). Lastly, note any atrophy of the lumbrical or thenar muscles, which can suggest nerve compression.

- **Palpate** each joint for tenderness. If there is finger lag with extension palpate the flexor tendon for a snapping with extension or the presence of a nodule. Either of these findings may suggest **trigger finger.**
- Also note **grip strength** and ability to fine pinch. Normal patients should be able to make a completely closed fist.
- **Heberden's nodes:** Hard, painless nodules on the dorsolateral aspects of the distal interphalangeal (DIP) joints and are characteristic of osteoarthritis (OA).
- **Bouchard's nodes:** Similar to Heberden's nodes, except found on the proximal interphalangeal (PIP) joints (also characteristic of OA).
- "Swan neck" deformity: Hyperextension of the PIP joint with fixed flexion of the DIP joint.
- "Boutonniere" deformity: Fixed flexion of the PIP joint with hyperextension of the DIP joint.
- Other findings include **tophi** (hard or soft uric acid deposits seen in chronic gout), **fingernail and cuticle abnormalities** (seen in psoriatic arthritis, dermatomyositis) and sclerodactyly (thin, tapered fingers with tight overlying skin and loss of soft tissue seen in scleroderma).

Wrists

- Passively flex, extend, and deviate the wrists medially (ulnarly) and laterally (radially). Normal range of motion for flexion is 80 degrees and extension is 70 degrees.
- Note any swelling, warmth, or tenderness along the joint.

Elbows

- Passively flex, extend, pronate, and supinate the forearms. Normal range of motion is extension to 0 degrees (hyperextension occurs with > minus 10 degrees extension) and flexion to 150 degrees (the thumb should be able to touch the shoulder). With the elbow flexed at 90 degrees, the forearms should supinate and pronate to 80 degrees.
- Palpate along the extensor surface of the ulna and over the olecranon bursa for **rheumatoid nodules.** These fleshy nodules are usually firm, nontender, and mobile with respect to the overlying skin. Gouty **tophi,** which often occur in the same area, are usually more firm.
- Palpation of the elbow joint is easier posteriorly and laterally as less soft tissue obscures the joint. Tenderness over the medial or lateral epicondyles should be noted.
- Finally, observe the **olecranon bursa** for any swelling, warmth or erythema.

Shoulders

- The shoulder is a highly mobile joint with normal flexion and abduction of up to 180 degrees.
- A brief screening test of shoulder range of motion is the **Apley Scratch Test.** It includes the following maneuvers: To evaluate external rotation and abduction ask the patient to touch the contralateral scapula by reaching behind the neck. To evaluate internal rotation and adduction ask the patient to touch the contralateral scapula by reaching behind the back.
- To evaluate the rotator cuff perform both **impingement and drop arm tests.** The **Neer impingement sign** can be elicited by passive forward flexion of the internally rotated arm while the examiner stabilizes the scapula. A positive test

produces pain with this maneuver. The drop arm test evaluates for a tear of the rotator cuff. The test is performed by placing the patient's shoulder in 90 degrees abduction. Have the patient slowly lower the arm to the side. The test is considered positive if the arm cannot be smoothly lowered to the side.

Neck

- Ask the patient to flex and extend the neck. Normal range of motion permits the chin to touch the chest. Ask the patient to turn his or her neck to the right then the left. Normal rotation is about 60 degrees. To evaluate lateral flexion, ask the patient to bring his or her ear toward each shoulder.
- Palpation of the spinous processes should be performed on the basis of the clinical history to assess for tenderness that can suggest infection, fracture or joint involvement. Examine for tender points in the paraspinal musculature.
- **Spurling's test** may be performed to help assess if radicular pain from the neck is present. The patient's neck is extended and rotated to the side of the pain and then firm pressure is applied to the top of the head pushing downwards. If radicular symptoms are present it suggests foraminal stenosis as the cause.
- Finally, RA can lead to atlantoaxial subluxation. Caution should be taken with passive range of motion testing in these patients.

Back

- Assess the curvature of the spine. The normal spine has three curves: Lumbar lordosis, thoracic spine kyphosis, and cervical lordosis. Identify the presence of abnormal lordosis, kyphosis, scoliosis, or list (lateral tilt of the spine).
- Palpate for any tenderness along the spine and paraspinal muscles. While the patient is standing, instruct him or her to bend forward, backward, right, and left.
- If spondyloarthropathy (see Chapter 15, Undifferentiated Spondyloarthritis) is suspected, perform the modified **Schober test.** With the patient standing, mark two midline points, one 10 cm above the lumbosacral junction (midline between the posterior iliac spines) and one 5 cm below the junction. The points will be 15 cm apart. Ask the patient to flex forward and measure the distance between the two points. In a normal individual, the span will increase by $\geq$4 cm.

Hips

- While the patient is lying supine on the examination table, passively flex one hip and knee while the other leg is held straight. Normal flexion is 120 degrees (the patient should be able to touch the heel to the buttock). While the hip and knee are flexed at a 90-degree angle, rotate the hip to measure hip external and internal rotation. Normal values are 45 degrees for each. Internal rotation is often limited with arthritis of the hip. Note any limitation, crepitus, or pain.
- A quick screening maneuver to assess the hip joint is the **FABER test:** Flexion, abduction, and external rotation of the hip are tested by exerting light downward pressure on the knee while the hip is flexed with the heel touching the opposite knee. Pain suggests hip or sacroiliac joint pathology.

Knees

- Note the alignment of the knees in standing including valgus or varus deformities.
- Palpate along the joint margins for tenderness and bony ridges (seen with OA). Palpate surrounding tendons and bursa.
- Passively flex and extend the knee while feeling for crepitus. The knee normally extends to 10 degrees of hyperextension and flexes to 135 degrees.

- Effusions are relatively easy to detect in the knee. Feel for joint effusion by palpating the medial and lateral aspects of the patella while using the other hand (placed proximal to the patella) to gently "milk" fluid toward the patella. One can also assess for fluid with the "bulge" sign: Observe for a "bulge" medial or lateral to the patella as pressure is applied from the opposite side.

Ankles
- Passively flex and extend the ankle (tibiotalar joint) to assess range of motion. Normal dorsiflexion (from the ankle at a 90-degree angle to the leg) is 20 degrees, and normal plantar flexion is 50 degrees.
- Then medially (varus) and laterally (valgus) deviate the calcaneus to elicit abnormalities of the subtalar joint motion. To test the midtarsal joint, stabilize the heel with one hand, then use the other hand to invert and evert the forefoot.
- In order to palpate the tibiotalar joint (ankle joint) the best approach is anteriorly with the foot in plantar flexion, as the dome of the talus nestled between the distal tibia and fibula becomes more exposed.
- Other common sources of pain in the ankle should be palpated and include the anterior talofibular ligament and the posterior tibialis/peroneal tendons.

Metatarsophalangeal Joints
- Ask the patient to plantar flex and dorsiflex the toes.
- Palpate each joint for tenderness, warmth and effusion.
- Observe for **hallux valgus,** lateral deviation of the great toe with respect to the first metatarsal. With hallux valgus, the head of the first metatarsal is more prominent and may enlarge on the medial side. Observe for tophi at the first metatarsophalangeal joint.

Arthrocentesis: Aspirating and Injecting Joints and Bursa

3

Rebecca Brinker and Leslie E. Kahl

INTRODUCTION

- Arthrocentesis is an essential tool for evaluating and treating articular disease.
- Acute monoarthritis necessitates immediate aspiration to rule out a septic joint.
- Do not inject steroids if there is still suspicion of a septic joint. **Rule out septic arthritis first.**
- Procedures on artificial joint replacements should ideally be done by the treating surgeon.
- Do not forget to check labs and to ask the patient about anticoagulants or antiplatelet therapy.

Indications

- Suspected crystalline disease.
- Suspected infection.
- Posttraumatic effusion (to rule out hemarthrosis).
- Undiagnosed acute monoarthritis.
- Monoarticular joint effusion in a patient with polyarticular inflammatory arthritis.
- Intra-articular injections (with steroids, anesthetic, contrast for arthrography or hyaluronidate derivatives).

Contraindications

- **Overlying cellulitis.**
- Patients predisposed to bleeding have a relative contraindication to arthrocentesis, that is, platelets <50,000, coagulopathy, or anticoagulant therapy.
- Contraindications to intra-articular injection with steroids include septic arthritis/bursitis, bacteremia, unstable joints, fractures, Charcot joint, prior failure to respond to injection, joint prosthesis, and tumor.

Possible Complications

- Bleeding (local hematoma or hemarthrosis).
- Iatrogenic infection (rare and is estimated to occur only in 1:50,000 procedures).
- Rupture of tendon or damage to periarticular structure.
- Nerve damage (e.g., median nerve atrophy following a steroid injection).
- Allergic reaction to the equipment or injected medications.
- Postinjection flare.
- Subcutaneous fat atrophy with steroid injections (more common with fluorinated steroids: Dexamethasone, betamethasone, and triamcinolone). Table 3-1 lists various steroids for intra-articular injection.

TABLE 3-1	STEROID PREPARATIONS FOR JOINT INJECTIONS	
Steroid	Concentration (mg/mL)	Dose (mg)
Hydrocortisone acetate	24	200
Dexamethasone acetate[a]	8	4
Methylprednisolone acetate	20, 40, 80	40
Triamcinolone hexacetonide[a]	20	40
Triamcinolone acetonide[a]	10, 40	40
Betamethasone acetate[a]	6	6
Prednisolone tebutate	20	40

[a]Fluorinated steroids.

- Skin discoloration at injection site (more common with fluorinated steroids).
- Hyperglycemia if systemic absorption of steroids is significant.
- Osteoporosis, avascular necrosis, and tissue fragility with chronic and frequent injections.

Equipment
- Iodine or chlorhexidine
- 3-, 5-, 10-, 30-, or 60-cc syringes
- 18-, 20-, 25-gauge needles
- 1% lidocaine
- Hemostat/Kelly clamp
- Gloves
- Gauze, bandages
- Alcohol pads
- Glass slides with coverslips
- Test tubes (ethylenediaminetetraacetic acid [EDTA] and heparinized)
- Blood culture bottles, culture swab
- Ballpoint pen

GENERAL APPROACH

- To access the joint space, palpate and define the anatomy of the joint. Mark the desired location of entry by applying pressure to the patient's skin with a retracted ballpoint pen. This will leave a circular impression on the skin.
- Put on your gloves (they do not have to be sterile).
- Clean the skin thoroughly and perform the procedure with aseptic technique.
- Using a 25-guage infiltrate 1% lidocaine into the skin and subcutaneous tissues for local anesthesia.
- Attach the appropriate gauge needle to the desired size syringe for joint aspiration.
- Using your previous skin mark and anatomic landmarks, carefully introduce the needle into the desired joint space. During needle advancement into the

TABLE 3-2	RECOMMENDED COMPOSITION OF INJECTATE BY JOINT SIZE	
Joint or Bursa	Methylprednisolone Acetate (mg)	1% Lidocaine (mL)
Trochanteric bursa	40	1
Knee, prepatellar bursa, trochanteric bursa	40	1
Anserine bursa	20	0.5
Ankle	20	1
Shoulder (anterior or posterior)	40	1
AC joint, subacromial bursa	20	None
Biceps tendonitis or epicondylitis	40	0.5
Elbow	40	1
Olecranon bursa	20	1
Wrist	20	0.5
MCP, PIP, MTP	10	None

AC, acromioclavicular; MCP, metacarpophalangeal; PIP, proximal interphalangeal; MTP, metatarsophalangeal.

joint, slightly pull back on the plunger of the syringe to create suction. Aspiration of synovial fluid should result.

- If injecting a steroid preparation after joint aspiration (Table 3-1 and Table 3-2), or if you require more than one syringe for removal of all the joint fluid, you may change the syringe while leaving the needle in the joint. A Kelly clamp/hemostat may be used to grasp and provide stability to the hub of the needle while unscrewing the syringe. Take great care not to withdraw or advance the remaining needle during the syringe exchange.
- If joint aspiration is unsuccessful or assistance is needed for anatomically complex joints, ultrasound guidance may be useful.
- If injecting superficial bursa, it is wise to enter the skin and bursa in a "Z" line to avoid establishing a drainage track.
- **It is recommended to limit steroid injections to—three to four injections per site per year.**
- After any arthrocentesis, record the amount of synovial fluid removed and grossly examine the fluid for viscosity, clarity, and color.
- If you desire to perform microscopic analysis, place a small drop of fluid onto a slide and apply a coverslip.
- Send the synovial fluid to the lab for cell count (in an EDTA lavender-top tube), routine Gram stain and culture, and crystal analysis. Glucose, protein, autoantibodies, pH, and complement levels from the fluid are rarely helpful and should not be ordered. Acid-fast bacilli, fungal cultures (in a culture bottle/swab), and cytology can be ordered if clinically indicated.

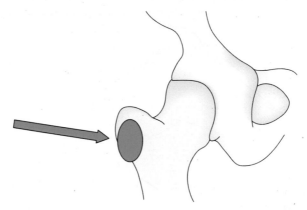

FIGURE 3-1. Anterior view of the hip for trochanteric bursitis.

HIP

- Aspiration and injection of the femoral acetabular joint is only done under ultrasound or radiographic guidance and therefore is not described in this chapter.
- The trochanteric bursa is a lubricating sac located between the femoral trochanteric process and the gluteus medius tendon on the lateral aspect of the hip. Point tenderness is often identified by the patient on top of the femoral trochanter. The bursa may be injected with the patient lying in the lateral decubitus position on the unaffected side. Insert the needle perpendicular to the skin into the site of maximal tenderness. You may feel resistance as you pass through the gluteus medius tendon as the needle advances to the underlying bursa and femoral trochanter (Fig. 3-1).

KNEE

- The knee joint is formed by the articulation of the femur, the tibia, and the patella (which lies in the femoral intercondylar groove). The joint space of the knee extends from the proximal tibia to the suprapatellar region below the quadriceps muscle. Therefore, the knee joint may be entered through the medial or lateral approach. Both are discussed here.
- **There should never be any resistance to knee injections.** If resistance is encountered you may be attempting the injection into a tendon or bone.

Lateral Suprapatellar Approach

- Position the patient supine on the table with the knee extended (some physicians prefer up to 90 degrees of flexion) and with the quadriceps tendon relaxed.
- Palpate the superior lateral aspect of the patella (approximately 2 o'clock on the left, and 10 o'clock on the right) and mark the skin one finger space superior and lateral to this location.
- Advance the needle into the joint space at approximately a 45-degree angle from the skin toward the underside of the superior lateral aspect of the patella (Fig. 3-2).

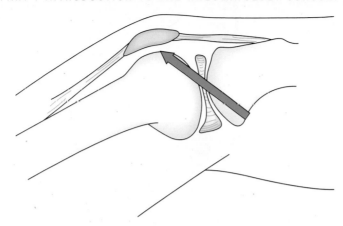

FIGURE 3-2. Medial view of the knee joint.

Medial Approach

- Position the patient supine on the table with the knee extended or flexed at up to 90 degrees and the quadriceps tendon relaxed.
- Palpate the medial patella and mark the skin medially at the base of the patella (9 o'clock on the left and 3 o'clock on the right).
- Advance the needle perpendicular to the skin. You may need to adjust inferiorly slightly depending on specific patient anatomy or presence of severe osteoarthritis (Fig. 3-2).

Prepatellar Bursa

- This bursa is located directly over the patella. Cystic swelling at this location represents bursitis.
- Position the patient in the supine position with the leg extended.
- Enter the bursa on the medial or lateral aspect of the bursa with the needle parallel to the bed.

Anserine Bursa

- This superficial bursa is located at the medial tibial plateau, about 3 cm below the medial joint line. Inflammation often results from abnormal gait.
- Position the patient supine on the table. Identify the anserine bursa and its point of maximal tenderness.
- While staying relatively superficial, enter the bursa perpendicular to the skin.

ANKLE

- The leg should be rested with the foot at a 90-degree angle. The tibialis anterior tendon and the medial malleolus should be identified.
- The needle should enter the skin medial to the tendon and lateral to the mid-superior portion of the malleolus. Direct the needle posteriorly to enter the joint space (Fig. 3-3).

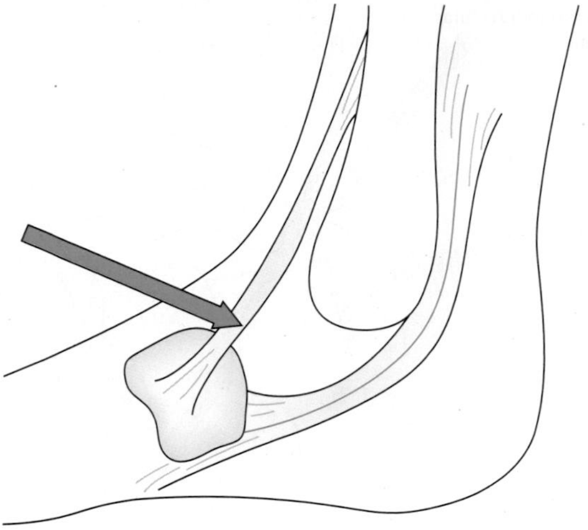

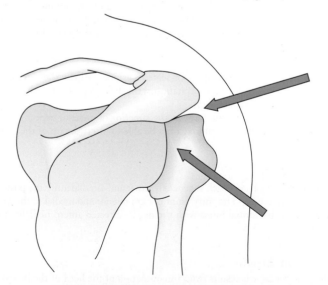

FIGURE 3-3. Medial view of the ankle joint.

SHOULDER

Posterior Approach

- With the patient sitting, palpate the posterior margin of the acromion.
- The needle is inserted and directed anteriorly 1 cm below and 1 cm medial to the posterior corner of the acromion. Direct the needle toward the coracoid process until bone is touched at the articular surface (Fig. 3-4).

FIGURE 3-4. Posterior view of the shoulder.

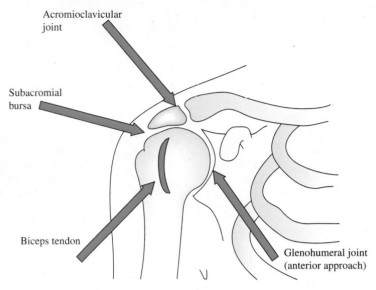

FIGURE 3-5. Anterior view of the shoulder.

Anterior Approach

- The patient should be sitting or supine with the affected shoulder internally rotated.
- The point medial to the head of the humerus and slightly inferior and lateral to the coracoid process should be located and marked. Introduce and direct the needle posteriorly. Redirect superiorly and laterally if bone is hit (Fig. 3-5).

Acromioclavicular Joint

- With the patient in the supine or seated position, palpate the clavicle and follow it distally to its lateral termination. This slight depression is the articulation of the acromioclavicular joint.
- Insert the needle into the joint at the superior or anterior aspect of the joint. This space is small and you may only be able to insert the tip of the needle into the space (Fig. 3-5).

Subacromial Bursa

- The posterolateral approach is generally easier and safer. Identify the posterior corner of the acromion. The entry point is 1 cm inferior and medial to this landmark.
- Enter the subacromial bursa with the needle directed anteromedially under the acromion (Fig. 3-5).

Biceps Tendon Sheath

- Bicipital tendonitis results from inflammation of the head of the biceps tendon as it passes through the bicipital groove in the humerus.

- With the patient sitting, externally rotate their relaxed arm. Palpate the biceps tendon in the bicipital groove. To confirm anatomy, flex and extend the patient's externally rotated arm to feel the tendon slide in the groove.
- When injecting, aim the needle superiorly to the tendon at a tangential angle. Take care to only inject around the tendon as injection into the tendon itself may result in tendon rupture. There should be no resistance to injection when done appropriately (Fig. 3-5).

ELBOW

- The elbow should be flexed at 90 degrees and the joint should be entered in the center of the triangle formed by the lateral epicondyle, radial head, and olecranon process.
- Insert the needle perpendicular to the skin at the joint.

Common Extensor Tendon

- **Lateral epicondylitis** ("tennis elbow") is caused by injury of the common extensor tendon at its insertion of the lateral epicondyle of the humerus.
- When injecting around this tendon, enter the skin directly over the prominence of the lateral epicondyle and perpendicular to the skin. Take care not to inject directly into the tendon (Fig. 3-6).

Common Flexor Tendon

- **Medial epicondylitis** (golfer's elbow) is caused by injury to the common flexor tendon at the medial epicondyle of the humerus.
- When injecting around this tendon enter half inch distal to the medial epicondyle. Take care not to inject directly into the tendon.

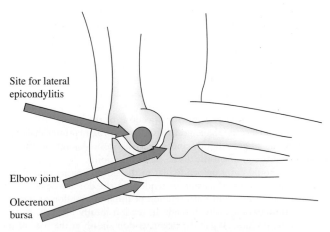

Site for lateral epicondylitis

Elbow joint

Olecrenon bursa

FIGURE 3-6. Lateral view of the elbow.

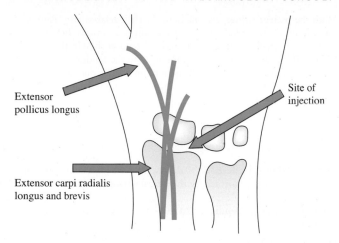

Extensor
pollicus longus

Site of
injection

Extensor carpi radialis
longus and brevis

FIGURE 3-7. Dorsal view of the right wrist.

Olecranon Bursa

- This superficial bursa is located at the extensor surface of the ulna distal to the olecranon process. Position the patient with their arm comfortably flexed or extended and supported.
- Enter the superficial bursa perpendicular to the skin in a "Z" line to avoid establishing a drainage track.
- Try to avoid areas of the elbow with callus as these areas harbor more bacteria.

WRIST

- Entry into the radiocarpal joint may be performed easily.
- Palpate the joint between the distal radius and the navicular bone. This is on the radial side of the second digit extensor tendon. Mark this joint accurately so as not to injure the extensor tendons of the first or second digits.
- Enter into the joint perpendicular to the wrist (Fig. 3-7).

HAND

- Use the smallest needle available for injections of the hand.
- To inject the metacarpophalangeal (MCP) and proximal interphalangeal (PIP) joints, flex the fingers slightly and inject the desired joint on the medial or lateral side of the joint on the dorsal half of the joint.
- The needle should enter perpendicular to the skin on either side of the finger.
- Take care not to injure the extensor tendon on the dorsal side of the finger.
- **Trigger finger** results from inflammation of the flexor tendon of the finger preventing it from passing easily through the tendon sheath. Place the patient's hand in the supine position. Inject the flexor tendon sheath at the base of the finger just distal to the metacarpal head. Take care not to inject directly into the tendon.

Synovial Fluid Analysis

4

Jeffrey Sparks and Leslie E. Kahl

GENERAL PRINCIPLES

- Synovial fluid analysis is useful in distinguishing between inflammatory, septic, noninflammatory, or hemorrhagic conditions.
- New effusions, suspected septic arthritis, and acutely tender, erythematous, and swollen single joints generally require arthrocentesis and synovial fluid analysis.
- Synovial fluid analysis includes: Gross inspection, microscopic inspection for crystals and birefringence, cell count and differential, Gram stain, and microbiologic cultures.
- Repeated unsuccessful arthrocenteses may require injection of a small amount of saline to analyze a diluted sample of synovial fluid, or aspiration with ultrasound or radiographic guidance.

Definitions

- Normal synovial fluid is an ultrafiltrate of plasma that contains small amounts of high molecular weight proteins (fibrinogen, complement, globulin) complexed with hyaluronan.
- Synovial fluid has viscoelastic properties, normally acting as a lubricant and shock absorber for the joint.
- Birefringence of synovial fluid crystals is evaluated by orientating the polarizer parallel to the long axis of the crystal. Positive birefringence is blue while negative birefringence is yellow. For example, monosodium urate crystals are needle shaped and have strongly negative birefringence, while calcium pyrophosphate dihydrate crystals are rhomboid shaped and have weakly positive birefringence.

Classification

- Many rheumatologic and nonrheumatologic conditions may disrupt the normal composition of synovial fluid.
- Other causes of effusions and synovial fluid abnormalities include: Trauma, hemarthrosis, recent arthroplasty, and prosthetic orthopedic devices.
- See Table 4-1 for general analysis of synovial fluid.
- See Table 4-2 for crystal analysis of synovial fluid.

TABLE 4-1	GENERAL ANALYSIS OF SYNOVIAL FLUID

Exam	Normal	Noninflammatory	Inflammatory	Septic
Viscosity	High	High	Low	Very low
Color	Colorless to straw colored	Straw colored to yellow	Yellow	Yellow or purulent
Clarity	Transparent	Transparent	Cloudy, rice bodies, black speckles[a]	Cloudy
WBCs/mm^3	<200	50–1,000	1,000–75,000	>50,000
Neutrophils	<25%	<25%	Often >50%	>85%
Differential diagnosis		OA, SLE, amyloidosis, osteonecrosis, Charcot's joint, trauma, tumors, ochronosis, Wilson's disease	RA, PsA, reactive arthritis, crystalline arthropathies, SLE, scleroderma, infectious (bacterial, tuberculous, viral, fungal)	Infectious (most often bacterial but also mycobacterial, viral, fungal)

[a]Rice bodies, seen in chronically inflamed joints, are composed of cellular debris, fibrin, and collagen precipitate. Black speckled fluid ("ground pepper sign") may result from the fragmentation of a prosthetic arthroplasty.

WBCs, white blood cells; OA, osteoarthritis; SLE, systemic lupus erythematosus; RA, rheumatoid arthritis; PsA, psoriatic arthritis.

TABLE 4-2	CRYSTAL ANALYSIS OF SYNOVIAL FLUID

Crystal Type	Disease	Morphology	Birefringence	Color
Monosodium urate	Gout	Needles	Negative	Yellow
CPPD	Pseudogout	Rhomboid, rods	Weakly positive	Blue
Cholesterol	OA, RA	Rectangles	Variable	Yellow, blue
Calcium oxalate	Renal disease	Bipyramidal	Positive	Blue
Hydroxyapatite	OA	Round, irregular	None	None

CPPD, calcium pyrophosphate dehydrate; OA, osteoarthritis; RA, rheumatoid arthritis.

Laboratory Evaluation of Rheumatic Diseases

Kristine A. Kuhn and Leslie E. Kahl

ERYTHROCYTE SEDIMENTATION RATE

General Principles

- Erythrocyte sedimentation rate (ESR) is the rate of erythrocytes settling in anticoagulated blood; it is a **nonspecific marker of tissue inflammation.** The presence of asymmetric macromolecules produced by the liver during inflammation promotes erythrocyte aggregation and increases the ESR.
- The ESR is affected by many conditions, some of which may be present in patients with rheumatologic diseases.
  - Noninflammatory conditions that tend to raise the ESR include anemia (except sickle cell anemia), renal disease (including nephrotic syndrome and glomerulonephritis), hypercholesterolemia, female sex, pregnancy, oral contraceptives, malignancy, thyroid disease, and increasing age.
  - Conditions that can lower the ESR include high-dose steroid use, sickle cell anemia, polycythemia, anisocytosis, spherocytosis, microcytosis, hepatic failure, and cachexia.
- The ESR is sometimes used to monitor the activity of inflammatory conditions such as systemic lupus erythematosus (SLE) and rheumatoid arthritis (RA), although other markers of disease activity such as clinical signs and symptoms and lab indicators of organ function are more useful.

Laboratory Assessment

- Anticoagulated whole blood is allowed to stand for one hour. The distance between the erythrocyte sediment and top of the tube in millimeters is the ESR.
- The presence of acute phase reactants makes the cells fall faster and raises that distance.

C-REACTIVE PROTEIN

General Principles

- C-reactive protein (CRP) is a beta globulin normally present in the serum in trace amounts. **Serum concentrations rapidly increase during inflammation** within 4 to 6 hours and normalize over a week.
- CRP is a component of the innate immune response whose major function is to recognize foreign pathogens and damaged cells by binding to phosphocholine surfaces. Activation of complement proteins or phagocytic cells follows.
- Similar to ESR, CRP levels are elevated in acute or chronic inflammatory states. Obesity, smoking, coronary artery disease, malignancy, and diabetes mellitus may also elevate CRP levels.

- The use of CRP levels in addition to the ESR in the rheumatic diseases is limited.
  - In patients with RA, a persistently elevated CRP level may be associated with radiographic progression of joint disease and with long-term disability.
  - CRP levels may also be useful in patients with SLE. In contrast to ESR, CRP levels are usually normal in active SLE except in chronic synovitis or acute serositis. In SLE patients with fever in whom synovitis or serositis can be excluded, elevated CRP levels suggest a bacterial source of inflammation and fever.

Laboratory Assessment

- Nephelometry and enzyme-linked immunosorbent assays (ELISAs) are used to measure CRP.
- Levels <0.2 mg/dL are normal and >1 mg/dL are consistent with active inflammation.

ANTINUCLEAR ANTIBODIES

General Principles

- Antinuclear antibodies (ANAs) are directed against nuclear antigens. The ANA pattern reflects different nuclear antigens targeted. Antibodies against specific nuclear antigens can be detected (see later) and have improved specificity for certain diseases.[1]
- ANAs can be useful in the diagnosis of many autoimmune diseases including SLE and other connective tissue diseases (CTDs).
  - The specificities and sensitivities of ANA titers vary for each disease and vary on the basis of the type of lab assay used. Therefore, one must be cautious in interpretation of ANA results.
  - Titers do not correlate with disease activity and remain fairly stable throughout the disease course. **There is no need to repeat the ANA once the diagnosis is clearly established.**
  - Testing should only be performed to support a suspected, specific clinical diagnosis.
  - **While the absence of an ANA virtually excludes a diagnosis of SLE, the presence of ANAs does not establish the diagnosis.**
- Some ANAs such as anti–double-stranded DNA (anti–dsDNA) antibodies are thought to contribute to disease pathogenesis by cross-reacting with self-antigens or forming immune complexes, while most ANAs are not considered pathogenic.

Laboratory Assessment

- ANAs are detected by indirect immunofluorescence or ELISA. Due to minor variations in assay protocols, the sensitivity and specificity varies on the basis of the assay used and the titer cut-off for a positive result.
  - Higher titers convey increased clinical significance but do not correlate with disease activity.
  - ANAs in healthy individuals tend to be of low titers.
- When indirect immunofluorescence is performed, most laboratories use the human epithelial HEp-2 cell line as the substrate.
- Several staining patterns have been described. With the exception of the centromere pattern, which is specific for limited systemic sclerosis (LSSc or

calcinosis, Raynaud's, esophageal dysmotility, sclerodactyly, and telangiectasias [CREST]), the ANA staining pattern is generally unhelpful because it is subject to observer interpretation.
- Specific ANAs are tested by ELISA.

Extractable Nuclear Antigens
- Extractable nuclear antigens (ENAs) are **specific antigenic targets for ANAs** that can be extracted from the nucleus.
- These include **anti-Smith (anti-Sm)**, which is included in the American College of Rheumatology (ACR) criteria for the diagnosis of SLE, and **anti-ribonucleoprotein (anti-RNP)**, which is specific for mixed connective tissue disease (MCTD). **Anti-Ro (anti-SSA)** and **anti-La (anti-SSB)**, associated with Sjögren's syndrome, subacute cutaneous lupus, and neonatal lupus, are also included in the ENA test battery.
- Patients with negative ANA titers will also have negative ENAs, although positive ANAs do not necessarily result in detectable antibodies to ENAs. A positive ANA in a patient with clinically suspected CTD should prompt one to test more specific ENAs.
- See Table 5-1 for a summary of specific ENAs and disease associations.

Other Antinuclear Antibodies
- **Anti-dsDNA, anti–Scl-70,** and **anti-histone** are other ANAs that can be associated with particular CTDs and carry prognostic information. These are also summarized in Table 5-1.

RHEUMATOID FACTOR

General Principles
- Rheumatoid factor (RF) is a **polyclonal antibody directed against the Fc portion of immunoglobulin** (Ig), most commonly IgM directed against IgG, although IgG and IgA isotypes of RF are also detected in sera.
- RF is associated with **chronic inflammatory diseases including RA** (see Table 5-1).
  - ○ RF has a sensitivity of 60% to 80% for RA and a specificity of about 70%.
  - ○ RF is also found elevated in Sjögren's syndrome, hepatitis C infection, multiple myeloma, interstitial lung disease, cryoglobulinemic vasculitis, and sarcoidosis, among other chronic inflammatory and infectious disorders. A small percentage of healthy individuals will have a positive RF.
- The role of RF in the pathogenesis of disease is unclear, although one hypothesis suggests that RF initiates immune complexes in the synovium, which activate, complement and release chemoattractants that recruit immune cells.

Laboratory Assessment
- RF is classically detected using a latex immunofixation test and reported as a titer.
- Newer methods, including nephelometry and ELISAs, report results in international units.
- The inverse ratio of the nephelometric result correlates roughly with the titer result; for example, 120 IU correlates roughly with a titer of 1:120.

TABLE 5-1 AUTOANTIBODIES AND THEIR ASSOCIATED DISEASES

Antibody	Disease Association	Comments
ANA	SLE, MCTD, SS, PM, DM, scleroderma	Nonspecific (present in 5% of population and prevalence increases with age). Sensitivities: SLE >95%, MCTD >95%, SS ~75%, PM/DM >75%, scleroderma 60%–90%, RA 15%–35%. Also present in other autoimmune disorders, cancer, and infections.[1]
Anti-centromere (pattern of ANA)	LSSc, or CREST	Sensitivities: LSSc 10%–50%. Associated with CREST.[1] May be observed in idiopathic Raynaud's 25%, but some will progress to developing CREST. Staining pattern is easily identifiable on ANA stain.
RF	RA	Nonspecific, prevalence increases with age (false-positive in up to 25% of subjects aged >70). Sensitivities: RA 60%–80%, SS 70%, viral hepatitis 25%, bacterial endocarditis 25%, chronic infection, sarcoidosis, malignancy, and cryoglobulinemia. In RA, may have loose correlation with clinical activity and predicts poorer prognosis and extraarticular disease.[2]
Anti-CCP	RA	Highly specific for RA approaching 99%; sensitivity parallels that for RF at ~70%. May be present years before clinically apparent disease. Presence indicates more severe disease with radiographic damage and extraarticular manifestations.[2,3]
Anti-dsDNA	SLE	Very specific for SLE, only 50%–80% sensitive. Associated with lupus nephritis and may correlate with disease activity in SLE.[1]
Anti-Sm	SLE	Very specific for SLE, only ~15% sensitive. Associated with lupus nephritis.[1]
Anti-Ro (SSA)	SS	Sensitivities: SS 70%, SLE 25%. Associated with sicca symptoms in other CTDs, extraglandular disease in SS, heart block in neonates with anti-Ro positive mothers. Correlates with SCLE rash, photosensitivity, or thrombocytopenia in SLE.[1]

TABLE 5-1 AUTOANTIBODIES AND THEIR ASSOCIATED DISEASES (Continued)

Antibody	Disease Association	Comments
Anti-La (SSB)	SS	Sensitivities: SS 40%, SLE 10%. Association with anti-Ro. Correlates with benign course in SLE if no other autoantibody present except ANA.[1]
Anti-U1RNP	MCTD	Detected in 100% of patients with MCTD.[1]
Anti-histone	DIL, SLE	Nonspecific. Sensitivities: DIL >90%, SLE >50%.
Anti–Scl-70 (Topoisomerase I)	Scleroderma	Very specific but only 15%–35% sensitive for diffuse systemic sclerosis. Associated with ILD as manifestation of SSc.[1]
Anti-RNA polymerase III	SSc	Very specific but only 20%–25% specific for scleroderma. These antibodies correlate with increased risk for malignant hypertension and renal crisis.[1]
c-ANCA	WG	Confirm positive values with anti-PR3. Very sensitive (>90%) and specific (99%) for active disease in fulminant WG but less sensitive in limited WG (50%). Questionable if levels correlate with disease activity. Less sensitive for MPA 25%, CSS 33%, and PAN 10%.
p-ANCA	CSS, MPA	Nonspecific; confirm positive finding with anti-MPO. Sensitivities for anti-MPO: CSS 50%, idiopathic crescentic glomerulonephritis 64%, MPA 58%, PAN 40%, WG 24%. Non–anti-MPO p-ANCA present in RA, SLE, PM/DM, relapsing polychondritis, APS, and other autoimmune diseases.
Anti–Jo-1	PM	25%–30% sensitive in PM. Predicts a constellation of deforming arthritis, "mechanic's hands," Raynaud's, and pulmonary fibrosis in DM and PM (also called anti-synthetase syndrome).[1]
Anti–Mi-2	DM	Found in 20%–30% of patients with DM. Associated with V-sign, shawl sign, cuticular overgrowth, good response to therapy and good prognosis.[4]

(continued)

| TABLE 5-1 | AUTOANTIBODIES AND THEIR ASSOCIATED DISEASES (*Continued*) |

Antibody	Disease Association	Comments
Anti-SRP	PM/DM	<5% sensitive in PM/DM. Associated with acute onset, severe weakness, palpitations, and poor prognosis.[4]
Lupus anticoagulant	Hypercoagulable states, APS	APA; screened for by detecting prolonged PTT or dRVVT that fails to correct with mixing studies and confirmed with phospholipid neutralization studies that confirm a phospholipid-dependent in vitro anticoagulant.[5]
Anti-cardiolipin antibody	Hypercoagulable states, APS	APA; association with thrombosis: IgG>>IgM>IgA. Titers tend to correspond with disease activity.
beta-2-GPI–dependent aCL	Hypercoagulable states, APS	A type of aCL that binds to complex of beta-2-GPI and cardiolipin. Positive values associated with higher risk of hypercoagulable states than non–beta-2-GPI–dependent aCL.
Cryoglobulins	HCV, LPD, CTD	Type I: Monoclonal Ig (usually IgM or IgG) that self-aggregate; may have RF activity, associated with LPD. Type II: Monoclonal Ig (usually IgM) with activity against polyclonal IgG (i.e., RF activity), most commonly idiopathic, may be associated with HCV or CTD. Type III: Polyclonal Ig (usually IgM) with activity against polyclonal IgG (i.e., RF activity), most commonly idiopathic, may be associated with HCV or CTD.

ANA, antinuclear antibody; SLE, systemic lupus erythematosus; MCTD, mixed connective tissue disease; SS, Sjögren's syndrome; PM, polymyositis; DM, dermatomyositis; DIL, drug-induced lupus; LSSc, limited systemic sclerosis; ILD, interstitial lung disease; SSc, systemic sclerosis; CREST, calcinosis, Raynaud's, esophageal dysmotility, sclerodactyly, and telangiectasias; RF, rheumatoid factor; RA, rheumatoid arthritis; anti-ccp, anti-cyclic citrullinated peptide; anti-dsDNA' anti–double-stranded DNA; anti-Sm, anti-Smith; SCLE, subacute cutaneous lupus erythematosus; RNP, ribonucleoprotein; MCTD, mixed connective tissue disease; ANCA, Antineutrophil cytoplasmic antibody; WG, Wegener's granulomatosis; PR3, proteinase 3; MPA, microscopic polyangiitis; CSS, Churg–Strauss syndrome; PAN, polyarteritis nodosa; MPO, myeloperoxidase; APS, antiphospholipid syndrome; anti-SRP, anti–signal recognition protein; PTT, partial thromboplastin time; dRVVT, dilute Russell viper venom time; GPI, glycoprotein I; aCL, anticardiolipin antibodies; HCV, hepatitis C virus; LPD, lymphoproliferative diseases; CTD, connective tissue disease.

ANTI-CITRULLINATED PROTEIN ANTIBODIES

General Principles

- Anti-citrullinated protein antibodies (ACPAs) include antibodies directed against **cyclic citrullinated peptide** (**CCP**), filaggrin, vimentin, and fibrinogen, among others yet unidentified. CCP is a synthetic peptide derived from filaggrin that confers high sensitivity and specificity when testing for antibodies in individuals with RA.
- These peptides/proteins are unique in that they contain citrulline, an amino acid formed by post-translational deimination of arginine.
- ACPAs are sensitive (70%) and highly specific (95%) for RA.[2]
- Anti-CCP antibodies have been detected in sera of patients with RA up to 10 years prior to the onset of disease. About one-third of patients with RA will be positive for these antibodies, but RF negative, on presentation.
- There is evidence that these antibodies contribute to disease pathogenesis as higher titers correlate with more erosive disease.[3] The stimuli for the induction of these antibodies and the mechanism by which they contribute to disease activity are under investigation.

Laboratory Assessment

- The only ACPA that is currently available for clinical testing is anti-CCP antibody.
- Newer generations of an ELISA with CCP have increased the specificity for RA.

ANTINEUTROPHIL CYTOPLASMIC ANTIBODIES

General Principles

- Antineutrophil cytoplasmic antibodies (ANCAs) are directed against cytoplasmic antigens in human neutrophils.
- ANCAs are not ANAs, although proximity of perinuclear-ANCA (p-ANCA) staining to the nucleus may be mistaken for an ANA. Hence, a positive ANA or p-ANCA may result in false-positive results for p-ANCA or ANA, respectively.
- Two distinct staining patterns have been described: Cytoplasmic-ANCA (c-ANCA) and p-ANCA.
  - c-ANCA is associated with Wegener's granulomatosis (WG) and p-ANCA is associated with Churg–Strauss syndrome (CSS), microscopic polyangiitis (MPA), and polyarteritis nodosa (PAN).
  - The specific antigen for most c-ANCA is proteinase 3 (PR3) and for most p-ANCA is myeloperoxidase (MPO).
  - PR3 is a protein present in azurophil granules in neutrophils and is involved in the function and activation of neutrophils. Antibodies to PR3 have high sensitivities and specificities for active, fulminant WG. It is believed that neutrophil modification by anti-PR3 antibodies in WG may account for some of the disease manifestations.
  - MPO is a protein involved in the generation of reactive oxygen species and in the modulation of macrophage function. Since p-ANCA and anti-MPO antibodies are present in a large number of diseases, their roles in pathogenesis are poorly understood.

- ANCAs are present in other inflammatory conditions, including autoimmune hepatitis, primary biliary cirrhosis, and ulcerative colitis. Further, they may be induced by certain infections such as Staphylococcus aureus and mycobacteria, and by drugs such as propylthiouracil and hydralazine.

Laboratory Assessment

- ANCAs are identified with indirect immunofluorescent staining assays using ethanol-fixed neutrophils.
- Testing for anti-PR3 and anti-MPO antibodies is performed by ELISAs at a reference lab.

MYOSITIS-SPECIFIC ANTIBODIES

- The three best-described **myositis-specific antibodies (MSAs)** are **anti–Jo-1** (directed to t-RNA histidyl synthetase), **anti–signal recognition protein (anti-SRP)**, and **anti–Mi-2**. Their sensitivities for inflammatory myopathies are low, ranging 25% to 30%.
- Specific MSA may be associated with certain clinical features and prognosis (see Table 5-1).[4]
- These antibodies are detected by ELISA.

ANTIPHOSPHOLIPID ANTIBODIES

General Principles

- Antiphospholipid antibodies (APAs) are directed against phospholipids and are associated with hypercoagulable and thrombotic states.
- APA is detected by assays for the **lupus anticoagulant (LAC), anticardiolipin antibodies (aCL), and false-positive serologies for syphilis.**
- Of the three APAs, **LAC has the strongest association with hypercoagulation.** The name LAC is derived from the fact that the antibody was first described in patients with SLE, and from its tendency to cause prolonged activated partial thromboplastin time (aPTT) that did not correct with the addition of normal plasma. We now know that LAC can be found in other CTDs or in isolation.[5]
- The association between aCL and hypercoagulable states is related to antibody titers and Ig isotype. As a general rule, increasing titers of aCL are associated with increasing risk of hypercoagulation and thrombosis. IgG aCL carry more risk than IgM aCL, and the risk with IgA aCL is questionable.
- Some aCL bind to complexes composed of phospholipids and beta-2-glycoprotein I (beta-2-GPI), a natural serum anticoagulant. Beta-2-GPI–dependent aCL are associated with increased risk of hypercoagulable states.

Laboratory Assessment

- LAC is identified in a stepwise manner using functional phospholipid-dependent clotting assays that reveal a coagulation inhibitor that is neutralized by phospholipids.[5]
  - First, phospholipid-dependent clotting assays such as a dilute prothrombin time, aPTT, kaolin clotting time, or a dilute Russell viper venom time (dRVVT) are drawn; prolonged times are considered positive results. Each

test has different sensitivities in detecting LAC, and **the use of more than one test is recommended.**

○ **The preferred screening test is an aPTT-based test** using silica as an activator in the presence of low levels of phospholipids. A prolonged time suggests the presence of LAC. Positive tests should then be confirmed with a dRVVT. In this assay, Russell viper venom activates factor X, which leads to the conversion of prothrombin to thrombin, dependent upon the presence of phospholipids. If a LAC is present, the phospholipids are unavailable and the dRVVT is prolonged.

○ **Mixing studies** are then performed on samples with prolonged times to exclude factor deficiencies. If a prolonged time corrects in mixing studies, the sample is further incubated in different temperatures to exclude a temperature-sensitive inhibitor of coagulation. A sample that does not correct with mixing studies or with variable-temperature incubation is identified as having an inhibitor of coagulation. This sample is then incubated with excessive phospholipids to characterize the inhibitor as either a phospholipid-dependent or a phospholipid-independent inhibitor. Excessive phospholipids neutralize the LAC and the prolonged times correct.

○ Although LAC is a phospholipid-dependent inhibitor of coagulation in laboratory assays, in vivo the LAC's interactions with phospholipid-rich endothelial and platelet surfaces are thought to activate both platelets and the coagulation cascade and result in hypercoagulation and thrombosis.

• **Serologic assays for syphilis such as the venereal disease research laboratory (VDRL) and rapid plasma reagin (RPR) tests detect cardiolipin phospholipids.** When VDRL or RPR is positive, perform a confirmatory test for antibodies against treponemes such as the fluorescent treponemal antibody absorbed (FTA-ABS) test. A false-positive test for syphilis identifies an APA; however, newer ELISAs for aCL have improved sensitivity and specificity and are the preferred method for detection.

• Antibodies to beta-2-GPI are detected by IgM and IgG specific ELISAs.

• Testing for all APAs can be influenced by anticoagulants and acute thrombotic events. Therefore, testing should be repeated in 6 weeks to verify results.

CRYOGLOBULINS

General Principles

• Immunoglobulins that are soluble at body temperature but reversibly precipitate at lower temperatures are known as cryoglobulins.

• Cryoglobulins are classified into three types depending on the characteristics of the immunoglobulins, and each type is associated with different diseases.

○ **Type I** cryoglobulins are monoclonal antibodies, usually of the IgM isotype. They do not typically activate complement. Type I cryoglobulins are typically observed in **lymphoproliferative disorders** and cause vasooclusive symptoms.

○ **Type II** cryoglobulins are a mixture of polyclonal IgG and monoclonal IgM antibodies, while **type III** cryoglobulins are polyclonal IgG and IgM antibodies. These are associated with **viral hepatitis and CTDs.** As they activate complement, types II and III cryoglobulins result in **small vessel vasculitis** symptoms.

Laboratory Assessment

- A cryocrit is obtained using a minimum of 10 to 20 mL of fresh venous blood that is drawn into prewarmed test tubes and transported to the lab in sand or water warmed to 37°C. The specimen is allowed to clot at 37°C for 30 to 60 minutes before centrifugation. The supernatant is then left at 4°C for as long as 7 days; types I and II usually precipitate within 24 hours, whereas type III may take days.
- Newer methods using electrophoresis can detect and quantify cryoglobulins, but preheated tubes and warm transportation are still required.

COMPLEMENT

General Principles

- The **complement cascade** involves >30 proteins and accounts for 15% of the globulin portion of plasma protein.
- Three pathways have been identified.
  - The **classical pathway** involves the opsonization and/or lysis of cells covered with antibodies to cell surface antigens.
  - The **alternative pathway** involves the nonspecific opsonization and/or lysis of foreign cells that lack cell membrane complement regulators.
  - The **mannose-binding lectin pathway** involves the opsonization and/or lysis of foreign cells with mannose groups on the cell membrane.
- The rheumatic diseases that involve immune complex formation and subsequent activation of the classic pathway include SLE, cryoglobulinemic vasculitis, and Henoch–Schönlein purpura.
- The **total hemolytic complement** activity is a functional assay that tests the integrity of the classical pathway. Low total hemolytic complement activity suggests a deficiency of ≥1 factors.
- **C3 and C4** are individual components of the complement cascade.
  - In SLE, low C3 and C4 complement levels may correlate with disease activity, especially in lupus nephritis.
  - Conversely, complement proteins may act as acute phase reactants and appear elevated during increased disease activity.
  - Not all patients have complement levels that correlate with disease activity, and the pattern of correlation may vary with each patient. Nevertheless, once a pattern is established in a particular patient, levels may be used to monitor disease activity.
  - Low C4 levels are present in patients with cryoglobulinemic vasculitis, reflective of complement activation by immune complex deposition.
- Congenital deficiencies in complements C1 and C4 increase the risk for SLE.

Laboratory Assessment

- Individual complement proteins such as C3 and C4 are measured by ELISA or nephelometry.
- Total hemolytic complement activity (CH50) is measured by adding diluted patient serum to antibody-coated sheep red blood cells (RBCs), and reported as the amount serum required to lyse 50% of the RBCs.

REFERENCES

1. Satoh M, Vázquez-Del Mercado M, Chan EK. Clinical interpretation of antinuclear antibody tests in systemic rheumatic diseases. *Mod Rheumatol.* 2009;19:219–228.
2. Nishimura K, Sugiyama D, Kogata Y, et al. Meta-analysis: diagnostic accuracy of anti-cyclic citrullinated peptide antibody and rheumatoid factor for rheumatoid arthritis. *Ann Intern Med.* 2007;146:797–808.
3. Berglin E, Johansson T, Sundin U, et al. Radiological outcome in rheumatoid arthritis is predicted by presence of antibodies against cyclic citrullinated peptide before and at disease onset, and by IgA-RF at disease onset. *Ann Rheum Dis.* 2006;65:453–458.
4. Mammen AL. Dermatomyositis and polymyositis: clinical presentation, autoantibodies, and pathogenesis. *Ann N Y Acad Sci.* 2010;1184:134–153.
5. Tripodi A. Testing for lupus anticoagulants: all that a clinician should know. *Lupus.* 2009;18:291–298.

Radiographic Imaging of Rheumatic Diseases

Ashwini Komarla and Leslie E. Kahl

APPROACH TO BONE AND JOINT RADIOGRAPHS

- The availability and technology behind imaging techniques has expanded greatly in recent years. Imaging can aid in diagnosis and provide objective assessment of disease severity and progression. Modalities useful in the assessment of rheumatologic conditions include conventional radiography, computed tomography (CT), magnetic resonance imaging (MRI), ultrasound, arthrography, angiography, radionuclide imaging, and bone densitometry.
- **Conventional radiographs are the initial imaging choice for most rheumatic conditions.** Radiography has the ability to demonstrate fine bone detail and detect small calcification, but it lacks the capacity to distinguish soft tissue structures.
  - Its poor sensitivity to soft tissue contrast does not allow direct visualization of inflamed synovial tissues, articular cartilage, bone marrow edema, or periarticular tendons.
  - In inflammatory arthritis, it can detect the osseous erosions and joint space narrowing that are the later irreversible sequelae of preceding synovitis. In this manner, plain radiographs can provide limited yet very valuable information about disease activity.
  - Despite its constraints, conventional radiography is universally available and inexpensive and remains the mainstay in the basic imaging of arthritis.
- A simplified systemic approach using the mnemonic ABCDS can be used to interpret bone and joint plain films.
  - *A* refers to joint alignment.
  - *B* refers to bone.
  - *C* refers to cartilage and joint space.
  - *D* refers to distribution.
  - *S* refers to soft tissue findings.
- Not all features described for each disease below are present at any one time, and no individual abnormality is pathognomonic. See Table 6-1 for commonly ordered radiographs for evaluation of arthritic joints and Table 6-2 for radiographic findings of common types of arthritis.

OSTEOARTHRITIS

- Primary osteoarthritis (OA) is the most common arthropathy.
- **The most characteristic findings are nonuniform joint space narrowing and formation of osteophytes,** also known as bone spurs. Joint involvement can be unilateral or bilateral.

TABLE 6-1	COMMONLY ORDERED RADIOGRAPHS FOR EVALUATION OF ARTHRITIC JOINTS

Hand
  Posteroanterior
  Norgaard (supinated oblique)
Foot
  Anteroposterior
  Lateral
Knee
  Standing anteroposterior
  Tunnel view (intercondylar notch view)
  Non-standing flexed lateral
	Hip
	  Anteroposterior
	  Frog-leg of affected hip
	Sacroiliac joint
	  Straight anteroposterior view
	  Anteroposterior: Modified Ferguson view
	Cervical spine
	  Lateral view in a flexed and extended position

- **Joint erosions commonly seen in inflammatory arthropathies are not present in OA.**
- Subchondral bone cysts or subchondral bone formation (sclerosis) is also associated with OA.
- OA most commonly affects the hands, feet, hips, knees, and the lumbar and cervical spine. Involvement of the shoulders, elbows, and ankles is uncommon unless there is a history of trauma or other preexisting disease.
- **OA most frequently targets the hand,** involving the distal interphalangeal (DIP) and proximal interphalangeal (PIP) joints.
  - **Bouchard's and Heberden's nodes** refer to osteophyte formation at the DIP and PIP joints, respectively.
  - There is usually sparing of the metacarpophalangeal (MCP) joints.
  - The first carpometacarpal or trapeziometacarpal is the typical site of degenerative abnormalities in the wrist.
  - Radial subluxation of the first metacarpal base is also common.
  - Without significant occupational trauma, degenerative arthropathy in other joints of the wrist, like the radiocarpal joint, should suggest a diagnosis other than primary OA.
- The most commonly affected joint in the **feet** is the first metatarsophalangeal (MTP) joint.
  - It is commonly associated with **hallux valgus** (lateral deviation of the tip of the first toe) or **hallux rigidus** (stiffness and painful restriction of dorsiflexion in the first MTP joint).
  - Dorsal osteophytes are characteristic of OA in the foot, and subchondral bone cyst formation is more common in the feet than in the hands.
- OA of the **knees** is common.
  - Bone growth may form and extend into the joint space when cartilage has been lost.
  - Joint space narrowing is usually asymmetric and **worse on the medial side,** although women often have lateral femorotibial disease. **Varus angulation** of the knee is the most common deformity, demonstrating more severe involvement of the medial femorotibial compartment than the lateral one.

TABLE 6-2   RADIOGRAPHIC FINDINGS OF COMMON TYPES OF ARTHRITIS

	RA	OA	PsA	Gout
Alignment	Affected early	Affected late	Affected late	Not affected
Erosions	Symmetric, marginal	None	Occur with bony proliferation	Asymmetric, with overhanging edges
Periarticular osteoporosis	Present	Absent	Absent	Absent
Joint space	Uniformly narrowed	Non-uniformly narrowed	Narrowed in severe cases	Preserved
Distribution	Symmetric, peripheral joints: Hands, wrists, feet, knees, and others, but spares lower spine	May be asymmetric, hands, hips, knees, lumbar and cervical spine	May be asymmetric, hands, wrists, feet, knees	Asymmetric, hands, feet
Soft tissue swelling	Present	Mild swelling	May be very swollen, "sausage digit"	Asymmetric when tophi are present (tophi are not radiopaque)

RA, rheumatoid arthritis; OA, osteoarthritis; PsA, psoriatic arthritis.

○ OA changes in the patellofemoral compartment are also common and can be seen either alone or in addition to medial femorotibial compartment disease.

○ Assessment of cartilage thinning is best provided on tunnel projection or **weight-bearing position radiographs.** Cartilage space narrowing is documented if the joint space width is less than 3 mm, narrower than half the width of the other articulation in the same knee or the same articulation in the other knee, or smaller on weight-bearing compared to non–weight-bearing radiographs. While joint space width has been shown to correlate with cartilage thickness, a decrease in the joint space can also occur as a result of meniscal degeneration.

○ Degenerative tears can be evaluated by MRI.

• OA of the **hip** may lead to significant disability.

○ **Most often cartilage loss is focal and usually involves the weight-bearing superolateral aspect of the joint,** leading to upward migration of the femoral head.

○ Diffuse loss of cartilage with axial migration of the femoral head is more commonly seen in inflammatory arthropathies and secondary OA from diseases like calcium pyrophosphate dihydrate (CPPD) deposition disease (pseudogout).

○ OA of the sacroiliac joint (SI) is extremely common in elderly patients. On radiography, it is characterized by joint space narrowing with a thin, distinct band of subchondral sclerosis, especially around the ilium.

○ Osteophytes may appear as radiodensities at the superior synovial aspect of the joint in the anteroposterior (AP) view.

• OA of the **spine** is commonly referred to as degenerative disk disease or spondylosis and involves osteoarthritic changes of the apophyseal joints between the vertebral bodies.

○ Disk space narrowing or apophyseal joint space narrowing and bone sclerosis are commonly seen.

○ A potentially important complication of severe degenerative disk disease is spondylolisthesis, which is movement of a vertebral body on the vertebral body below it or on the sacrum. Movement occurs either forward (anterolisthesis) or backward (posterolisthesis).

RHEUMATOID ARTHRITIS

• Rheumatoid arthritis (RA) is **the most common systemic inflammatory rheumatologic disease.**

○ The distribution of arthritis is usually bilateral and symmetric in the small joints but unilateral in large joints. RA also affects the appendicular skeleton and cervical spine.

○ **Joint changes are most frequently seen in hands, feet, knees, and hips,** and less commonly in the shoulder and elbow joints.

• Radiographs show periarticular soft tissue swelling and joint malalignment.

• **The earliest radiographic change in RA is symmetric soft tissue swelling** around the involved joints in the hands and feet, with juxta-articular osteoporosis often present.

- Soft tissue swelling is caused by **joint effusion, synovial proliferation, and periarticular soft tissue edema.**
- In the hand, the MCP and PIP joints are involved.
- Soft tissue atrophy and subcutaneous rheumatoid nodules develop in the later stages of the disease.
- Early marginal erosions are often subtle.
- Bony structures commonly have **marginal erosions** initially that may develop into severe subchondral bone erosions.
  - New bone formation is not a feature of RA.
  - Erosions first appear where the articular cartilage is absent or thinnest and may be subtle (first appearing as a disruption of the white cortical line).
  - In the wrist, early erosions often occur at the waist of the capitate, the articulation of the hamate with the base of the fifth metacarpal, and the ulnar styloid.
  - Later in the disease course, the MCPs and PIPs are uniformly involved and all the carpal bones may be affected as a unit.
- **Subluxations and dislocations** such as ulnar deviation at the MCP joints are common.
- **Osteopenia** due to hyperemia from chronic joint inflammation starts in the juxta-articular region and progresses to generalized osteoporosis.
- **Subchondral cysts** are also common. They appear as radiolucent areas in the bone. Occasionally, very large cystic lesions are found in the bones of the elbow, hip, and knee joints, predisposing to pathologic fractures.
- **Joint space narrowing** is diffuse and uniform due to the progressive destruction of articular cartilage. With increasing cartilage damage, the joint space may become partially or completely obliterated by fibrous **ankylosis** and eventually bony ankylosis can develop. This most characteristically occurs in the wrist and the midfoot.
- In RA, the **feet** are almost as commonly involved as the hands.
  - In general, the feet are evaluated with posteroanterior and lateral views.
  - As in the hands, early involvement of the feet results in juxta-articular osteoporosis and erosion of the bare areas at the metatarsal heads.
  - The **lateral aspect of the head of the fifth metatarsal is usually involved first.** The heads of other metatarsals generally erode in a medial to lateral direction.
  - At later stages of the disease, there are **lateral subluxations of the proximal phalanges** and uniform **loss of the MTP joint cartilage space.** This leads to forefoot deformities such as **hallux valgus, hammer toes, cock up deformities of the MTP joints, fibular deviation of the toes, and plantar subluxation of the metatarsal heads.**
- MRI, with its superior soft tissue contrast, offers a greater sensitivity for the detection of some of the early changes of RA.
  - Inflammatory changes such as joint effusions, acute synovitis, pannus, and synovial sheath effusions can be recognized with MRI.
  - The synovial membrane can be seen on MRI depending on the imaging sequence and the nature of the tissue.
  - MRI is also the preferred method of imaging musculoskeletal complications of RA, such as tendon ruptures, ischemic necrosis, insufficiency fractures, and cervical spinal cord compression.

ANKYLOSING SPONDYLITIS

- Ankylosing spondylitis (AS) **primarily affects the axial skeleton and less commonly the appendicular skeleton.**
- It is **more ossifying than erosive** in comparison to other inflammatory arthropathies.
- The axial distribution of disease and the classic "**bamboo spine**" changes are the two features that make the radiographic diagnosis relatively easy.
- Bone density is usually normal before ankylosis and becomes osteoporotic after ankylosis.
- AS involves the SI joints and spine, especially the lumbar spine. The hips and glenohumeral joints are the most common extra-spinal locations of disease. Peripheral joints are usually only mildly involved.
- Subluxations, as seen in RA and psoriatic arthritis (PsA), are not seen in AS.
- **The first abnormalities usually seen are in the SI joints.**
  - The SI joints are commonly involved bilaterally and symmetrically and **often fuse completely.**
  - Erosions and sclerosis are mild and sometimes subtle.
  - Abnormalities are usually more prominent on the iliac side of the articulation.
  - Subchondral bone resorption with loss of definition of the articular margins, superficial osseous erosions, and osteoporosis are interspersed with focal areas of bony sclerosis. This can progress to complete intra-articular bone fusion with disappearance of the prior periarticular sclerosis.
  - The modified Ferguson view provides a better assessment of the SI joints than standard AP views of the pelvis.
  - CT and MRI define the complex anatomy of the SI joints better than conventional radiographs and are more sensitive to early changes. However, most patients with clinical sacroiliitis can be diagnosed with high-quality radiographs.
- The lumbosacral and thoracolumbar junctions are the usual sites of initial spine involvement, with changes progressing in a caudocranial direction.
  - Osteitis of the anterior portion of the discovertebral junction is a common initial finding.
  - On lateral radiographs, the **vertebrae often look "squared."** This is due to erosions at the anterosuperior and anteroinferior vertebral margins leading to loss of the normal concavity of the anterior facet of the vertebral body.
  - Bony sclerosis adjacent to sites of erosion can produce a "**shiny corner sign**" on radiographs.
  - Ossification of the outer fibers of the annulus fibrosus of the intervertebral disk leads to vertically oriented bony outgrowths that are called **syndesmophytes.**
  - The anterior longitudinal ligaments are the first visible sites of ossification.
  - With disease progression, the extensive syndesmophyte formation bridges intervertebral disks producing a smooth vertical spinal contour labeled as "**bamboo spine.**"
  - Erosions of the odontoid process may occur in cases of cervical spine AS and result in **atlantoaxial subluxation.**
  - **Enthesitis,** bony proliferation and inflammation at sites of tendon and ligament insertion, is notable in AS and other seronegative spondyloarthropathies.

PSORIATIC ARTHRITIS

- PsA affects the **axial and appendicular skeleton.** An asymmetric bilateral or unilateral polyarthritis is the most common presentation, but PsA can follow varying patterns.
- PsA differs from RA radiographically in many important ways, particularly with regard to **periosteal bone proliferation and normal bone mineralization.**
- In decreasing order of frequency, PsA involves the hands, feet, SI joints, and spine. **DIP joint involvement in the hands also differentiates PsA from RA.**
- Periarticular soft tissue swelling can be striking in the hands and feet. The swelling often extends beyond the joint into the soft tissue in the digit, forming a "sausage digit", which is very characteristic of this disease.
- The arthritis **may be very erosive.**
  - In severe cases, erosions can destroy large portions of the underlying bone and give the appearance of a widened joint space.
  - In severe cases, the ends of the bones involved become pointy and produce **"pencil-in-cup"** deformities.
  - **Acroosteolysis and resorption of the distal phalanges** of the hands and feet is characteristic of PsA.
  - **Bony proliferation is also relatively unique to PsA.** It occurs adjacent to areas of erosions, along the shafts of the bones, across joints, and at tendinous and ligamentous insertion sites. Initial bone proliferation appears fluffy and spiculated.
  - The radiographic changes of PsA in the feet are similar to those in the hands. In particular, involvement is seen at the posterior and inferior aspects of the calcaneus, sites of tendinous insertion.
- **SI joint involvement** on radiographs is found in 30% to 50% of patients with PsA.
  - It is usually bilateral and may or may not be symmetric.
  - Erosions and bone proliferation are the usual findings and are more common on the iliac side.
  - Bony ankylosis may occur in the SI joints, but it is much less frequent than in AS.
  - Spondylitis usually occurs along with SI joint involvement.
- Large, bulky, and unilateral or asymmetric **paravertebral ossification** is a characteristic finding in PsA, but the ossification may also appear as thin and curvilinear densities.
- The cervical spine may be involved with **atlantoaxial subluxation** similar to that in RA and AS.

REACTIVE ARTHRITIS (REITER'S SYNDROME)

- Many of the radiographic findings in reactive arthritis (ReA) are indistinguishable from those in PsA.
- As in PsA, **bone erosions, bone proliferation, uniform joint space narrowing, ligamentous and tendinous ossification, a bilateral asymmetric distribution, fusiform soft tissue swelling, and lack of osteopenia are common in ReA.**
- However, ReA has a **different distribution** with a predilection to the lower extremities. It affects the feet, ankles, knees, and SI joints with less frequent involvement in the hands, hips, and spine.

- **Joint ankylosis is less common** than in PsA, but heel changes may be more prominent than in PsA.
- Clinical correlations are particularly important in differentiating ReA from PsA.

SYSTEMIC LUPUS ERYTHEMATOSUS

- Characteristic radiographic findings of systemic lupus erythematosus (SLE) include **deforming nonerosive arthritis and osteonecrosis.**
- Unlike other inflammatory arthropathies, there are **no erosions or joint space loss** in SLE. However, **subluxations and dislocations are often seen** in SLE.
- The arthropathy is most commonly seen in the hands, wrists, hips, knees, and shoulders. Symmetric involvement of the hands is typical, but the specific type of deformity varies.
- **Bone infarcts or osteonecrosis** can occur as a result of chronic steroid use or, less commonly, vasculitis. The femoral heads, femoral condyles, tibial plateaus, humeral heads, and tali are the sites most frequently involved in osteonecrosis.

CALCIUM PYROPHOSPHATE DIHYDRATE DEPOSITION DISEASE

- CPPD deposition disease is **the most common crystalline arthropathy** and affects about 5% of the elderly population.
- The radiographic spectrum of disease ranges from subtle to striking, but certain features are constant.
  - **The hallmark of CPPD deposition disease is chondrocalcinosis,** the deposition of calcium salts in cartilage.
  - This finding is quite specific for CPPD deposition disease, and is **most commonly seen in the knee menisci and the triangular fibrocartilage of the wrist.** Other sites that are affected are the hips, pubic symphysis, and spine.
  - The presence of chondrocalcinosis is **not necessary to make the diagnosis of CPPD arthritis,** and conversely, some patients with chondrocalcinosis are asymptomatic.
- Features of CPPD arthropathy are uniform **joint space loss and sclerosis** with or without radiographically detectable intra-articular or periarticular calcifications.
  - This is similar to OA, but the joints affected differ.
  - The pattern of distribution is bilateral and usually symmetric with the patellofemoral, radiocarpal, and MCP joints often involved.
- Like OA, there are **subchondral cysts,** but they are typically more prominent in CPPD deposition disease.
  - CPPD cysts appear as clusters of coalescent lucencies of variable size and shape with indistinct margins.
  - This radiologic appearance is not usually seen in OA.
- As with other nonrheumatoid arthritides, **bone mineralization is normal.**
- CPPD arthropathy may be associated with rapid subchondral bone collapse leading to fragmentation with intra-articular loose bodies, resembling neuropathic osteoarthropathy.

- During acute attacks of pseudogout, the usual radiographic findings are soft tissue swelling and joint effusion. Chondrocalcinosis may or may not be present.

GOUT

- Chronic tophaceous gout is an asymmetric and erosive process with a polyarticular distribution that most commonly involves the feet (especially with first MTP joint) early, and hands, wrists, elbows, and knees later.
- Although **tophi are not radiopaque unless they calcify,** their effects on the surrounding tissues allow for radiographic detection.
  - ○ Periarticular tophi produce "punched-out" lesions in the adjacent bone.
  - ○ Bone proliferation next to these lesions produces "overhanging edges."
- Since tophaceous gout does not involve the cartilage directly, **joint space is preserved.**
- This and **preserved bone mineralization** allow differentiation from RA and other inflammatory arthropathies.
- The radiographic findings in acute gouty arthritis are nonspecific and include soft tissue swelling, joint effusion, and periarticular osteopenia.
- When the acute arthritic attack subsides, the bone remineralizes, and the more chronic, slowly progressive bony changes described above may develop.
- In severe cases, gout can lead to secondary OA, disuse osteopenia, and occasionally mutilating arthritis.

SEPTIC ARTHRITIS

- No single radiographic feature distinguishes septic arthritis from the other arthropathies.
- Typically, the history and physical exam lead one to suspect the diagnosis.
- The possibility of the superinfection of an already abnormal joint further complicates the picture.
- **When there is clinical suspicion of septic arthritis, joint aspiration should be performed as soon as possible** to confirm diagnosis and determine specific treatment.
- Radiographic findings are relatively nonspecific.
  - ○ **Soft tissue swelling** around the joint is the earliest finding, followed by **marginal erosions.**
  - ○ The synovial hyperemia and early disuse atrophy may result in **periarticular osteopenia.**
  - ○ Nongonococcal septic arthritis is typically monoarticular, with a **rapidly progressive** radiologic course.
  - ○ Destruction of the central cartilage and subchondral cortex causes central erosion with **loss of the cortical white line from the articular surfaces.** This is especially suggestive of the diagnosis.
  - ○ Without proper treatment, deformities progress and **ankylosis** can develop.
- The most commonly involved joints are the knee and hip.
- Although radiologic findings are not specific to certain organisms, generally nongonococcal bacterial arthritis is characterized by rapid destruction of bone and articular cartilage with preservation of bone mineralization.

- **Gonococcal arthritis rarely produces severe bony changes.**
- **Tuberculous arthritis** is characterized by juxta-articular osteoporosis, marginal erosions, and absent or mild joint space narrowing (Phemister's triad).
- The radiographic manifestations of fungal arthritis are similar to the manifestations of tuberculosis.
- The MRI appearance of septic arthritis is also nonspecific, as similar findings can be seen in inflammatory arthritis and early neuropathic joints. MRI can be used to determine complications of septic arthritis, such as abscesses and osteomyelitis.
- Radionuclide imaging is also not specific in differentiating septic arthritis from inflammatory arthritis but is useful in ruling out osteomyelitis.

Rheumatologic Emergencies

Reeti Joshi and Leslie E. Kahl

R heumatologic emergencies, albeit uncommon, present diagnostic challenges and require prompt action.[1] This chapter highlights common rheumatologic emergencies.

INFECTIOUS ARTHRITIS

- The differential diagnosis of **acute monoarthritis** must always include infectious (septic) arthritis. Fever and other constitutional signs are usually present; however, they may be absent in immunosuppressed or geriatric population.
- The common mimics of septic arthritis include acute gout or pseudogout, reactive arthritis, hemarthrosis, and primary or metastatic bone tumors.
- The diagnosis of septic arthritis is made unequivocally by **synovial fluid analysis.**
  - The fluid is sent for cell count and crystals (in a heparinized, lavender-top tube), Gram stain and culture (in plain/red-top tube/culture media).
  - **Synovial fluid white blood cell (WBC) counts more than 50,000 are associated with septic joint;** however, partially treated infections or immunosuppression may be associated with lower cell counts.
- **Therapy should not be delayed while awaiting confirmatory diagnosis** as septic arthritis has a mortality rate of about 10% and serious sequelae including sepsis and joint destruction. Risk factors include delay in diagnosis >3 days, increasing age, diabetes mellitus, and immunosuppression.
- **Joints with orthopedic hardware warrant urgent surgical consultation.**
- **Empiric antibiotic treatment** should include staphylococcal (including methicillin-resistant *Staphylococcus aureus* [MRSA]) and streptococcal coverage. Specific coverage for *Salmonella, Pasteurella,* and Gram-negative organisms is to be provided on a case-by-case basis.
- Duration of therapy is guided by culture and sensitivity and is usually 3 to 4 weeks.
- See Chapter 32, Infectious Arthritis for a full discussion.

GIANT CELL ARTHRITIS

- Giant cell arthritis (GCA) or temporal arthritis (TA) is a primary **systemic vasculitis affecting large vessels distal to aortic arch.** It is an often overlooked rheumatologic emergency—given the risk of sudden and permanent vision loss.
- The clinical presentation includes **jaw claudication, headache** (present in about two-thirds of the patients), **scalp tenderness, and nodularity along the temporal** arteries. **Visual changes** including acute, usually unilateral, vision loss may occur.

- It is often associated with **polymyalgia rheumatica**, which is characterized by aching and stiffness of hips and shoulder girdle muscles. It may include symptoms of fever and symmetrical arthralgias in shoulder, hip, neck, and torso.
- When the diagnosis of GCA is suspected, especially when associated with symptoms of transient visual loss, blurry vision, diplopia, light scotomas, and/or visual field narrowing, **initiate treatment with oral prednisone at 1 mg/kg/day** and then proceed with other evaluation.
- Definitive diagnosis requires a **temporal artery biopsy.**
  - As vessel involvement may be patchy, obtaining an adequate length of affected tissue is essential.
  - **Biopsy will still show characteristic histologic abnormalities after as much as 2 weeks of high-dose steroid therapy.**
- In suspected cases, a **temporal artery ultrasound** may be useful when done by a center experienced in its use.[2] A halo around the vessel indicates edema along the vessel wall and is a specific but insensitive finding. This halo resolves 2 to 3 weeks after therapy.
- Lab studies usually show a **high erythrocyte sedimentation rate** (ESR) (>50) or C-reactive protein (CRP), anemia and elevated alkaline phosphatase.
- Symptoms often rapidly resolve with steroid initiation.
- See Chapter 22, Giant Cell Arthritis and Polymyalgia Rheumatica for a full discussion.

SCLERODERMA RENAL CRISIS

- Scleroderma renal crisis (SRC) is a severe, sometimes life-threatening complication that occurs in approximately 10% to 15% of patients with diffuse scleroderma.
- SRC is characterized by **rapidly progressive azotemia, malignant hypertension, microangiopathic hemolytic anemia, and thrombocytopenia.**
- Approximately 10% of patients are normotensive at presentation but demonstrate these manifestations as well.
- Features of hypertensive encephalopathy including seizures may be present as well.
- **Risk factors** include diffuse scleroderma, rapidly progressive skin disease, presence of RNA polymerase III antibodies, presence of new pleural effusion or congestive heart failure, cool ambient temperatures, and use of cocaine, corticosteroids, or cyclosporine.
- Differentiating true SRC from thrombotic thrombocytopenic purpura (TTP) is critical as the treatments are different.
- The pathogenesis of SRC reflects a severe vasculopathy leading to ischemic **activation of the renin–angiotensin system.**
- Treatment involves blood pressure (BP) control starting with the use of **short-acting angiotensin-converting enzyme (ACE) inhibitors** such as captopril (initiate at 25 mg bid and titrate to maximum of 50 mg PO tid). Once the patient is stabilized, long-acting ACE inhibitors may be used.
- **ACE inhibitors must always be used** even in the face of deteriorating renal function with the goal of normalizing BP. Angiotensin receptor blockers (ARBs) and direct renin inhibitors have a theoretical benefit; corticosteroids, plasma exchanges and immunosuppressants have no benefits.
- For patients intolerant of ACE inhibitors, ARBs may be effective.

- **Avoid intravenous (IV) antihypertensives,** such as nitroprusside and labetalol, and all nephrotoxins. Calcium channel blockers can be added to the regimen of ACE inhibitor if necessary for BP control.
- Dialysis may be necessary for those patients with severe acute kidney injury.
- See Chapter 38 Scleroderma for a full discussion.

CERVICAL SPINE ABNORMALITIES IN RHEUMATOID ARTHRITIS

- Cervical spine involvement is a common manifestation of rheumatoid arthritis (RA). **Neurologic deficits** can occur even in the absence of pain and, when present, should be addressed urgently.
- The atlantoaxial joint is the second most commonly involved joint in RA after the MCP joints.
- **C1–C2 instability** may result from tenosynovitis of the transverse ligament of C1, erosion of the odontoid process, ligament laxity, ligament rupture, or apophyseal joint erosion.
- Approximately 10% to 85% patients with RA have neck pain and radiographic evidence of instability while approximately 10% to 60% will have neurologic deficits.
- **Risk factors** include seropositivity, steroid use, rheumatoid nodules, and erosive disease.
- The lesions most likely to lead to myelopathy are nonfixed atlantoaxial anterior subluxation or downward/upward subluxation of the C1–C2 facet joints. Cranial settling (also known as basilar invagination) in which the odontoid process pushes up into the foramen magnum may also occur.
- **Clinical features** include headaches (compression of greater occipital branch of cranial nerve II), loss of pain or touch over trigeminal nerve, sleep apnea, downbeat nystagmus and internuclear ophthalmoplegia, facial diplegia and dysphagia (cranial nerve IX dysfunction), and myelopathy.
- **Radiographic changes** of the C1–C2 joints are common but do not always correlate with neurologic deficits.
  - Appropriate radiographs include cross-table lateral and **dynamic flexion and extension views** with calculation of anterior atlanto-dens interval (ADI).
  - ADI >9 mm is associated with neurologic injury and requires fusion and wiring.
  - MRI can provide additional information about cord compression, bone destruction and the presence of pannus.
- Most severe instability occurs in flexion and the main goal is to prevent flexion operatively with fusion or nonoperatively with an orthosis (Headmaster Cervical Collar).
- Neurologic symptoms should be addressed with a neurosurgical evaluation for possible stabilization procedures.
- In addition, patients with cervical spine arthritis are at increased risk of traumatic injury during intubation and should be appropriately managed perioperatively.

CRICOARYTENOID ARTHRITIS

- Cricoarytenoid arthritis (CA) is a rare complication reported in RA patients. It is often asymptomatic and more common in women.

- Clinical symptoms and signs include **hoarseness, inspiratory stridor, sensation of foreign body in throat, dyspnea, and wheezing.** These findings **may be mistaken for asthma.**
- **Fiberoptic laryngoscope with CT or MRI** can be used to make the diagnosis.
- Nonurgent patients can be managed by local or systemic steroids.
- Surgical treatment is done only after failure of medical management. When patients present with acute airway obstruction from CA, intubation is difficult and tracheostomy and arytenoidectomy may be needed.

SUBGLOTTIC STENOSIS

- Subglottic stenosis is partial or complete narrowing of the subglottic area presenting as **stridor, hoarseness, brassy voice, or acute respiratory distress.**
- Although acquired causes are commonly trauma, surgery and malignancy, this can be seen in **antineutrophil cytoplasmic antibody (ANCA)-associated vasculitis** (Wegener's granulomatosis), **relapsing polychondritis, sarcoidosis, and infections** including diphtheria, syphilis and tuberculosis. It may occur in Wegener's granulomatosis even when the disease is clinically silent.
- Diagnosis is made by **fiberoptic laryngoscopy with MRI/CT scan. Flow volume loops showing fixed obstruction** and virtual bronchoscopy may also be useful.
- Although systemic immunosuppression can help, **glucocorticoids and intratracheal dilatation with intralesional steroids** are necessary in clinically significant disease.

Transverse Myelitis

- Transverse myelitis develops as an acute or subacute **inflammatory disorder of the spinal cord.**
- Most cases occur following an infection or immunization. In addition, transverse myelitis **can be associated with systemic lupus erythematosus (SLE), other collagen vascular diseases, Sjögren's syndrome, Behçet's disease, antiphospholipid syndrome, multiple sclerosis (MS), and sarcoidosis.**
- Symptoms of transverse myelitis may include focal neck and back pain, paresthesias, **weakness, sensory loss, urinary retention or incontinence, fecal incontinence,** and fever.
  - ○ **Symptoms typically start in the lower extremities and ascend.**
  - ○ The disease usually progresses over hours to days and varies in severity from mild neurologic involvement to functional transection of the spinal cord.
- Diagnostic workup includes **urgent spinal MRI, brain MRI** (to evaluate for MS), and **cerebral spinal fluid (CSF) analysis.** MRI of the spinal cord reveals variable spinal edema and signal enhancement.
- Obtaining normal CSF is useful to rule out acute infections. Alternatively, pleocytosis, elevated protein, and decreased glucose may be present.
- Treatment of transverse myelitis has not been well researched; however, **high-dose IV corticosteroids** are usually initiated within 24 hours of diagnosis.

CAUDA EQUINA SYNDROME

- Cauda equina syndrome is a rare complication of the seronegative spondyloarthropathies (related to arachnoiditis), in particular ankylosing spondylitis (AS), lumbar disk rupture, spinal or epidural anesthesia, or mass lesions from malignancies or infections.

- In patients with AS, symptoms may be slowly progressive. Cauda equina syndrome from any cause, however, has the potential for rapid onset and progression.
- Symptoms include **severe low back pain, rectal pain, and pain in both legs.**
  - In addition, with progressive disease patients can develop **saddle anesthesia** with **loss of bladder and bowel control,** poor anal sphincter tone, and impotence.
  - Patients may also develop variable lower extremity areflexia and asymmetric leg weakness or loss of sensation.
- Cauda equina syndrome should be **distinguished from sciatica or plexopathy,** which do not involve symptoms of incontinence or impotence.
- **MRI** can help confirm the diagnosis, and **urgent neurosurgical consultation** is required to prevent irreversible neurologic changes.
- **Steroids and localized radiation** treatment may be beneficial with lesions caused by malignancies.

PULMONARY HEMORRHAGE

- Pulmonary hemorrhage can be a complication of several rheumatologic and nonrheumatologic diseases including ANCA-associated vasculitis and other pulmonary renal syndromes, antiphospholipid antibody syndrome (APS), Behçet's syndrome, cryoglobulinemia, mixed connective tissue disease, polymyositis, RA, scleroderma, and SLE.
- Common presenting signs and symptoms include **progressive dyspnea with hypoxemia, hemoptysis,** radiographic appearance of **alveolar or interstitial infiltrates, and anemia** or a **drop in hemoglobin** level of 1.5 to 4 g/dL.
- Hypoxia and hemoptysis may be absent in one-third of the patients.
- Correction of hypoxemia and appropriate control of airway (possibly requiring intubation and mechanical ventilation) and correction of coagulopathies should be addressed immediately.
- Obtain **early consult with a pulmonologist** to assess the need for **urgent bronchoscopy** to help refine the diagnosis.
- Demonstration of active bleeding or hemosiderin-laden macrophages in bronchoalveolar lavage or sputum helps confirm the diagnosis of pulmonary hemorrhage.
- Other possible etiologies include uremia, congestive heart failure, infection, pulmonary infarction, pulmonary hypertension, and coagulopathy.
- Laboratory evaluation should include routine chemistries, liver function tests, complete blood count, and coagulation studies as well as antinuclear antibodies, antiglomerular basement membrane antibody, ANCA, and complement levels (C3, C4, and CH50).
- Lung (or other involved tissue) biopsy may be required for a definitive diagnosis.
- In addition to supportive treatment, target specific therapies at the underlying disorder. Pharmacologic therapy may involve a combination of corticosteroids (usually in high IV doses), cytotoxic agents, and sometimes plasmapheresis.

INTESTINAL INFARCTION

- Intestinal infarction is a rare complication associated with **SLE and polyarthritis nodosa.** The disease is manifested by diffuse vasculitis of the mesenteric blood vessels.

- Patients typically present with symptoms of an acute abdomen, which may be masked however by corticosteroids or may occur late in the clinical presentation.
- MRI may be useful in making the diagnosis.
- **Emergent surgical exploration and resection** is important, but overall prognosis is poor.

CATASTROPHIC ANTIPHOSPHOLIPID SYNDROME

- Catastrophic antiphospholipid syndrome (CAPS) is the most severe presentation of APS with **acute multiorgan involvement and vascular microthrombi.**
- The diagnosis of "definite CAPS" is made by **histopathologic diagnosis, high-titer antiphospholipid (APL) antibodies** and failure of three or more organ systems in 1 week. Less than three organ system involvement is considered as "probable APS."
- Differential diagnosis includes TTP/hemolytic-uremic syndrome (HUS), disseminated intravascular coagulation (DIC), hemolysis, elevated liver enzymes, low platelet count (HELLP) syndrome, sepsis and heparin-induced thrombocytopenia.
- Fortunately this form only affects about 1% of APS patients. Infection is thought to be a trigger.
- Mortality rate is high at around 30% but can be reduced with a combination of **anticoagulants, IV immunoglobulin, steroids, and plasma exchange.**
- Selected cases may benefit from cyclophosphamide. Rituximab trials for CAPS are under way.
- Patients who recover do relatively well on continued anticoagulation.
- See Chapter 39, for full discussion of the Antiphospholipid Syndrome.

REFERENCES

1. Solobodin G, Hussein A, Rozenbaum M, et al. The emergency room in systemic rheumatic diseases. *Emerg Med J.* 2006;23:667–671.
2. Meisner R, Labrapoulos N, Gasparis A, et al. How to diagnose giant cell arthritis. Int Angiol. 2011;30:58–63.

Regional Pain Syndromes 8

Michael L. Sams and Leslie E. Kahl

GENERAL PRINCIPLES

- Regional pain syndrome refers to pain localized to one area of the body and not caused by systemic disease. It encompasses many common musculoskeletal sources of pain.
- These syndromes (also called **soft tissue rheumatic pain syndromes**) occur frequently. They include disorders of bone, cartilage, ligament, muscle, tendon, enthesis (sites where tendons attach to bone), bursa, fascia, and nerve.

Etiology and Pathogenesis

- Regional pain syndromes may be caused by **trauma, injury from overuse, or degeneration with aging.**
- Consider infections, fractures, or other serious problems (e.g., deep venous thrombosis in a patient with leg pain) in patients who develop regional pain while in the hospital.

DIAGNOSIS

Clinical Presentation

History

- History and physical examination are usually enough to make a diagnosis and **exclude systemic diseases** such as cancer, infection, and arthritis (inflammatory and noninflammatory) that may present as regional pain. Signs and symptoms of a systemic process include weight loss, fever, rash, bilateral symptoms, and synovitis (Table 8-1) and should lead to further investigation.
- Question patients about the location and characteristics of their pain, radiation of the pain, duration, presence of numbness or tingling, their ability to function, precipitating events, aggravating and ameliorating factors, underlying diseases and systemic complaints. It may be helpful to ask the patient to locate the pain with one finger.

Physical Examination

- The physical examination should include **inspection** (looking for atrophy, asymmetry, alignment, swelling, erythema), **palpation** (warmth, crepitus, point tenderness), evaluation of **active and passive ranges of motion,** and a **neurologic examination.**
- Specific maneuvers exist to help identify involvement of specific structures.
- Always **compare** to the other side and examine at least one joint above and below the suspected involved joint as too focused an examination may miss abnormalities in other parts of the body or **sources of referred pain.**

TABLE 8-1	FEATURES THAT SUGGEST SYSTEMIC DISEASE
Fever, chills	Pulse abnormalities
Weight loss	Lymphadenopathy
Skin color changes	Neurologic deficits
Bilateral involvement	Muscle wasting or atrophy
Joint warmth, swelling, or tenderness (synovitis)	Laboratory abnormalities

Diagnostic Testing

Laboratories
- **Order laboratory tests only if there is suspicion of systemic disease.**
- In particular, tests such as erythrocyte sedimentation rate (ESR), rheumatoid factor (RF), and antinuclear antibodies (ANAs) have a low predictive value in the general population. Abnormal results may be seen in patients with diseases other than inflammatory arthritis or in healthy persons.

Imaging
- **Imaging is rarely indicated** at the initial evaluation.
- Problems of tendons, bursae, or nerves are not detected by plain radiographs.
- Osteoarthritis (OA) is a very common finding on plain radiographs but may be misleading as in the case of patients with OA of the knee on radiographs but knee pain due to anserine bursitis.
- Consider imaging in patients with a history of trauma, atypical symptoms, lack of improvement or if surgery is planned.

Electrodiagnostic Testing
Electromyogram/nerve conduction velocities (EMG/NCV) may be helpful in confirming nerve compression or involvement, especially if surgery is planned.

TREATMENT

- Most regional pain syndromes improve with **conservative treatment.** Table 8-2 presents a general guideline for managing regional pain syndromes.
- Some patients benefit from **assistive devices** such as splints.

TABLE 8-2	GUIDELINES FOR MANAGEMENT OF REGIONAL PAIN SYNDROMES

Exclude systemic disease with history and physical examination
Recognize aggravating and ameliorating factors
Provide an explanation of the problem and the likely outcome to the patient
Provide relief from pain
In patients who do not improve, consider other diagnoses and referral

- A referral to **physical or occupational therapy** to increase flexibility, strength, endurance, improve alignment and receive education may help.
- **Heat or cold application** may also be beneficial.
- When needed, treat pain with medications; however, exercises, physical modalities, and splinting are often more helpful. Medications include nonsteroidal antiinflammatory drugs (NSAIDs), acetaminophen, muscle relaxants, and opiate analgesics.
- Some conditions improve with intralesional injections of lidocaine or corticosteroids.
- Reassure patients that with time, most regional pain syndromes improve.

NECK PAIN

GENERAL PRINCIPLES

- Neck pain is less common than lower back pain but still affects one-third of the population at some time. **The majority of neck pain is not serious and most cases are nonspecific.**
- Pain may be due to involvement of the spine or surrounding soft tissues, spinal cord, or nerve roots, or referred from other structures or organs (Table 8-3).

Etiology and Pathogenesis

- Most causes of neck pain are benign and are due to strain/sprain in young adults or OA in an older population. However, **suspect a serious cause of neck**

TABLE 8-3	CAUSES OF NECK PAIN

Soft tissue disorders
    Nonspecific neck pain (muscle strain, sprain, spasm)
    Whiplash injury

Arthritis[a]
    OA and cervical spondylosis
    Degenerative disk disease with disk herniation
    RA
    AS
    Juvenile RA

Bone disease[a]
    Fracture (due to trauma or osteoporosis) or dislocation
    Metastatic lesions
    Osteomyelitis

Other
    Meningitis
    Septic discitis
    Thyroiditis
    Referred from intrathoracic or intra-abdominal disease

———
[a]May be associated with signs and symptoms due to radiculopathy or myelopathy.
OA, osteoarthritis; RA, rheumatoid arthritis; AS, ankylosing spondylitis.

pain (e.g., meningitis, epidural abscess, septic discitis, vertebral osteomyelitis, or metastatic lesions) in patients with a history of fever, intravenous drug use, weight loss, progressive neurologic findings, or cancer.

- **Sprains/strains** of the cervical spine are common, especially in the young. They may produce pain and are often the result of a maintained abnormal posture, trauma or overuse of muscles. **Whiplash** is a subtype of sprain/strain resulting after an acceleration/deceleration injury.
- In addition to causing strains and sprains, trauma can result in **fractures.**
- **Spasm** of the cervical musculature is a common component of pain after an acute or chronic injury of the spine and may account for a substantial portion of the pain.
- The neck is frequently involved in **arthritis,** both noninflammatory (OA) and inflammatory (rheumatoid arthritis [RA], ankylosing spondylitis [AS]).
  - ○ **OA/spondylosis** is a common cause of chronic neck pain in adults and the elderly.
    - ▪ Spondylosis results from the **degeneration of the disk,** leading to loss of disk height and creating abnormal mechanics with resultant OA of the anterior (vertebral body) and posterior (facet) portions of the intervertebral joints.
    - ▪ Bulging of the disk as well as vertebral subluxation can also occur with this process.
    - ▪ Osteophytes can result and together with the loss of disk height, can lead to mechanical pain and **compression of nerve roots.**
  - ○ **RA** causes an **erosive synovitis** that frequently involves the neck in addition to peripheral joints.
    - ▪ The synovitis and bony changes may encroach on the nerve roots.
    - ▪ Ligament involvement leads to laxity, instability and **C1–C2 subluxation.** Acute subluxation causes severe pain and may compress the cord and become life threatening. Subluxation may be spontaneous or follow mild trauma, so maintain a high index of suspicion with RA patients who develop neck pain. In the worst cases this can lead to **impingement of the spinal cord.** Many patients may have radiographic evidence of subluxation but be asymptomatic.
  - ○ **AS** also affects the cervical spine, usually following progressive involvement of the lumbar and thoracic spine. The cervical spine becomes stiff and fractures may occur even with mild trauma.
- **Cervical radiculopathy** is due to encroachment on a nerve root as it exits its intervertebral foramen. It can result from many causes including herniated disk, degenerative disk disease and OA/spondylosis. Compression of the nerve root can lead to **neck pain and sensory changes that radiate into the arm.** In more severe cases it can cause motor weakness. Symptoms vary with the root involved (Table 8-4).
- **Cervical spine stenosis** denotes narrowing of the central canal and can lead to **myelopathy,** which is less common than radiculopathy but more serious. It can result from both congenital causes and spondylosis. Spondylosis leads to osteophytes, protruding disks and thickening of the ligamentum flavum that cause narrowing of the canal and can compress the spinal arteries. Initially patients may have localized neck and arm pain due to radicular involvement. However, if the narrowing is more central it may lead to myelopathy with upper motor neuron signs in the legs.

TABLE 8-4	NEUROLOGIC FINDINGS IN CERVICAL RADICULOPATHY		
Nerve Root	Sensory Loss	Motor Loss	Reflex Loss
C5	Neck to lateral shoulder, upper arm	Deltoid	Biceps
C6	Lateral arm to thumb, index finger	Biceps	Brachioradialis
C7	Dorsal and palmar forearm, middle finger	Triceps	Triceps
C8	Medial forearm, ring, middle fingers	Finger flexion	—

- Less common causes of pain include **thoracic outlet syndrome,** which is due to compression of the neurovascular bundle as it exits the neck. Compression may occur at several sites including between the anterior and middle scalene muscles, the first rib and the clavicle or on a cervical rib.
- Other less common causes include **brachial plexopathy and fibromyalgia.**
- **Nonmusculoskeletal causes** of pain include angina, aortic dissection, thyroiditis, and peritonsillar/retropharyngeal abscess.

DIAGNOSIS

Clinical Presentation

History
- A good history should focus on the basic questions used to assess musculoskeletal pain. The answers to onset, location, duration, symptom quality, radiation, symmetry, sensory changes, motor changes, aggravating, and relieving factors help to identify the source of pain.
- The presence of pain in other joints and other systemic symptoms are important to decipher if there is a systemic process.
- A typical history of **spasm/strain** includes pain localized to the neck with symptoms of muscle spasm. Typical inciting events are trauma, poor posture, and overuse. It is more common in the young.
- Neck pain with or without radiculopathy in an older adult is likely due to **spondylosis/OA.**
- Neck pain that radiates into the arm in a dermatomal pattern with associated numbness and paresthesia is highly suggestive of **cervical radiculopathy.** Weakness may or may not be present.
- Clinical manifestations of **cervical myelopathy** include weakness and incoordination of the hands, lower extremity weakness and gait disturbances. Incontinence is a late finding.
- Patients with **RA** or **AS** present with symptoms of the disease in other joints. They will complain of **morning stiffness** that may take more than an hour to resolve.
- Patients with **thoracic outlet obstruction** will likely have neurologic symptoms in multiple dermatomes in addition to neck pain. Symptoms can be aggravated by overhead activities.

- Other important questions include a **history of drug use, infection, or fever** to identify a potential epidural abscess or septic discitis. A history of trauma to suggest fracture, diffuse pain to suggest fibromyalgia, headache and fever to suggest meningitis, or a history of cancer to suggest metastasis.

Physical Examination

- The physical examination of the patient with neck pain should include cervical **range of motion in all planes** (which normally decreases with age). In RA patients, limit range of motion testing to active range and not passive, given the risk of subluxation.
- Palpation for spinous process tenderness is important to detect osteomyelitis and fracture, but it is often also present due to mechanical problems. Tender spots and muscle spasms may be noted in neck paraspinal muscles.
- A **neurologic examination** is crucial to detect the presence of radiculopathy and myelopathy. Radicular compression may lead to sensory changes, weakness, and diminished reflexes depending on the severity in a dermatomal pattern. **Neurologic defects may not be detected with mild radiculopathy.** As spondylosis can be extensive, more than one cervical root level can be involved. Important findings suggesting myelopathy include upper and lower extremity weakness with hyperreflexia/spasticity and a Babinski sign in the lower extremities.
- **Spurling test** is helpful to assess if symptoms in the arm may be related to radiculopathy. The test is performed with cervical extension and rotation to the suspected side while providing axial pressure. This compresses the neural foramina on that side, thereby aggravating nerve compression.
- **Lhermitte sign** is the sensation of an electric shock down the spine and into the arms and legs with cervical extension. It may be present in cervical cord compression.
- **Roos hyperabduction/external rotation test** is used to assess for thoracic outlet syndrome. The arm is abducted to 90 degrees and externally rotated to 90 degrees and maintained in this position for 1 minute. The patient opens and closes the hand throughout this time. It is considered positive if it provokes the pain and paresthesias.

Diagnostic Testing

Imaging

- Consider imaging in patients with neck pain after trauma or with neurologic findings and in cases of suspected fractures, metastatic lesions, or infections.
- Plain films may identify osteophytes and intervertebral space narrowing that suggests disk degeneration. **Oblique views** may show narrowing of neural foramina. Occasionally, a cervical rib may be noted which could support a diagnosis of thoracic outlet syndrome.
- **Open mouth and lateral flexion/extension radiographs** may be needed to evaluate the atlantoaxial joint for subluxation in RA. If not conclusive, computed CT can be ordered.
- **CT and MRI** are more accurate in cases of suspected tumor or infection.
- MRI is the best technique to identify the cause and location of root impingement.
- Radiographic abnormalities are extremely common in the elderly and correlate poorly with symptoms.

Electrodiagnostic Testing
- Nerve conduction studies may be used to document the nerve root involved, but are seldom necessary unless surgery is contemplated.
- They also may be helpful in determining if the location of nerve compression is outside of the neck.

TREATMENT

- Most mechanical causes of neck pain will resolve with time and **conservative treatment.**
- **Strain/sprain:** These cases may improve with heat application or rest and usually resolve with time. Education on posture, avoidance of repetitive motion or strengthening may help to treat the underlying cause.
- Treatment of neck **OA** is conservative. Some activity restriction is beneficial. Soft cervical collars may provide symptomatic relief. **Use rigid cervical collars only in cases with instability and under close supervision.** NSAIDs are helpful, and local injections and cervical traction are sometimes used. Symptoms may recur periodically with stress of the degenerated structures.
- **Myelopathy:** Progressive myelopathy requires **urgent surgical decompression.**
- **Pharmacologic therapy** includes NSAIDs, acetaminophen, muscle relaxants, opiate analgesics, and gabapentin, depending on the symptoms that are present. Opiates should be used with caution as they can be habit forming and are ideally used only with acute pain.
- **Epidural corticosteroid injections** may be used for cervical radiculopathy.
- **Physical therapy** can be beneficial to educate the patient on appropriate posture to reduce stress/compression on the involved structures. Patients can be instructed on appropriate exercise to strengthen the involved structures and to improve range of motion. Ultrasound and electrical stimulation can also be performed which may help to provide some pain relief.
- Specific indications for surgery include bowel/bladder incontinence, worsening neurologic function, progressive myelopathy and intractable pain and radicular symptoms.[1]

LOW BACK PAIN

GENERAL PRINCIPLES

- Low back pain is one of the most common problems people experience. It is the **second most common reason to seek medical care** (after upper respiratory problems) and is the **most common cause of disability in young workers.**
- Most patients improve with **conservative treatment** over time, so education and reassurance are important to prevent unnecessary testing and anxiety.
- About 1% of patients who present with new-onset back pain have systemic diseases (cancer, infection, inflammatory disease).

Etiology and Pathogenesis
- Many different conditions cause low back pain (Table 8-5).
- **Mechanical disorders** (muscle sprain, herniated nucleus pulposus, OA) are by far the most common causes of back pain. **Sprains** may result from overuse,

TABLE 8-5 DIFFERENTIAL DIAGNOSIS OF LOW BACK PAIN

Mechanical low back pain (97%)
   Idiopathic low back pain (lumbago, lumbar strain)
   Degenerative disk disease
   Osteoarthritis
   Spondylosis
   Herniated disk
   Spinal stenosis
   Spondylolysis
   Spondylolisthesis
   Trauma
   Osteoporotic fracture

Neoplasia (<1%)
   Metastatic lesions
   Multiple myeloma
   Lymphoma and leukemia
   Primary vertebral tumors
   Spinal cord tumors

Infection (<1%)
   Osteomyelitis
   Paraspinous abscess
   Epidural abscess
   Septic discitis
   Bacterial endocarditis

Rheumatic diseases (<1%)
   AS
   PsA
   ReA
   Inflammatory bowel disease–related arthritis

Visceral disease and referred pain (<1%)
   Aortic aneurysm
      GI disease (pancreatitis, cholecystitis)
      Genitourinary (nephrolithiasis, pyelonephritis, pelvic inflammatory
         disease)
   Hip disease
   Sacroiliac joint—controversial if not part of an inflammatory arthropathy

---
AS, ankylosing spondylitis; PsA, psoriatic arthritis; ReA, reactive arthritis; GI, gastrointestinal.

trauma, or poor body mechanics. **Herniated disks** can compress a nerve root(s) as they exit, or occur more centrally and cause cord compression, depending on the size of the herniated fragment. As in the neck, **spondylosis** can occur as well, leading to compression of nerve roots or myelopathy.

- **Spondylolysis** is a defect of the pars interarticularis that can occur in young patients who are active in sports that require frequent extension, flexion, and rotation of the lumbar spine.

- **Spondylolisthesis** results from a bilateral defect of the pars interarticularis that allows the vertebral body to slip forward relative to the rest of the spine. It may be caused by congenital, developmental or degenerative causes.
- **Cauda equina** syndrome is the compression of the nerve roots as they exit the distal spinal cord. The nerves can be compressed by any mechanism that narrows the spinal canal. It is a **surgical emergency.**
- **Inflammatory diseases** that can cause low back pain include AS, inflammatory bowel disease–related arthritis, reactive arthritis (ReA), and psoriatic arthritis (PsA). Lumbar spine involvement in RA is rare.
- **Cancer** may present as a metastasis or a local tumor. In a study of >2000 patients with low back pain, no cancer was found in any patient aged <50 years without a history of cancer, unexplained weight loss, or failure of conservative therapy.[2] The pain may be due to damage of the bone and joints themselves, or to compression of neurologic structures.
- **Infectious causes** of low back pain include osteomyelitis, epidural abscess, and septic discitis. Predisposing conditions include intravenous (IV) drug use, concomitant infection, and endocarditis.
- Other visceral disorders can cause **pain referred to the back** and include abdominal aortic aneurysm and dissection, pancreatitis, cholecystitis, pyelonephritis, nephrolithiasis, and pelvic inflammatory disease.

DIAGNOSIS

Clinical Presentation

History

- **A careful history and physical examination are often enough to identify systemic disease** (Table 8-6).
- Inquire about the nature of the pain, aggravating and relieving factors and neurologic symptoms.
- Clues to **cancer** in the history are age >50 years, history of cancer, unexplained weight loss, lack of relief with bed rest, duration of pain and failure to improve over 1 month, and nocturnal pain.
- Fever, concomitant infections and a history of IV drug use suggest **infection** (spinal osteomyelitis, discitis.) Also suspect infection in patients who develop low back pain while hospitalized.
- Morning stiffness of >1 hour with improvement with exercise, and onset before the age of 40 years, suggests **AS.**
- **Disk herniation** may cause sciatica: pain, numbness, and paresthesias radiating to the lower extremity below the knee.
- Bowel or bladder dysfunction, saddle anesthesia, and bilateral lower extremity weakness are signs of **spinal cord compression** (**cauda equina syndrome**). Patients with these symptoms should undergo immediate imaging and surgical referral (see Chapter 7, Rheumatologic Emergencies).
- Symptoms of **spinal stenosis** due to degeneration/spondylosis mimic those of vascular insufficiency and are often referred to as **neurogenic claudication.** There is typically pain in the bilateral buttocks and thighs with walking upright, as this position causes lumbar extension which narrows the spinal canal. The pain is better when patients lean forward to increase lumbar flexion, as happens when walking with a shopping cart. The pain resolves after a very brief period

of sitting down, in contrast to the pain of vascular claudication, which may take much longer to resolve.

- **Spondylolisthesis** and **spondylolysis** are often aggravated by lumbar extension. Radicular symptoms are not typically present.
- A history of older age, female sex, thin build, and prednisone use may suggest **osteoporosis with a compression fracture.**
- Inquire about non-lumbar spine-related symptoms of RA, ReA and inflammatory bowel disease associated arthritis if an inflammatory cause is suspected.
- A history of vascular disease may suggest abdominal aortic aneurysm or vascular claudication.

Physical Examination

- Lumbar **range of motion** should be assessed in all planes. Often pain will be worse in flexion with a herniated disk. Pain is likely to be worse in extension with spondylolysis and spinal stenosis. Other sources of back pain can limit range and cause pain in multiple directions.
- Localized tenderness over the midline is seen in **vertebral fractures** due to osteoporosis, metastatic disease, multiple myeloma or osteomyelitis. Spinal tenderness can also be present from mechanical causes. Tenderness in the paraspinal muscles may represent spasm or a muscle strain.
- The **general physical examination** may provide clues to underlying systemic disease. Fevers (infection, inflammatory disease, cancer), murmurs (endocarditis), breast masses (metastases), pulsatile abdominal masses, and pulse abnormalities (aortic aneurysm) are important findings.
- The **neurologic examination** should identify spinal nerve root involvement or cord symptoms (Table 8-7). Sphincter tone and saddle anesthesia should be assessed if suspecting cauda equina.
- A positive **straight-leg raising test** suggests nerve root compression. The test is performed with the patient supine, and the leg is raised with the knee fully extended. A positive test reproduces pain radiating below the knee when the leg is raised. Compare the excursion of the straight-leg raise from one side to other. The involved side will have less range of motion. Low back pain without radiation below the knee does not constitute a positive test.
- **Schober's test** should be performed to help assess for limited flexion with suspected spondyloarthropathy (see Chapter 2, Rheumatologic Joint Examination).

Diagnostic Testing

Laboratories
Laboratory tests (e.g., ESR, CRP, UA, CBC, cultures) may occasionally help exclude systemic disease.

Imaging
- Plain radiographs are overused. They are recommended only for patients with **fever, unexplained weight loss, history of cancer, neurologic deficits, alcohol or injection-drug abuse, and trauma.**
- **CT scans and MRI** are more sensitive than plain radiographs. However, they often reveal abnormalities even in asymptomatic adults. On MRI, up to 40%

TABLE 8-6	EVALUATION OF SELECTED CAUSES OF LOW BACK PAIN					
	Idiopathic Low Back Pain	Herniated Disk	Spinal Stenosis	AS	Metastases	Spinal Infection
Characteristics of pain	Dull, lower back; may radiate to buttocks; improves with rest	Sudden, sharp, intense; radiates below the knee (sciatica); usually unilateral	Pseudoclaudication: Bilateral pain (buttocks, thighs, legs) brought on by standing or walking and relieved by sitting or flexing spine	Insidious, chronic, worse in the morning, improves with exercise	Chronic, severe, not improved with bed rest.	Severe, sharp; may radiate to thighs
History	History of lifting or straining	History of lifting or straining	Occurs in patients >60 years with degenerative disease of the spine	Occurs in patients <40 years; may have family history, or history of uveitis or axial arthritis	Age >50 years, history of cancer, weight loss, failure of conservative management	Immunocompromised patients; history of IV drug abuse, alcohol abuse, infections; fever not always present
Physical examination	May have pain with movement or in certain positions; neurologic examination is normal	Pain radiating down the leg with straight-leg raise; may have altered dermatomal sensation, weakness or decreased reflexes; 95% S1 root	May have sensory, motor, and reflex abnormalities	Decreased range of motion, arthritis	May show evidence of primary tumor; rule out spinal cord compression in patients with neurologic findings	Neurologic findings present and depend on the level of involvement

Lab studies	None needed	None needed	None needed	ESR often elevated; HLA-B27 may be present but is not a good screening test	ESR may be elevated	ESR often elevated; positive blood cultures, leukocytosis not always present
Imaging	None needed	MRI recommended in patients with neurologic deficits	MRI may be needed for diagnosis	Radiographs may show sacroiliitis; "bamboo spine" is a late finding	CT or MRI; emergent imaging needed in suspected cord compression	MRI indicated

AS, ankylosing spondylitis; IV, intravenous; ESR, erythrocyte sedimentation rate.

TABLE 8-7	NEUROLOGIC FINDINGS IN LUMBAR SPINAL NERVE ROOT INVOLVEMENT		
Nerve Root	Sensory Loss	Motor Loss	Reflex Loss
L4	Lateral thigh, medial leg to medial malleolus	Knee extension, thigh adduction, foot dorsiflexion	Knee
L5	Posterolateral thigh, lateral leg to dorsal foot	Great toe extension and foot dorsiflexion	—
S1	Posterior leg, lateral, and plantar foot	Plantar flexion of great toe and foot	Ankle

of young, asymptomatic volunteers have herniated disks and >90% of subjects >60 years have degenerative disks. **CT and MRI should be reserved for cases with a strong suspicion of cancer or infection or for patients with persistent neurologic deficits.**

- A **bone scan** may reveal a stress injury at the pars interarticularis in a young active adult.

TREATMENT

- Most patients improve with **conservative treatment** over time, so education and reassurance are important to prevent unnecessary testing and anxiety.
- Acetaminophen, NSAIDs, and muscle relaxants are effective for idiopathic acute low back pain. Opioids may be required. Gabapentin may be needed for pain from nerve compression.
- **Physical therapy** may be useful for patients with persistent pain. Patients may benefit from strengthening of abdominal and back muscles as well as education on rest and body mechanics.
- Encourage patients to return rapidly to their normal activities, but avoidance of heavy lifting may be prudent until the pain improves.
- Patients with herniated disks may require short-term opioids for pain control.
- **Bed rest does not accelerate recovery** in idiopathic low back pain or sciatica.
- Patients should be reassured that pain resolves in most cases within 12 weeks.
- Spinal stenosis may also benefit from NSAIDs, but the prognosis for relief of symptoms is not so good.
- **Surgical evaluation** should be immediate in patients with cord/cauda equina compression or progressive neurologic deficits. Patients with spinal stenosis and persistent, disabling pain and patients with herniated disks and persistent sciatica with neurologic findings may benefit from surgical referral.
- Chronic lower back pain is difficult to manage and sometimes requires a multidisciplinary approach to address rehabilitation, depression, or substance abuse.

SHOULDER PAIN

GENERAL PRINCIPLES

- Shoulder pain is the second most common musculoskeletal complaint after low back pain.
- The shoulder is exceedingly mobile at the expense of some stability. Stability is provided by the glenoid fossa, labrum ligaments, and rotator cuff. Hence damage of these structures can reduce stability and lead to further injury and pain.
- The **rotator cuff** is composed of the tendons of the supraspinatus, infraspinatus, teres minor, and subscapularis muscles, and attaches to the humeral tuberosities. The supraspinatus location between the acromion and the humeral head explains why pain from rotator cuff disease worsens with elevation of the arm (**impingement**).
- The shoulder is made up of four joints that are typically affected in different types of arthritis: glenohumeral joint (affected in RA, calcium pyrophosphate deposition disease [CPPD], septic arthritis, and OA), acromioclavicular (OA), sternoclavicular (AS, septic arthritis), and scapulothoracic.

Etiology and Pathogenesis

- There are many causes of shoulder pain (Table 8-8).
- **Impingement** is caused by impingement of the rotator cuff and/or subacromial bursa on the under surface of the acromion and/or acromioclavicular ligament.
  - ○ The acromion and ligament form an arch over the humeral head, and the supraspinatus and bursa lie between the humeral head and this arch.
  - ○ When reaching up, especially with shoulder in internal rotation these structures are opposed to each other.
  - ○ Normally the rotator cuff helps to stabilize the humeral head in the glenoid fossa, but with injury, weakness or tendinopathy of the rotator cuff the humeral head may translate superiorly during overhead activities leading to impingement.
  - ○ Scapular muscle weakness may also contribute to impingement.
- **Rotator cuff tendinopathy is the most common cause of shoulder pain.** It may be acute or chronic and may be associated with calcium deposits in the tendon (calcific tendinitis). It may be due to overuse, mild trauma, age-related degeneration, and osteophytes on the inferior portion of the acromion.
- **Subacromial bursitis** may be associated with rotator cuff tendinitis or other abnormal mechanics that cause impingement of the bursa against the acromion or coracoacromial ligament.
- **Rotator cuff tears** may be partial or complete and may be due to trauma or the result of gradual degeneration. Complete tears cause inability to abduct the shoulder.
- **Bicipital tendinitis** can result from overuse, especially in laborers or weight lifters. A bicep tendon tear may occur in an older adult.
- **Adhesive capsulitis** ("frozen shoulder") is an inflammation of the shoulder capsule that causes generalized pain with severe loss of active and passive ranges of motion. It may be due to diabetes, inflammatory arthritis, or prolonged shoulder immobilization.
- **Acromioclavicular OA** may occur with chronic repetitive irritation.
- **Instability** may occur secondary to injury of the ligaments through trauma, including dislocation. It may also be due to a primary laxity of the patient's connective tissue. The end result can be pain from impingement.

TABLE 8-8	CAUSES OF SHOULDER PAIN

Periarticular disorders
  Rotator cuff tendinitis
  Calcific tendinitis
  Rotator cuff tear
  Subacromial bursitis
  Bicipital tendinitis
  Adhesive capsulitis

Articular disorders
  Inflammatory arthritis (RA)
  Glenohumeral arthritis
  Acromioclavicular arthritis
  Sternoclavicular arthritis
  Septic arthritis
  Osteonecrosis (of humeral head)
  Fractures, dislocations

Neurovascular diseases (usually have neurovascular symptoms)
  Brachial plexopathy
  Suprascapular nerve entrapment
  Thoracic outlet syndrome

Referred pain (should be suspected in cases with normal range of motion)
  Cervical spine disease
  Intrathoracic or intra-abdominal disease

Other
  PMR (usually bilateral)
  Fibromyalgia
  Reflex sympathetic dystrophy

RA, rheumatoid arthritis; PMR, polymyalgia rheumatica.

DIAGNOSIS

Clinical Presentation

History

- **Impingement/subacromial bursitis/rotator cuff tendinopathy:** Pain is usually over the lateral deltoid and worsens with overhead activity. Night pain due to difficulty positioning the painful shoulder is common.
- **Rotator cuff tendon tears:** Complete tears cause inability to actively abduct the shoulder.
- **Biceps tendinopathy** usually causes anterior shoulder pain.
- **Adhesive capsulitis** causes a painful shoulder with loss of range of motion. Patients will complain of difficulty reaching behind their backs to put on a shirt or reaching overhead to comb their hair.
- **Acromioclavicular (AC) arthritis** causes pain over the AC joint that is aggravated by reaching across the body or overhead.

Physical Examination

- **Both passive and active ranges of motion** should be assessed. In adhesive capsulitis passive and active ranges will be decreased, whereas in many other shoulder disorders active range will be decreased, but passive range will be normal or near normal.
- Palpation of the subacromial space should be performed to assess for bursitis or supraspinatus tenderness. The subscapularis can be palpated anteriorly just inferiolaterally to the coracoid process. The infraspinatus and teres minor can be palpated posteriorly and inferiorly to the acromion. Also palpate the acromioclavicular joint for tenderness.
- The **impingement sign** is typically positive in supraspinatus tendinopathy, impingement, and subacromial bursitis (but may also be seen in other shoulder diseases). The sign is elicited by passively forward flexing the patient's internally rotated arm with the examiner holding down the scapula with the other hand. This produces pain in cases of impingement.
- The **drop arm** test is positive with a large rotator cuff tear. It is performed by placing the arm at 90 degrees abduction and instructing the patient to lower it slowly to the side. The test is positive when the patient is unable to perform the motion smoothly.
- **Biceps tendinitis** is suspected when the bicipital groove along the anterior humeral head is tender on palpation. Pain with supination of the forearm against resistance or forward flexion of the externally rotated arm against resistance is seen.
- Have the patient horizontally adduct the arm across the chest to stress the AC joint. Pain at the AC joint suggests that this joint is irritated.

Diagnostic Testing

Imaging

- Plain films are needed if the history and physical examination suggest a dislocation, fracture, or a primary/metastatic tumor.
- MRI (or ultrasound) may distinguish between partial and complete rotator cuff tears.

TREATMENT

- Treatment of **rotator cuff/bursitis/impingement injuries** includes rest and specific exercises to strengthen the rotator cuff and improve range of motion. Prolonged immobilization of the shoulder in any shoulder disease should be avoided as it may cause adhesive capsulitis. NSAIDs and local anesthetic with corticosteroid injections are also used. Surgery may be needed to address the impingement.
- **Biceps tendinitis** is treated with rest and rotator cuff strengthening as is rotator cuff tendinitis.
- **Adhesive capsulitis** treatment is with physical therapy for aggressive range of motion, injections, and occasionally surgery.
- The AC joint may be injected if needed and surgery may be performed if conservative treatment does not help.
- Surgery is necessary to repair complete rotator cuff tears.

ELBOW PAIN

GENERAL PRINCIPLES

- Elbow pain is usually caused by **periarticular disorders.**
- The elbow joint is frequently involved in RA but rarely in OA.

Etiology and Pathogenesis

- **Olecranon bursitis** may be septic or idiopathic, due to inflammatory conditions (RA, gout), or trauma. It can be caused by repetitive low-pressure trauma, such as frequently resting on the olecranon. The bursa is located just proximal to the olecranon.
- **Lateral and medial epicondylitis** are known as tennis and golfer's elbow, respectively, but may be due to any type of activity. Lateral epicondylitis is more common. They occur at the origin of the common extensor tendon (lateral epicondylitis) and flexor tendons (medial epicondylitis). The name is somewhat of a misnomer as the pathologic process is a degeneration of the tendon due to overuse. This misnomer applies to tendinitis throughout the body. Actual inflammation is rare and microscopic tearing and scarring may be present.
- The biceps and triceps tendons and the **epicondylitis** muscles can also produce pain with overuse.
- **Ulnar nerve entrapment** occurs at the cubital tunnel where the nerve passes through. The nerve can become irritated by direct pressure, repetitive motion, osteophytes, and prolonged elbow flexion.
- Other causes of pain include septic arthritis, RA, gout, pseudogout, and compression of the posterior interosseous nerve just distal to the posterior elbow as it passes through the supinator.

Clinical Presentation

History

- **Olecranon bursitis** can begin acutely or chronically. If it is infectious it will be quite painful. Patients will complain of a visible swelling posteriorly that will vary in the amount of pain present depending on the cause.
- Patients with medial or lateral **epicondylitis** will complain of pain localized to the respective epicondyle. Pain is aggravated with repetitive use of the hand. They may often occur in laborers.
- **Ulnar nerve compression** will produce symptoms of posteromedial elbow soreness that is aggravated by resting on the medial elbow. Tingling will be noted in the fourth and fifth digits. Complaints of numbness may be present. Weakness is possible.
- Gout pain will be acute with complaints of swelling. RA will involve other joints. A septic joint will be quite painful with fever present.
- **Posterior interosseous nerve entrapment** may produce complaints of posterolateral elbow pain and occasionally numbness/tingling in the lateral forearm and hand. Weakness of the wrist and finger extensors is expected.

Physical Examination

- Begin the examination by noting flexion, extension, supination, and pronation **range of motion.** Palpate the major tendons at their origins or insertions for tenderness. Visually inspect for joint or bursa swelling, warmth, and erythema.

- **Olecranon bursitis** presents with swelling over the posterior elbow. The surrounding area may be swollen, warm, and erythematous in septic bursitis. Septic bursitis usually does not compromise elbow mobility as a septic elbow joint does. Septic bursitis should be aspirated (taking care to avoid penetrating into the elbow joint).
- **Lateral epicondylitis** presents with tenderness localized to the lateral epicondyle at the insertion of the common extensor tendon. Pain is exacerbated by resisted wrist extension as well as resisted middle finger extension.
- **Medial epicondylitis** is diagnosed by tenderness over the medial epicondyle at the insertion of the flexor tendons and by painful resisted wrist flexion and forearm pronation.
- Percussion of the ulnar nerve in the cubital tunnel and prolonged elbow flexion will produce pain and paresthesia in **ulnar nerve entrapment.** Check the sensation in the fourth and fifth digits.
- **Posterior interosseous nerve entrapment** symptoms can be aggravated with resisted supination with the elbow at 90 degrees and fully flexed. There will be tenderness 5 to 6 cm distal to the lateral epicondyle over the supinator. Weakness is present on testing wrist and finger extension.

TREATMENT

- Non-septic **olecranon bursitis** due to trauma can be treated with NSAIDs, avoiding aggravating activity and a compression strap. It may need aspiration. It can be injected with corticosteroids but may recur. Septic bursitis should be treated with antibiotics and may need to be aspirated daily. Surgery may be required.
- Treatment of **lateral and medial epicondylitis** includes rest and avoidance of exacerbating activities. NSAIDs may be helpful for both conditions. A tennis elbow strap may be beneficial. Corticosteroid injections may be needed for short-term relief, if an inflammatory component is suspected. The injection should not be directly into the tendon. Surgery to debride degenerative portions of the tendon is an option if conservative treatment fails.
- **Ulnar nerve entrapment** can be treated conservatively with the use of an elbow pad. The pad cushions the posteromedial elbow during the day to reduce pressure on the cubital tunnel. At night the pad can be rotated so that it is anterior in the cubital fossa. This placement prevents excessive elbow flexion at night. Occasionally, ulnar nerve transposition is required.
- **Posterior interosseous nerve compression** can be treated with rest from offending motions. If symptoms do not improve then surgery for decompression is possible.

HAND AND WRIST PAIN

GENERAL PRINCIPLES

- The hand and wrist are frequently affected by arthritis, both inflammatory (RA, lupus, PsA) and noninflammatory (OA). The presence or absence of synovitis, joint deformities, and the specific joints involved may lead to a diagnosis.
- OA typically affects the proximal and distal interphalangeal joints and the first carpometacarpal (CMC) joints.

- RA affects the wrist, metacarpophalangeal (MCP), and the proximal interphalangeal joints, sparing the distal interphalangeal joints and the first CMC.
- Hand and wrist pain may also be due to periarticular disorders and infections.
- Unilateral pain is often due to trauma, overuse or infection; consider arthritis or systemic diseases in patients with bilateral pain.

Etiology and Pathogenesis

- **Carpal tunnel syndrome** (CTS) is a very common cause of hand pain. The median nerve and the flexor tendons pass through a tunnel at the wrist limited by the carpal bones and the transverse carpal ligament. CTS may be idiopathic but is also seen in pregnancy, RA, diabetes, obesity, and myxedema and with disorders that encroach on the nerve (osteophytes, tophi, amyloid deposits).
- The **ulnar nerve,** as discussed earlier, may become entrapped at the elbow, causing hand pain and numbness or paresthesias of the ulnar side of the ring and little fingers. Compression of the ulnar nerve at the wrist causes similar symptoms and may be due to trauma or fracture of the carpal or fifth metacarpal bones.
- **De Quervain's tenosynovitis** is the inflammation of the extensor pollicis brevis and abductor pollicis longus tendons at the level of the radial styloid that causes pain, tenderness, and occasionally swelling of that area. It may be due to repetitive thumb pinching while moving the wrist.
- **Tenosynovitis and tendinopathy** may also occur in other flexor and extensor tendons. Localized pain and tenderness on palpation and with resisted movement are seen. Tenosynovitis/tendinopathy may be due to overuse, trauma, RA or may be idiopathic.
- **Infectious tenosynovitis** may be seen in gonococcal arthritis and as a result of puncture wounds.
- **Ganglions** are the most common soft tissue tumors of the hand and wrist. They are mucin-filled cysts that arise from adjacent tendon sheaths or joint capsules. They usually appear on the dorsal aspect and are painless but may limit movement if large.
- **Trigger finger** is a common cause of hand pain and discomfort. Trigger finger is due to thickening of the retinacular pulley in the palm or a fibrous nodule on the tendon that interferes with flexion. The thumb, ring, and long fingers are most commonly affected. Corticosteroid injections or surgery are helpful.
- **Dupuytren's contracture** is a thickening and shortening of the palmar fascia that results in visible thickening and cording of the palm that is usually painless. The ring finger is affected most frequently. It may be idiopathic and is also seen in diabetics or in patients with chronic alcohol abuse.

Clinical Presentation

History

- **CTS:** Pain and tingling of the hand is characteristic but may extend to the wrist, forearm, arm, and sometimes, shoulder. Numbness and paresthesias are felt in the distribution of the median nerve (thumb, index, and middle fingers; radial aspect of ring finger). The hand may be weak and clumsy and feel swollen. Bilateral disease is common. Women are affected more frequently.
- Patients with **de Quervain's tenosynovitis** will complain of radial-sided wrist pain that is worse with gripping tightly.

- **Tendinopathy** presents with pain localized to a tendon that is aggravated by activity and relieved with rest.
- Patients with **infectious tenosynovitis** will complain of significant pain and swelling along the tendon. They are likely to complain of fever, depending on the acuity of the infection.
- Patients with **trigger finger** note painful clicking on the palmar aspect, and locking of the finger in flexion. These symptoms may be intermittent.

Physical Examination
- To diagnose **CTS** the examination should identify median nerve involvement and exclude cervical or brachial plexus abnormalities. Weakness and atrophy of the thenar muscles are usually late findings. Tinel and Phalen's signs may be present but are neither sensitive nor specific. **Tinel's sign** is distal paresthesias produced by sharp tapping over the median nerve at the wrist. **Phalen's sign** is reproduction of symptoms when the wrists are held flexed against each other. The **"flick" sign** may be more accurate: When asked "What do you actually do with your hand(s) when the symptoms are at their worst?" patients with CTS do a flicking movement with their hand(s) similar to how someone would shake water off their hands.[3]
- **Finkelstein's test** is positive in de **Quervain's tenosynovitis** when passive ulnar deviation of the wrist while the fingers are flexed over the thumb reproduces pain.
- Tenosynovitis /tendinopathy can be diagnosed by localized pain and tenderness on palpation and with resisted movements. Infectious tenosynovitis will display edema, warmth, and erythema with likely surrounding cellulitis and drainage.
- On examination of **trigger finger,** difficulty extending the finger from flexion is noted. A palpable nodule may be felt.
- **Dupuytren's** presents with a lump in the hand and difficulty extending the fingers. The contraction worsens with time.

Diagnostic Testing
Imaging
Order radiographs in patients with hand trauma and visible abnormalities of the joints.

Electrodiagnostics
Nerve conduction studies are usually diagnostic in unclear cases of CTS.

TREATMENT

- Treatment of **CTS** begins with conservative measures including nighttime splinting in a wrist cock-up splint, rest, and NSAIDs. Careful injection with corticosteroids is helpful. Surgical release of the transverse carpal ligament is beneficial if conservative measures fail.
- **De Quervain's tenosynovitis** responds to rest, splinting, and NSAIDs. Surgery or corticosteroid injection may be indicated in refractory cases.
- **Tenosynovitis and tendinopathy** are treated with rest, ice, and NSAIDs.
- **Infectious tenosynovitis** requires drainage and antibiotics.
- **Dupuytren's contracture** benefits from stretching and corticosteroid injections in the initial stages, but surgery may be needed to release chronic contractures.

- **Ganglions** are treated with aspiration and surgical excision if they limit motion or are cosmetically unacceptable.
- Corticosteroid injections or surgery is helpful for **trigger finger.**

HIP PAIN

GENERAL PRINCIPLES

- Hip pain is a very common complaint and may be due to articular and periarticular disorders, or may be referred from other structures (Table 8-9).
- Different disorders cause pain in different areas around the hip joint, which may be useful for diagnosis. Ask the patient to point to the location of maximal pain.

Etiology and Pathogenesis
- **Hip OA** is a very common cause of hip pain and increases with age. True hip joint arthritis usually causes **pain in the anterior groin** that worsens with weight bearing (see Chapter 11, Osteoarthritis).
- Lumbosacral spine and sacroiliac (SI) joint disease cause **buttock pain,** as do spinal stenosis and vascular insufficiency.

TABLE 8-9	CAUSES OF HIP PAIN

Articular disorders
  Noninflammatory
    OA
    Osteonecrosis (AVN) of the femoral head
    Fracture
    Labral tear
    Hip impingement
  Inflammatory
    Seronegative spondyloarthropathies
    Septic arthritis
    Juvenile RA
    RA (usually late in the disease)

Periarticular disorders
  Trochanteric bursitis
  Ischiogluteal bursitis
  Iliopsoas bursitis
  Septic bursitis

Referred pain
  Lumbar spine OA and sciatica
  Spinal stenosis
  Sacroiliitis
  Knee disorders
  Vascular insufficiency
  Meralgia paresthetica

OA, osteoarthritis; AVN, avascular necrosis; RA, rheumatoid arthritis.

- The hip joint is affected in RA (usually late in the disease) and in juvenile RA and the seronegative spondyloarthropathies.
- **Fractures** of the femoral neck are common in elderly women with osteoporosis and may occur after a fall.
- **Avascular necrosis (AVN)** commonly affects the hip joint. Refer patients with fractures and osteonecrosis for orthopedic consultation.
- **Trochanteric bursitis** is very common and causes **lateral hip pain** that may radiate down the thigh and can be severe. It is more common in the elderly and is often associated with OA of the lumbar spine or hip.
- **Ischiogluteal bursitis** is caused by trauma or prolonged sitting on hard surfaces. It results in **pain over the ischium.**
- **Iliopsoas bursitis** is caused by inflammation of the bursa located between the hip joint and the overlying psoas muscle. **Anterior thigh and groin pain** are present.
- **Meralgia paresthetica** is caused by compression of the lateral femoral cutaneous nerve at the groin. This condition is seen in pregnant or obese patients, and in people who wear tight garments or heavy belts. Eliminating the source of compression and, occasionally, corticosteroid injections are useful.
- **Labral tears** of the hip are more common in young active patients. They may occur with trauma or insidiously. Patients complain of **groin pain** that is worsened with activity.
- **Piriformis syndrome** is a compression of the sciatic nerve as it passes deep to or through the piriformis and can cause **pain in the buttock** with numbness and tingling in the leg in a non-dermatomal pattern.

DIAGNOSIS

Clinical Presentation

History

- **Hip arthritis** will cause pain in the groin that is aggravated with weight-bearing activities. Patients will also note decreased range of motion when attempting to sit with legs crossed.
- OA of the lumbar spine can refer pain to the buttock and patients will often complain that this is hip pain.
- **AVN** of the hip will present with groin pain that is aggravated with weight bearing.
- Patients with **trochanteric bursitis** will complain of pain that is worse with lying on the affected side. They often note pain when they first stand up that improves after walking for a few minutes but, may worsen if they walk for a prolonged period.
- In **ischiogluteal bursitis** the pain is over the buttocks, may radiate down the thigh, and is worse with sitting. As this is the origin of the hamstring muscles differential diagnosis includes hamstring tendinopathy.
- **Meralgia paresthetica** causes anterior or lateral thigh pain that can be accompanied by numbness or paresthesias.
- **Labral tears** typically cause chronic hip pain in a younger patient that often is difficult to diagnose. Activity aggravates symptoms.
- **Piriformis syndrome** presents with complaints of buttock pain with paresthesia and pain in the posterior leg.

Physical Examination
- Hip arthritis is identified by decreased range of motion and pain in the groin with combined flexion/adduction and internal rotation. Combined flexion/abduction/external rotation (**FABER test**) can also illicit pain in the groin.
- Pain originating in the hip joint in general will be aggravated by combined flexion/internal rotation and adduction. The FABER test will also provoke symptoms.
- On examination of **trochanteric bursitis,** localized tenderness with palpation of the trochanteric area (the uppermost area with the patient lying on his or her side) and pain with resisted abduction are seen.
- **Iliopsoas bursitis** is identified by a combination of pain with palpation or with hyperextension or with resisted flexion. Ischiogluteal bursitis is noted with palpation over the ischium.
- **Labral tear** symptoms can be elicited with the FABER test.
- In **piriformis syndrome** the posterior buttock will be tender and stretching of the piriformis muscle may aggravate the symptoms.

Diagnostic Testing

Imaging
- Imaging is reserved for cases of trauma and suspected fracture, for patients with hip pain and risk factors for AVN (corticosteroid use, alcohol abuse), and for patients with chronic hip pain.
- MRI is useful to establish the presence of a labral tear.

TREATMENT

- **Trochanteric bursitis** treatment consists of stretching exercises, weight loss, and NSAIDs. Injection of the trochanteric bursa area with lidocaine and corticosteroids is a relatively simple procedure and may bring relief.
- Both **ischiogluteal and iliopsoas bursitis** respond to conservative measures of rest, NSAIDs and, potentially, corticosteroid injections.
- **Meralgia paresthetica** can be addressed by eliminating the source of compression. Occasionally, corticosteroid injections are useful.
- **Labral tears** can be treated with arthroscopic surgery.[4]
- **Piriformis syndrome** is treated with stretching, massage and, if recalcitrant, surgery.

KNEE PAIN

GENERAL PRINCIPLES

- Knee pain is a very common complaint and can be due to articular or periarticular disorders (Table 8-10).
- Common arthritides such as OA, RA, and gout frequently affect the knee.

Etiology and Pathogenesis
- **Knee OA** is a very common cause of knee pain. It is insidious in onset, but often has its origins after trauma earlier in life that damaged the normal cartilage or created abnormal mechanics in the knee.

TABLE 8-10 CAUSES OF KNEE PAIN

Articular disorders
  Noninflammatory
    OA
    Internal derangement (due to meniscal cartilage or cruciate ligament injuries)
    Osteonecrosis (AVN)
    Fracture
  Inflammatory
    RA
    Gout and calcium pyrophosphate deposition disease
    Seronegative spondyloarthropathies
    Viral arthritis
    Septic arthritis
Periarticular disorders
  Bursitis (anserine, prepatellar, infrapatellar)
  Tendinitis (patellar, quadriceps)
  Patellofemoral pain syndrome
  Popliteal cysts

OA, osteoarthritis; AVN, avascular necrosis; RA, rheumatoid arthritis.

- There are multiple intra-articular structures (articular cartilage, meniscal cartilage, cruciate ligaments) that may degenerate with age, overuse, or trauma and lead to internal derangement.
- Knee pain may be **referred from hip disorders.**
- **Anserine bursitis** derives its name from the pes anserinus, composed of the conjoined tendons of the sartorius, gracilis, and semitendinosus muscles that insert in the medial proximal tibia. The associated bursa often becomes inflamed, causing medial knee pain. Anserine bursitis often coexists with knee OA or occurs with athletic activity.
- **Prepatellar bursitis** causes pain (and occasionally erythema, warmth, and swelling) anterior to the patella and is common in people who spend a lot of time on their knees. This bursitis is occasionally septic, so send fluid for cultures. **Infrapatellar bursitis** presents similarly to prepatellar bursitis.
- **Tendinopathy:** Degeneration of the tendons around the knee may occur with overuse. Tendinitis may occur with inflammatory arthritis.
- **Patellar tendinopathy** is seen in young athletes who engage in repetitive jumping or kicking (jumper's knee). Pain is over the patellar tendon.
- **Popliteal tendinopathy** causes posterolateral knee pain.
- The quadriceps and patellar **tendons may rupture** due to trauma and repetitive injuries and in patients with RA and lupus and those who are receiving corticosteroids. Sudden pain and inability to extend the knee result.
- **Iliotibial band syndrome** is due to friction as the band passes over the lateral femoral condyle with flexion and extension. Repeated motions such as running promote repetitive friction. Excessive pronation may increase the amount of stress on the band as it passes over the condyle.

- **Patellofemoral pain** is thought to be due to malalignment (poor positioning of the patella) as it moves up and down the trochlear groove of the femur during flexion and extension. Softening of the cartilage with some non–full thickness breakdown may occur resulting in **chondromalacia patellae.**
- **Popliteal cysts** (Baker's cysts) may be asymptomatic or cause swelling in the popliteal fossa area. Cysts may be seen in patients with OA or RA and often communicate with the knee joint cavity. Large popliteal cysts may rupture and cause pain, swelling, and erythema of the calf, mimicking venous thrombosis.
- **Osgood–Schlatter disease** is seen in adolescents and presents with pain at the site of the insertion of the patellar tendon to the tibial tuberosity.
- **Osteochondritis dissecans** occurs most often in the teenage years and is due to focal necrosis of the subchondral bone. The overlying cartilage is thereby fragile and fragments of cartilage and bone can break off and form a loose body in the joint. It usually occurs in patients involved in athletics.
- Other less common causes of knee pain can include a **synovial plica,** which can be irritated and cause anteromedial knee pain. **Pigmented villonodular synovitis** is an overgrowth of the synovial lining of a joint and can occur in the knee. It leads to vague knee pain and swelling.

DIAGNOSIS

Clinical Presentation

History

- **OA** symptoms include brief morning stiffness and pain with use.
- Suspect **internal derangement** in patients, often young adults, who complain of "locking" or "catching" sensations after trauma (particularly sports injuries). Commonly they will report acute, painful swelling (due to hemarthrosis) at the time of injury. They may also note the knee giving way with pivoting after an anterior cruciate ligament tear.
- Medial knee pain occurs with **anserine bursitis.** Young patients are typically active in athletics. Pain is noted with using stairs and may improve after a few minutes of activity.
- Lateral knee pain occurs with **iliotibial band syndrome.** It is typical in runners and bikers.
- Anterior knee pain aggravated by activity can reflect **patellofemoral pain.** It is characterized by pain in the patellar region that is worse with using stairs and running. Brief stiffness after prolonged sitting is common. **Osgood–Schlatter's** may be causing the pain in a pubertal male who is involved in sports. **Patellar tendinopathy** can cause anterior knee pain with activity as well.
- Posterior knee pain can result from hamstring tendinitis, popliteal tendinitis, or Baker's cyst.
- Knee pain occurs in **osteochondritis dissecans.** There may be symptoms of catching or limited range of motion if a loose body is present.

Physical Examination

- On physical examination of the **osteoarthritic knee,** tenderness along the joint line, small effusions, and crepitus may be found. There may be decreased range of motion (see Chapter 11, Osteoarthritis).

- Specific maneuvers on physical examination may detect damage to the internal structures with internal derangement.
- Palpation is helpful in locating the specific structure involved.
- **Arthrocentesis** is relatively simple to perform on the knee and should be done in cases of monoarthritis to exclude infection, crystal-induced arthritis, or hemarthrosis.
- The **anserine bursa** is point tender to palpation just inferior to the medial joint line. Swelling is not usually appreciated.
- **Prepatellar bursitis** will present as a large swelling anterior to the patella. It may be red and warm suggesting possible infection. Arthrocentesis can help to establish the presence of infection.
- The popliteal tendon will be tender to palpation in the posteriolateral knee with tendinopathy. Resisted knee flexion with the tibia externally rotated may reproduce pain.
- In **iliotibial band syndrome** there is point tenderness over the band at the lateral condyle of the femur. Swelling is not typically present.
- **Patellofemoral pain** can be identified by palpating for tenderness on the posterior surface of the patella while the knee is extended and the quadriceps are relaxed. The pain can also be reproduced when the patella is held immobile while the patient contracts the quadriceps muscle.
- Tenderness and a prominent size of the tibial tuberosities will be noticed with **Osgood–Schlatter disease.**
- With the patient lying prone with both knees extended a swelling in the popliteal fossa will be notable if **Baker's cyst** is evident.
- A painful **plica** may be palpated medial to the medial border of the patella.

Diagnostic Testing
Imaging

- In general, reserve imaging for post-traumatic pain and for patients with chronic pain. Ligament and meniscal tears are noted with MRI.
- **Ultrasound** can be used to diagnose **Baker's cyst** and to rule out more serious pathology, such as a popliteal artery aneurysm or a soft tissue tumor.
- Plain films can identify **osteochondritis dissecans.** Then MRI can be used to determine the extent and stability of the lesion.
- **Pigmented villonodular synovitis** can be identified on MRI.

TREATMENT

- **Anserine bursitis** treatment includes rest, ice, and stretching. If symptoms do not improve then corticosteroid injections can be helpful.
- In **prepatellar bursitis,** recommend avoiding kneeling to help resolve the bursitis. However, aspiration may be needed in cases with abundant fluid. Surgical excision may be necessary for frequent recurrences.
- **Patellar tendinitis** treatment is rest, ice application, and stretching exercises. Corticosteroid injections are contraindicated due to the risk of tendon rupture.
- **Popliteal tendinopathy** responds to hamstring strengthening. Be sure to rule out an acute ligamentous injury to the knee if the injury is traumatic.
- Treatment of **rupture** of the patellar tendon and quadriceps tendon is surgery.

- **Iliotibial band syndrome** is treated by rest, physical therapy, orthotics, and stretching of the band. Corticosteroid injections may be needed if no improvement occurs with therapy. Surgery is a last resort.
- **Patellofemoral pain** is treated initially with rest from aggravating activities. Gradual pain-free strengthening of the quadriceps muscle and hip abductors is recommended. Orthotics may help improve knee alignment in those with increased pronation. Patellofemoral supports may provide some patients relief.
- Treatment of **Osgood–Schlatter** syndrome is rest from offending athletic activities. It usually resolves as the patient grows older.
- A symptomatic **Baker's cyst** can be treated with aspiration and injection of the knee joint with corticosteroids.
- Treatment of **osteochondritis dissecans** can be conservative or surgical depending on the extent of the lesion.
- Treatment of **pigmented villonodular synovitis** is surgical removal of the overgrown synovium; however, it can recur.
- Treatment of a painful **plica** involves quadriceps strengthening and hamstring stretching. Surgery can be performed to remove the plica if it does not improve.

ANKLE AND FOOT PAIN

GENERAL PRINCIPLES

- Ankle and foot pain are common problems and may be due to periarticular disorders, arthritis, or trauma, and are often worsened by **inappropriate footwear.**
- The history and physical examination usually lead to a diagnosis. A history of diabetes, peripheral neuropathy, or peripheral vascular disease is particularly important.

Etiology and Pathogenesis

- Arthritis frequently affects the ankle and foot. **OA spares** the ankle but often involves the first metatarsophalangeal (MTP) joint causing lateral deviation (**hallux valgus** or **bunion**). Bunions are more common in women.
- **RA** affects the ankle and forefoot in most of the patients. Bilateral ankle pain and synovitis and forefoot pain usually accompanies other joint involvement.
- The first MTP is the most commonly affected joint in acute **gout.**
- Motor, sensory, and autonomic neuropathies (seen in diabetic and other peripheral neuropathies) may lead to ankle and foot pain and severe deformity in **neuropathic arthropathy (Charcot joint).**
- **Ankle sprains** are very common in outpatients and usually follow ankle inversion after a misstep or fall.
- **Stress fractures** are common causes of foot pain and occur as a result of overuse. They are often seen in dancers, runners, or military recruits and affect the second or third metatarsals most frequently.
- **Plantar fasciitis** is the most common cause of plantar foot pain and is due to inflammation of the plantar fascia at its insertion into the calcaneus. It may be idiopathic or due to overuse, and is sometimes seen in patients with seronegative spondyloarthropathies.
- **Achilles tendinitis** occurs when the Achilles tendon becomes inflamed due to trauma or overuse (dancers, runners). Heel pain due to Achilles tendon

enthesopathy is characteristic of the seronegative spondyloarthropathies. The **tendon may rupture** due to trauma, or spontaneously in patients taking corticosteroids or quinolone antibiotics. Injection of the Achilles tendon with corticosteroids may also lead to rupture. Patients with tendon rupture have difficulty walking and foot dorsiflexion.

- Inflammation of the **retrocalcaneal bursa** may be difficult to distinguish from Achilles tendinitis.
- **Posterior tibial tendinitis** causes pain along the tendon near the medial malleolus.
- **Peroneal tendinitis** causes pain anterior to the lateral malleolus.
- **Tarsal tunnel syndrome** is characterized by pain, numbness, and paresthesias of the sole. The posterior tibial nerve is compressed at the flexor retinaculum, posterior to the medial malleolus.
- **Morton's neuroma** is due to compression of an interdigital nerve, most commonly between the third and fourth toes. It causes forefoot pain and numbness and tingling of these toes. It occurs more frequently in middle-aged women and is exacerbated by walking and by wearing narrow shoes or high heels.
- **Metatarsalgia** (pain arising from the metatarsal heads) may be due to high heels, everted foot, arthritis, trauma, or deformities, and is quite common.

DIAGNOSIS

Clinical Presentation

History

- **Stress fractures** become more painful as an activity continues.
- **Plantar fasciitis** causes pain that is worse in the morning, especially when the patient first stands up. Pain may also occur after prolonged standing or walking and may be severe.
- **Tendinitis** is often most painful when beginning an activity and then becomes less painful as the area "warms up."
- Patients often feel a pop as if they have been "shot" when the Achilles ruptures.

Physical Examination

- The physical examination should include inspection (looking for deformities, abnormal calluses), palpation (of tender areas), testing of sensation, and evaluation of distal pulses.
- **Examine the patient's footwear.** Signs of abnormal (or unilateral) wear or frequent use of high heels or narrow pointed shoes are important clues.
- Tophi and deformities at the first MTP joint may be seen in chronic **gout.**
- **Ankle sprains** will present with edema and tenderness to palpation over the ligament(s) involved. Valgus and varus testing is provocative for ligament injury.
- Palpation of the involved bone will produce tenderness with a **stress fracture.**
- Tenderness over the distal edge of the plantar surface of the calcaneus will be present in **plantar fasciitis.**
- Tenderness over the tendon will be present with Achilles tendinitis.
- Tenderness just proximal to the insertion of the Achilles and between the tendon and the calcaneus will be present with **retrocalcaneal bursitis.** However, it is difficult to distinguish the two.

- **Rupture of the Achilles tendon** can be noted as an anatomical defect, but also by the **Thompson test.** The patient lies prone with the knee extended. Squeezing the calf muscle will cause plantar flexion if the tendon is intact. If the tendon is ruptured, plantar flexion will not occur.
- In **tarsal tunnel syndrome** tapping over the nerve as it passes around the medial malleolus may reproduce symptoms. The area may be tender to palpation.
- Squeezing the metatarsal heads together can aggravate the pain of **Morton's neuroma.**
- Palpation over the metatarsal heads reveals tenderness in **metatarsalgia.**

Diagnostic Testing

Imaging

- Radiographs are rarely useful except in cases of trauma.
- According to the Ottawa guidelines for ankle sprains, **obtain radiographs** to rule out fracture in patients with medial or lateral malleolar tenderness or with inability to bear weight after the event or in the emergency department (ED).
- The Ottawa guidelines for foot injuries recommend plain films to rule out fracture if there is pain in the midfoot after the injury and if any of the following are present: There is tenderness at the base of the fifth metatarsal or the navicular, or if the patient cannot bear weight after the event or in the ED.
- Radiographs sometimes do not detect stress fractures. Bone scan or MRI may be used for diagnosis.

Electrodiagnostic Testing

When considering surgery for tarsal tunnel syndrome, electrodiagnostic testing will help confirm the diagnosis.

TREATMENT

- Treatment of foot and ankle pain is conservative. Rest, stretching exercises, and NSAIDs are frequently used.
- **Orthoses and appropriate footwear** are an essential part of care in many cases. Assistance from podiatrists and orthotists is invaluable.
- A shoe with a wide toe box provides symptomatic relief for **bunions,** but surgery is often performed for cosmetic reasons.
- **Stress fracture** treatment is usually conservative.
- **Ankle sprains** are initially treated with rest, ice, compression, and elevation followed by gradually increasing range of motion and strengthening exercises.
- **Plantar fasciitis** is treated with stretching of the calf muscles, heel inserts/ orthotics and NSAIDs. Occasionally corticosteroid injections are used.
- Treatment of **Achilles tendinitis** is conservative, but rupture requires surgical evaluation. Retrocalcaneal bursitis treatment involves rest and NSAIDs.
- **Posterior tibial and peroneal tendinopathy** respond well to rest. Arch supports/orthotics help to decrease pronation and the stress that it causes on these tendons.
- In **tarsal tunnel syndrome** corticosteroid injections are helpful but should be done carefully. If excessive pronation is present, orthotics should be provided. Surgical decompression may be needed.

- Properly fitting footwear with sufficient width or a metatarsal pad is helpful in treating **Morton's neuroma**. Corticosteroid injections are sometimes used for relief. Some patients require surgery.
- Proper footwear and a metatarsal pad are helpful in treating **metatarsalgia**.

REFERENCES

1. Furman MB, Simon J. Cervical disc disease: treatment and medication. Last accessed 02/01/2012 http://emedicine.medscape.com/article/305720-treatment
2. Deyo RA, Weinstein JN. Low back pain. *N Engl J Med.* 2001;344:363–370.
3. Shoen RP, Moskowitz RW, Goldberg VM. *Soft Tissue Rheumatic Pain: Recognition, Management, Prevention.* 3rd ed. Philadelphia, PA: Lea & Febiger; 1996.
4. Kamath AF, Componovo R, Baldwin K, et al. Hip arthroscopy for labral tears: review of clinical outcomes with 4.8-year mean follow-up. *Am J Sports Med.* 2009;37:1721–1727.

Drugs Used for the Treatment of Rheumatic Diseases

9

Alfred H.J. Kim and Leslie E. Kahl

GENERAL PRINCIPLES

- While rheumatologic diseases encompass a wide range of organ systems, there are a relatively limited number of drug classes for treatment.
- The main classes of medications used in rheumatology include:
  - ○ Analgesics
  - ○ Salicylates/Non-steroidal anti-inflammatory drugs (NSAIDs)/Cyclooxygenase-2 (COX-2) inhibitors
  - ○ Glucocorticoids (GCs)
  - ○ Disease-modifying antirheumatic drugs (DMARDs)
  - ○ Biologics
  - ○ Gout medications
    - ■ Antihyperuricemics
    - ■ Antiinflammatory
  - ○ Osteoporosis medications

ANALGESICS

- Analgesics largely **reduce pain,** not inflammation. Consequently, their use is limited in rheumatology as many diseases are strongly inflammatory.
- Analgesics are very useful for **osteoarthritis (OA)** given their minimal side effect profiles.
- Medications
  - ○ **Acetaminophen**
    - ■ **Dosage:** 325 to 650 mg PO q4 to 6 hours or 1000 mg PO q6 to 8 hours. Limit to 4 g/24 hours in liver-competent patients and ≤2 g/24 hours with hepatic insufficiency.
    - ■ **Mechanism:** Largely unclear, although it inhibits prostaglandin synthesis in central nervous system (CNS). There may also be inhibition of COX isoenzymes.
    - ■ **Side effects:** It is generally well tolerated. Combination with hepatotoxicity agents, such as ethanol, potentiates hepatotoxicity. It can increase INR when large doses are given with warfarin.
    - ■ **Contraindications/precautions:** Chronic alcohol use, liver disease, glucose-6-phosphate dehydrogenase (G6PD) deficiency.
  - ○ **Tramadol**
    - ■ **Dosage:** 50 to 100 mg PO q4 to 6 hours.
    - ■ **Mechanism:** It binds to μ-opiate receptors in CNS, inhibiting ascending pain pathways, and also inhibits norepinephrine and serotonin reuptake.

- **Side effects:** Somnolence, dizziness, headache, nausea, vomiting.
- **Contraindications/precautions:** History of alcohol or drug use, chronic respiratory disease, liver disease, concomitant use of tricyclic antidepressants (TCAs), monoamine oxidase inhibitors (MAOIs), or selective serotonin reuptake inhibitors (SSRIs), seizure disorder.
- **Tramadol has a synergistic effect on pain when combined with acetaminophen.** They are often prescribed together.

SALICYLATES/NSAIDS/COX-II INHIBITORS

- Used for antiinflammatory, antipyretic, and analgesic purposes.
- These drugs work by **inhibiting cyclooxygenase** (COX), with other unidentified mechanisms likely contributing to effect.
- Salicylates and NSAIDs block COX-I and COX-II nonspecifically, while COX-II inhibitors predictably inhibit only COX-II.
- COX converts arachidonic acid to prostaglandins, leukotrienes, or thromboxanes, leading to a complex response involving both pro- and antiinflammatory actions.
- COX-II is an inducible enzyme that leads to a proinflammatory phenotype.
- Adverse effects seen with salicylates and NSAIDs are diverse, including
  - **Gastrointestinal (GI):** Gastritis and ulcer formation which can lead to perforation (particularly with age >65, smoking, higher duration and dose of NSAIDs; risk=1%/patient year).
  - **Renal:** Hypertension, hyperkalemia, reduction in efficacy of diuretics and antihypertensives, edema (due to vasoconstriction and water and sodium retention), rarely interstitial nephritis (with long-term, chronic use).
  - **CNS:** Headaches, aseptic meningitis, tinnitus (with ASA), altered mental status, aseptic meningitis.
  - **Hepatic:** Transaminitis, Reye's syndrome in children with viral illness.
  - **Hematologic:** Impaired platelet aggregation (reversible except with salicylates), anemia (usually from GI blood loss).
  - **Hypersensitivity reactions: Samter's triad of nasal polyps, asthma, and hypersensitivity to all NSAIDs** is due to excessive leukotriene production after NSAID administration. Other hypersensitivity reactions, such as rash, can also occur separately from Samter's triad.
- **COX-II inhibitors reduce GI events by 20%–40%, and do not inhibit platelet aggregation.** Renal and hypersensitivity reactions equal to NSAIDs.
- See Table 9-1 for a list of medications.

GLUCOCORTICOIDS

- GCs, also referred to as corticosteroids or steroids, remain one of the most effective antiinflammatory and immunosuppressive medications, and also possess significant toxicity with prolonged use.
- Patients taking alternate day GC therapy, low dose prednisone (<5 mg/day), or GCs less than 3 weeks usually do not have suppression of the hypothalamic/pituitary axis (HPA). Anyone who is on ≥20 mg/day or has clinical Cushing's syndrome is assumed to have HPA axis suppression. Otherwise, there is variable suppression of the HPA axis.

TABLE 9-1   NSAIDS AND SELECTIVE COX-2 INHIBITORS

Classification	Drug	Dosage (PO, adult dose unless indicated)
Carboxylic acid: acetylated[a]	Aspirin	2400–5400 mg/day in 4 divided doses
Carboxylic acid: nonacetylated salicylates[a]	Salsalate	3 g/day in 2–3 divided doses
	Diflunisal	500–1500 mg/day in 2 divided doses
	Choline salicylate	870–1740 mg/dose given qid
	Choline magnesium trisalicylate	1–3 g/day in 2–3 divided doses
Carboxylic acid: acetic acids	Etodolac	Immediate release: 800–1200 mg/day in 2–4 divided doses
		Sustained release: 400–1000 mg once daily
	Diclofenac	Immediate release: 100–200 mg/day in 2–3 divided doses
		Sustained release: 100–200 mg once daily
	Diclofenac and misoprostol[b]	150–200 mg/day (diclofenac) in 3 divided doses
	Indomethacin	Immediate release: 50–200 mg/day in 2–3 divided doses
		Sustained release: 75 mg once or twice daily
	Ketorolac[c]	PO: 10 mg q4–6h; IM/IV: 30–60 mg × 1, followed by 15–30 mg q6h
	Nabumetone	1000–2000 mg in 1–2 divided doses
Propionic acids	Fenoprofen	900–3200 mg/day in 3–4 divided doses
	Flurbiprofen	200–300 mg/day in 2–4 divided doses
	Ibuprofen	OTC dose: 200–400 mg q4–6h; prescription dose: 1200–3200 mg/day in 3–4 divided doses
	Ketoprofen	OTC dose: 12.5 mg q4–6h; prescription dose: 150–300 mg/day in 3–4 divided doses
		Extended release: 200 mg once daily

TABLE 9-1   NSAIDS AND SELECTIVE COX-2 INHIBITORS (*Continued*)

Classification	Drug	Dosage (PO, adult dose unless indicated)
	Naproxen	Immediate release: 500–1500 mg/day in 2–3 divided doses Extended release: 750–1500 mg once daily
	Naproxen sodium	OTC: 220 mg bid–tid; prescription: 550–1375 mg/day in 2–3 divided doses; may increase to 1650 mg/day for limited periods of time only
	Oxaprozin	600–1800 mg/day; doses <1200 mg/day in 1–2 divided doses; doses >1200 mg/day in 2–3 divided doses
Fenamates	Meclofenamate	200–400 mg/day in 3–4 divided doses
	Mefenamic acid[d]	250 mg q6h
Oxicams	Meloxicam	7.5–15 mg once daily
	Piroxicam	10–20 mg/day
Selective COX-2 inhibitors[e]	Celecoxib[e]	OA: 100–200 mg/day in 1–2 doses; RA: 200–400 mg/day in 2 divided doses

[a]Salicylate level may be used to monitor therapy (target level is 15–30 mg/dL).
[b]Risk of gastric ulcer is decreased relative to other traditional NSAIDs.
[c]Not indicated for use exceeding 5 days due to increased risk of side effects including GI bleed; adjust dose based on weight and age.
[d]Not indicated for use exceeding 1 week.
[e]Caution in patients with a history of hypersensitivity to sulfonamides.

- Medications
  - **Prednisone (PO), prednisolone (PO), hydrocortisol (PO/IM/IV), methylprednisolone (IV/intraarticular), dexamethasone (PO/IV/IM), triamcinolone (intraarticular)** (see Table 9-2 for equivalent doses of GCs).[1]
    - **Dosage:** Highly dependent on disease and clinical situation (Table 9-3).[2]
    - **Mechanism:** Effects are pleiotropic and include: Inhibition of leukocyte trafficking, restriction of leukocyte access to inflamed tissue, attenuated production of inflammatory humoral mediators and inhibition of various functions of leukocytes, fibroblasts, and endothelial cells.
    - **Side effects:** Adverse effects are **usually seen with doses ≥10 mg/day** and may impact the following systems:
      - Musculoskeletal (secondary osteoporosis, myopathy).
      - Endocrine (hyperglycemia, weight gain, iatrogenic Cushing's syndrome).
      - Cardiovascular (dyslipidemia, hypertension).

| TABLE 9-2 | COMPARISON OF REPRESENTATIVE CORTICOSTEROID PREPARATIONS |

	Approximate Equivalent Dose[a], mg	Relative Anti-inflammatory Activity	Relative Mineralo-corticoid Activity	Duration of Action, Hours
Cortisol[b]	20	1	1	8–12
Cortisone acetate	25	0.8	0.8	8–12
Hydrocortisone	20	1	1	8–12
Prednisone	5	4	0.8	12–36
Prednisolone	5	4	0.8	12–36
Methylprednisolone	4	5	0.5	12–36
Triamcinolone	4	5	0	12–36
Fludrocortisone[c]	—	10	125	12–36
Dexamethasone	0.75	30	0	36–72

[a]Equivalent dose shown is for oral or IV administration. Relative potency for intra-articular or intramuscular administration may vary considerably.
[b]Data for cortisol, endogenous corticosteroid hormone, are included for comparison with synthetic preparations listed.
[c]Fludrocortisone is not used for anti-inflammatory effect.

  □ Dermatologic (acne, purpura and cutaneous atrophy due to catabolic effects).
  □ Ophthalmologic (cataract, glaucoma).
  □ Infectious (overall relative risk of infection is 2.0, but is dose-dependent).
  □ Psychological (psychosis, minor mood disturbances).
  ■ **Contraindications/precautions:** Systemic infection (especially fungal), heart failure (due to fluid retention), diabetes mellitus (hyperglycemia), hepatic impairment, acute myocardial infarction (risk of myocardial rupture), myasthenia gravis (exacerbation of symptoms may occur).
  ■ **Special considerations:** For patients with suspected HPA axis suppression, GCs must be tapered off gradually, not discontinued abruptly, to allow for recovery of the HPA axis. Additionally, those undergoing major surgery may need stress-dose GCs until 48 hours postoperatively and should be monitored for signs of adrenal insufficiency.

DISEASE-MODIFYING ANTIRHEUMATIC DRUGS

  • This group of medications has both anti-inflammatory and immunomodulatory effects, with highly variable clinical responses.
  • They are usually used as steroid-sparing therapy, and have a slow onset of action.
  • There is a high rate of discontinuation due to lack of efficacy or drug toxicity.

TABLE 9-3	APPROXIMATE DOSAGES OF GLUCOCORTICOIDS FOR VARIOUS CLINICAL SITUATIONS AND POTENTIAL ADVERSE EFFECTS		
Terminology	Dosage[a]	Clinical Application	Adverse Effects
Low	≤7.5	Maintenance therapy	Few
Medium	>7.5 to ≤30	Initial therapy for mild to moderate disease such as rash or arthritis.	Dose-dependent and considerable if treatment given for longer periods of time
High	>30 to ≤100	Initial therapy for moderate to severe (non–life-threatening) disease such as nephritis or vasculitis.	Cannot be administered for long-term therapy due to severe side effects
Very High	>100	Initially given in severe, acute and/or life-threatening exacerbations of rheumatic diseases	Cannot be administered for long-term therapy due to dramatic side effects
Pulse therapy	>250 for one or several days	Particularly severe and/or potentially life-threatening forms of rheumatic diseases	High proportion of cases have a relatively low incidence of side effects

[a]Dosage is given in milligrams of prednisone equivalent per day.

Adapted from: Buttgereit F, Burmester G-R. Glucocorticoids. In: Klippel JH, Stone JH, Crofford LJ, White PH, eds. *Primer on the Rheumatic Diseases.* New York: Springer Science+Business Media; 2008:644–650.

- Medications
  - Hydroxychloroquine
    - **Dosage:** 4 to 6 mg/kg/day, which is usually 200 to 400 mg PO qday. The 400 mg dose can be split into 200 mg bid.
    - **Mechanism:** It inhibits neutrophil trafficking and complement-dependent antigen–antibody responses. It also interferes with lysosomal enzymes.
    - **Onset of action:** 4 to 6 weeks.
    - **Side effects:** This drug is generally well tolerated, but some patients may have indigestion or hypersensitivity rash; retinopathy and bone marrow suppression are rare complications.
    - **Contraindications/precautions:** It carries a **boxed warning** for use by experienced physicians only. History of hypersensitivity or visual changes on related therapy, G6PD deficiency, psoriasis (may worsen on therapy),

macular degeneration are contraindications to its use. Food and Drug Administration (FDA) **pregnancy category: C** (animal reproduction studies have shown an adverse effect on the fetus and there are no adequate and well-controlled studies in humans, but potential benefits may warrant use of the drug in pregnant women despite potential risks).

- **Monitoring:** Ophthalmologic examination is required q6 to 60 months (depending on dose, length of therapy, age, and baseline retinal health).

○ Methotrexate
- **Dosage:** Start with 10 to 15 mg/week (PO/IM/SC), and increase 5 mg q2 to 4 weeks as needed to a maximum of 20 to 25 mg/week.
- **Mechanism:** It inhibits dihydrofolate reductase, acting as folate antimetabolite that inhibits DNA synthesis.
- **Onset of action:** 3 to 6 weeks, but additional improvement can be seen up to 12 weeks.
- **Side effects:** Anorexia, nausea, diarrhea, stomatitis, transaminitis are not rare, and all can be reduced with administration of folic acid 1 mg daily; pneumonitis and infection are much less common.
- **Contraindications/precautions:** There is a **boxed warning** for acute renal failure, bone marrow suppression, dermatologic reactions (including toxic epidermal necrolysis), diarrhea/stomatitis, hepatotoxicity, lymphomas, infections, pneumonitis, and ascites/pleural effusions (reduced eliminationof methotrexate). Chronic alcohol use is a contraindication. **FDA pregnancy category: D** (positive evidence of human fetal risk based on adverse reaction data from investigational or marketing experience or studies in humans, but potential benefits may warrant use of the drug in pregnant women despite potential risks), and breastfeeding is contraindicated.
- **Monitoring:** A baseline complete metabolic profile (CMP), complete blood count (CBC), and chest radiographs are required. CMP and CBC should be done q2 to 4 weeks for first 3 months, then q8 to 12 weeks next 3 to 6 months, then q12 weeks afterward. Liver biopsy should be performed if persistent hepatic function profile (HFP) abnormalities, alcoholism, or chronic hepatitis B or C, and pulmonary function tests if lung toxicity suspected.

○ Leflunomide
- **Dosage:** 10 to 20 mg PO qday.
- **Mechanism:** It inhibits dihydroorotate dehydrogenase, inhibiting de novo pyrimidine synthesis.
- **Onset of action:** 4 to 8 weeks.
- **Side effects:** These include diarrhea, alopecia, hepatitis, rash, infection, hypertension, and headache.
- **Contraindications/precautions:** There is a **boxed warning** for severe liver injury. Renal or hepatic impairment, chronic alcohol use, and preexisting bone marrow suppression are contraindications to its use. **It is teratogenic; FDA pregnancy category: X** (Studies in animals or humans have demonstrated fetal abnormalities and/or there is positive evidence of human fetal risk based on adverse reaction data from investigational or marketing experience, and **the risks involved in use of the drug in pregnant women clearly outweigh potential benefits**).
- **Monitoring:** Screen for pregnancy and tuberculosis prior to therapy. Baseline CMP and CBC are required. Blood pressure, CMP, phosphate

(leflunomide can occasionally increase renal excretion of phosphate), and CBC should be monitored q4 weeks for first 6 months, then q12 weeks. Discontinue leflunomide and initiate cholestyramine therapy if alanine aminotransferase ALT ≥2 times upper limit of normal (ULN) or other serious adverse effects occur.

○ **Sulfasalazine**
  - **Dosage:** Start with 500 to 1000 mg PO daily, increasing weekly as needed to 2 to 3 g/day divided in 2 equal doses.
  - **Mechanism:** This drug interferes with prostaglandin synthesis.
  - **Onset of action:** 8 to 12 weeks.
  - **Side effects:** Headache, rash, anorexia, dyspepsia, nausea, vomiting, reversible oligospermia, dizziness, bone marrow suppression, transaminitis may all occur. GI symptoms are less common with the enteric-coated form of the drug.
  - **Contraindications/precautions:** Sulfa allergy, G6PD deficiency, renal or hepatic impairment, GI or genitourinary (GU) obstruction. **FDA pregnancy category: B** (animal reproduction studies have failed to demonstrate a risk to the fetus and there are no adequate and well-controlled studies in pregnant women or animal studies have shown an adverse effect, but adequate and well-controlled studies in pregnant women have failed to demonstrate a risk to the fetus in any trimester).
  - **Monitoring:** Baseline CMP and CBC are required, and should be repeated q2 weeks for first 3 months, then q4 weeks for the next 3 months, then q12 weeks afterward.

○ **Azathioprine**
  - **Dosage:** Start with 1 mg/kg/day PO daily or divided bid for 6 to 8 weeks, then increase by 0.5 mg/kg q4 weeks as needed until response or up to a maximum of 2.5 mg/kg/day.
  - **Mechanism:** This drug antagonizes purine metabolism, with 6-thioguanine nucleotides mediating most of the effects.
  - **Onset of action:** 6 to 8 weeks.
  - **Side effects:** Leukopenia, nausea, vomiting, diarrhea, myalgia, malaise, dizziness, hepatotoxicity, and HFP abnormalities may all occur and are usually dose-dependent.
  - **Contraindications/precautions: Boxed warning** for use by experienced physicians only and increased risk of neoplasia. History of treatment with alkylating agents. **FDA pregnancy category: D.**
  - **Monitoring:** Thiopurine methyltransferase (TPMT) genotyping or phenotyping prior to therapy can help guide initial dosing. CBC and CMP should be done at baseline. CBC should be repeated qweekly during first month, q2 weeks during months 2 and 3, then qmonthly, with CMP q3 months.

○ **Mycophenolate mofetil**
  - **Dosage:** Start with 500 mg PO bid, and increase by 1000 mg q3 to 4 weeks as needed to a maximum dose of 1500 mg PO bid.
  - **Mechanism:** This drug inhibits inosine monophosphate dehydrogenase (IMPDH), which inhibits de novo guanosine nucleotide synthesis, thereby reducing lymphocyte proliferation.
  - **Onset of action:** Unknown.
  - **Side effects:** The most common adverse effect is nausea. The following may also occur: Hypertension or hypotension, edema, chest pain, tachycardia,

pain, headache, insomnia, infection, dizziness, anxiety, hyperglycemia, hypercholesterolemia, hypomagnesemia, hypokalemia, abdominal pain with nausea and vomiting, diarrhea and/or constipation, dyspepsia, bone marrow suppression, acute renal failure, dyspnea, pleural effusion.

- **Contraindications/precautions:** There is a **boxed warning** for use by experienced physicians only. The drug is associated with increased risk of infections, lymphoma, and skin malignancy; **FDA pregnancy category: D.** It should be used with caution in peptic ulcer disease and renal impairment.
- **Monitoring:** CBC is required at baseline and qweekly during first month, q2 weeks during months 2 and 3, then qmonthly. CMP is done at baseline and then q3 months.

○ Cyclophosphamide
  - **Dosage:** Dose and route of administration are highly dependent on disease severity, and must be administered with the input of a rheumatologist. If PO, 1 to 2 mg/kg/day qAM is the usual starting dose; if IV, 0.25 to 1.0 g/m^2 qmonthly.
  - **Mechanism:** This is an alkylating agent, interfering with DNA synthesis.
  - **Onset of action:** 4 to 7 days.
  - **Side effects:** Alopecia, sterility, nausea, vomiting, diarrhea, mucositis/stomatitis, **acute hemorrhagic cystitis** (reduced with concurrent administration of Mesna IV), bone marrow suppression, headache, rash, and **bladder transitional cell carcinoma** may all occur.
  - **Contraindications/precautions:** Depressed bone marrow function, renal or hepatic impairment and infection are contraindications to its use; **FDA pregnancy category: D.**
  - **Monitoring:** CBC, CMP, and urinalysis (UA) are required at baseline and at least qweekly until the dose is stable, then qmonthly. Lymphopenia is common and is not an indication to reduce dose. Neutropenia should be avoided by dose reduction.

○ Cyclosporine
  - **Dosage:** For rheumatoid arthritis (RA), start with 2.5 mg/kg/day PO divided twice daily, increasing by 0.5 to 0.75 mg/kg/day after 8 weeks. Additional dosage increases can be done again at 12 weeks as needed to a maximum of 4 mg/kg/day. For lupus nephritis, start at 4 mg/kg/day for 1 month, then reduce by 0.5 mg/kg/day q2 weeks to maintenance dose of 2.5 to 3 mg/kg/day.
  - **Mechanism:** This drug inhibits interleukin (IL)-2 production and release from T lymphocytes.
  - **Onset of action:** 4 to 12 weeks.
  - **Side effects:** Common adverse effects include hypertension and edema. Headache, hirsutism, hypertriglyceridemia, nausea, diarrhea, dyspepsia, tremor, renal failure, and infection may also occur.
  - **Contraindications/precautions:** There is a **boxed warning** for use by experienced physicians only. Patients should be monitored for development of hypertension, infection, malignancy (lymphoma and skin), nephrotoxicity, and skin cancer. **FDA pregnancy category: C.**
  - **Monitoring:** Baseline studies should include blood pressure and creatinine. Thereafter, monitor creatinine q2 weeks for the first 3 months, then qmonthly. If hypertension develops, decrease dose by 25 to 50%; if hypertension persists, discontinue the drug. No additional benefit has been seen in monitoring cyclosporine levels.

BIOLOGICS

- Biologics represent a novel class of therapeutics that take advantage of modern recombinant protein engineering techniques that selectively block a pathway important in immunity.
- Biologics have revolutionized the treatment of many rheumatic conditions, leading to response rates that have been unmatched with prior therapies. This class has also occasionally reactivated prior infections that have lead to significant morbidity and mortality.
- Prior to initiating any biologic, ensure patient is **up-to-date with vaccinations** and **screened for tuberculosis (TB), hepatitis B, and hepatitis C. Live virus vaccines are contraindicated once a biologic has been initiated.** Biologic use is discouraged with any of these infections.
- **Anti-tumor necrosis factor (TNF) therapies**
  - Etanercept
    - **Dosage:** The usual dose is 50 mg SC qweek, can be split into 25 mg SC 2x/week. It is usually given with low-dose methotrexate, leflunomide, or azathioprine to improve efficacy of the biologic.
    - **Mechanism:** It is a soluble TNF receptor linked to the Fc portion of human IgG1, limiting amount of TNF-α that can bind to endogenous TNF receptors.
    - **Onset of action:** 1 to 2 weeks
    - **Side effects:** Injection site reactions, headache, infections (including TB), lymphoma, antinuclear antibody (ANA) positivity and drug-induced lupus may occur.
    - **Contraindications/precautions:** There is a **boxed warning** for infection, malignancy, and TB. Use only with extreme caution with infection (hepatitis B can reactivate), alcoholic hepatitis, heart failure, demyelinating disease/optic neuritis, or concurrent use of anakinra.
  - Adalimumab
    - **Dosage:** The usual dose is 50 mg SC q2 weeks, but it can be used 50 mg SC qweekly. It is usually given with low-dose methotrexate, leflunomide, or azathioprine to improve efficacy of the biologic.
    - **Mechanism:** It is a human anti-TNF monoclonal antibody (mAb) leading to TNF-α inhibition.
    - **Onset of action:** 4 to 6 weeks
    - **Side effects:** Injection site reactions, headache, infections (including TB), lymphoma, rash, ANA positivity, drug-induced lupus can all occur.
    - **Contraindications/precautions:** There is a **boxed warning** for infection, malignancy, and TB. Use only with extreme caution with infection (hepatitis B can reactivate), demyelinating disease/optic neuritis, heart failure, bone marrow abnormalities, or concurrent use of anakinra.
  - Infliximab
    - **Dosage:** Start with 3 mg/kg IV at 0, 2, and 6 weeks, then every 8 weeks afterward. Dosing can range from 3 to 10 mg/kg repeated 4 to 8 weeks. It is usually given with low-dose methotrexate, leflunomide, or azathioprine for improved efficacy of biologic.
    - **Mechanism:** It is a chimeric anti-TNF mAb leading to TNF-α inhibition.
    - **Onset of action:** 2 to 3 weeks

- **Side effects:** Infusion reactions may occur acutely. Headache, nausea, vomiting, diarrhea, infections (including TB), lymphoma, rash, ANA positivity, and drug-induced lupus also occur.
- **Contraindications/precautions:** There is a **boxed warning** for infection, malignancy, and TB. Use with extreme caution with infection (hepatitis B can reactivate), demyclinating disease/optic neuritis, heart failure (with doses >5 mg/kg), bone marrow abnormalities, or concurrent use of anakinra, seizure disorder.

○ **Certolizumab pegol**
- **Dosage:** Start with 400 mg SC at weeks 0, 2, 4, then 200 mg SC q4 weeks.
- **Mechanism:** It contains PEGylated humanized anti-TNF F(ab) fragments leading to TNF-α inhibition. It is usually given with an oral DMARD.
- **Onset of action:** <8 weeks
- **Side effects:** Injection site reactions, headache, nausea, infections (including TB), rash, ANA positivity, drug-induced lupus may occur.
- **Contraindications/precautions:** There is a **boxed warning** for infection, malignancy, and TB. Use only with extreme caution with infection (hepatitis B can reactivate), demyelinating disease/optic neuritis, heart failure, bone marrow abnormalities, or concurrent use of biologic agents.

○ **Golimumab**
- **Dosage:** It is given 50 mg SC qmonthly. Methotrexate is used as an adjunct for RA and DMARDs are optional for psoriatic arthritis, ankylosing spondylitis.
- **Mechanism:** It is a human anti-TNF mAb leading to TNF-α inhibition.
- **Onset of action:** <8 weeks
- **Side effects:** Injection site reactions, headache, nausea, infections (including TB), lymphoma, rash, ANA positivity, drug-induced lupus may occur.
- **Contraindications/precautions:** There is a **boxed warning** for infection, malignancy, and TB. Use only with extreme caution with infection (hepatitis B can reactivate), demyelinating disease/optic neuritis, heart failure, bone marrow abnormalities, or concurrent use of biologic agents.

- **B cell modulating agents**
○ **Rituximab**
- **Dosage:** Infuse 1 g IV at 0 and 2 weeks, then again q6 to 12 months. Redosing usually occurs when the patient relapses, though some studies suggest a preset q6-month regimen may work better. Monitoring B cell levels in blood is not useful.
- **Mechanism:** It is a chimeric CD20 mAb leading to peripheral B cell depletion.
- **Onset of action:** Unknown.
- **Side effects:** Headache, fever, infusion reactions, rash, nausea, abdominal pain, bone marrow suppression (especially in RA patients), weakness, infection, and cough may all occur. There are rare but well-documented reports of JC virus reactivation leading to progressive multifocal leukoencephalopathy (PML).
- **Contraindications/precautions:** There is a **boxed warning** for infusion reactions, mucocutaneous reactions, and PML. Use only with extreme caution with infection (hepatitis B can reactivate) and history of cardiovascular disease. Bowel obstruction and perforation have also been reported. **No live vaccines should be administered.**

- ○ **Belimumab**
  - ▪ **Dosage:** Start with 10 mg/kg IV q2 weeks for the first 3 doses, then q4 weeks afterward.
  - ▪ **Mechanism:** This is a human IgG1λ monoclonal antibody to human B lymphocyte stimulator (BLyS). BLyS is a major survival signal for B cells, and BLyS blockade attenuates B cell survival.
  - ▪ **Onset of action:** Unknown.
  - ▪ **Side effects:** Infection, chest pain/shortness of breath, depression, anxiety, suicide, infusion reactions, abdominal pain, nausea/vomiting, diarrhea, migraine headache, nasopharyngitis, bronchitis, leukopenia may occur.
  - ▪ **Contraindications/precautions:** Do not redose if the patient has had a prior anaphylactic reaction. **FDA pregnancy category: C. Live vaccines should not be administered 30 days prior or concurrently** with belimumab.
  - ▪ **Monitoring:** Guidelines for monitoring this new therapy had not yet been established at the time of publication.
- • **T cell modulating agents**
  - ○ **Abetacept**
    - ▪ **Dosage:** The dose of this IV medication is weight dependent: <60 kg: 500 mg; 60 to 100 kg: 750 mg; >100 kg: 1000 mg. Administer it at 0, 2, and 4 weeks, then q4 weeks.
    - ▪ **Mechanism:** It is a fusion protein composed of Fc fragment and extracellular domain of CTLA-4. It prevents T cell costimulation and activation.
    - ▪ **Onset of action:** 3 to 6 months
    - ▪ **Side effects:** Headache, nausea, infection, hypertension, and exacerbations of COPD may occur.
    - ▪ **Contraindications/precautions:** Caution with malignancy, infections, COPD, and concurrent use of biologics.
- • **Interleukin (IL)-1 blockade**
  - ○ **Anakinra**
    - ▪ **Dosage:** Dispense as 100 mg SC qday.
    - ▪ **Mechanism:** It is a recombinant IL-1 receptor antagonist, leading to IL-1 inhibition.
    - ▪ **Onset of action:** <1 week
    - ▪ **Side effects:** Headache, infusion site reactions, infection, nausea, vomiting, diarrhea, abdominal pain, neutropenia, and flu-like syndrome may occur.
    - ▪ **Contraindications/precautions:** Caution with renal impairment, malignancy, infections, asthma, bone marrow suppression, and concurrent use of other biologics.
- • **Interleukin (IL)-6 blockade**
  - ○ **Tocilizumab**
    - ▪ **Dosage:** Start with 4 mg/kg q4 weeks. The dose can increase to 8 mg/kg, up to 800 mg/infusion.
    - ▪ **Mechanism:** It is a humanized IL-6 receptor mAb, leading to IL-6 inhibition.
    - ▪ **Onset of action:** <2 weeks.
    - ▪ **Side effects:** Headache, infusion reactions, infection, nausea, vomiting, diarrhea, abdominal pain, hepatotoxicity, rash, hypertriglyceridemia, and **GI perforation** (especially with concurrent NSAID use) may occur.

- **Contraindications/precautions:** There is a **boxed warning** for infections, including TB. Avoid use in patients taking NSAIDs, or with a history of diverticulosis or peptic ulcer disease, active hepatic disease, or hepatic impairment. Patients should be monitored for bone marrow suppression and demyelinating disease. Avoid concurrent use with other biologics.
- **Monitoring:** CBC, CMP, and lipid panel should be checked at baseline and q4 to 8 weeks (lipid panel can be checked q6 months following initiation).
  - □ If transaminases >1–3× ULN, reduce dose to 4 mg/kg or hold therapy until they normalize. If transaminases >3–5× ULN, discontinue until they are <3× ULN, then resume at 4 mg/kg. If increases persistent, permanently discontinue therapy. If transaminases >5× ULN, discontinue therapy.
  - □ If absolute neutrophil count (ANC) 500–1000 cells/mm^3, hold therapy until ANC >1000 cell/mm^3 and restart at 4 mg/kg. If ANC <500 cells/mm^3, discontinue therapy.
  - □ If platelets 50,000–100,000 cells/mm^3, hold therapy until platelets >100,000 cell/mm^3 and restart at 4 mg/kg. If platelets <50,000 cells/mm^3, discontinue therapy.

GOUT MEDICATIONS

- Understanding which medications should be used during **flares** versus **maintenance periods** is the key to treating gout (see Chapter 13, Gout).
- In general, drugs used for acute flares possess antiinflammatory activity, while maintenance drugs work on reducing uric acid levels either by reducing uric acid synthesis (xanthine oxidase inhibitors) or increasing uric acid excretion (uricosuric agents).
- Medications
  - ○ **Glucocorticoids** (see Glucocorticoids above)
  - ○ **NSAIDs/COX-II inhibitors** (see NSAIDs/COX-II inhibitors above)
    - **Avoid use of aspirin** due to the paradoxical effect of salicylates on serum urate (uric acid retention at low doses and uricosuria at high doses).
  - ○ **Colchicine**
    - **Dosage:** Flare treatment—start with 1.2 mg PO, followed by 0.6 mg PO 1 hour later. Then 0.6 mg PO bid for the next one or two days, followed by several days of 0.6 mg PO qday. Prophylaxis—0.6 mg PO qday or bid.
    - **Mechanism:** Colchicine inhibits β-tubulin polymerization into microtubules, preventing activation, degranulation, and migration of neutrophils. It may also interfere with assembly of the inflammasome.
    - **Side effects:** Abdominal pain, nausea, vomiting, diarrhea, pharyngolaryngeal pain, hepatotoxicity, bone marrow suppression, myotoxicity (including rhabdomyolysis) may occur, and are generally dose-related.
    - **Contraindications/precautions:** Avoid use when concurrently administered with strong CYO3A4 inhibitors or P-glycoprotein in presence of hepatic or renal impairment. Use caution with renal and liver impairment, bone marrow dysfunction, use of protease inhibitors, cyclosporine, diltiazem, verapamil, fibrates, and statins.
  - ○ **Anakinra** (off-label use; see also under Biologics: IL-1 blockade above)
    - **Dosage:** 100 mg SC qday for 3 days.

○ **Allopurinol**
  - **Dosage:** The range is 200 to 800 mg PO qday, and dose is adjusted to maintain serum uric acid <6 mg/dL. Doses >300 mg should be divided into two doses. **Do not begin therapy during acute gouty flares. If a flare occurs in a patient already taking allopurinol, continue allopurinol.**
  - **Mechanism:** It inhibits xanthine oxidase, thereby reducing uric acid production.
  - **Side effects:** Rash may occur, and may be associated with life-threatening complications of **toxic epidermal necrolysis and allopurinol hypersensitivity syndrome** (AHS) which presents as rash, fever, hepatitis, eosinophilia, and acute renal failure. Gout flare, diarrhea, nausea, hepatotoxicity, rare bone marrow suppression may also occur.
  - **Contraindications/precautions:** Use with caution with renal and liver impairment, bone marrow dysfunction, use of angiotensin converting enzyme (ACE) inhibitors or diuretics (due to increased risk of hypersensitivity), amoxicillin or ampicillin (due to rash risk), or azathioprine or mercaptopurine.
○ **Febuxostat**
  - **Dosage:** The range is 40 to 80 mg PO qday. **Do not begin therapy during acute gouty flares. If a flare occurs in a patient already taking febuxostat, continue febuxostat.**
  - **Mechanism:** It inhibits xanthine oxidase, thereby reducing uric acid production. Unlike allopurinol, it is not a purine base analogue.
  - **Side effects:** Hepatotoxicity, nausea, arthralgia, gout flare, and rash may occur.
  - **Contraindications/precautions:** Use with caution with severe renal and liver impairment, cardiovascular disease, or azathioprine or mercaptopurine.
  - **Monitoring:** Obtain CMP at baseline, 2 and 4 months after initiation.
○ **Probenecid**
  - **Dosage:** Start at 250 mg PO bid for 1 week, then either 250 to 500 mg/day or 500 mg/month up to a maximum dose of 2 to 3 grams/day. **Do not begin therapy during acute gouty flares. If a flare occurs in a patient already taking probenecid, continue probenecid.**
  - **Mechanism:** This is a uricosuric drug, which competitively inhibits reabsorption of uric acid at the proximal convoluted tubule.
  - **Side effects:** Rash, gout flare, GI intolerance, and uric acid stone formation may occur.
  - **Contraindications/precautions:** Use with caution with renal impairment, peptic ulcer disease, and concurrent use of penicillins and salicylates.

OSTEOPOROSIS MEDICATIONS

- Virtually all patients with rheumatic diseases are at risk for osteoporosis, especially those on long-term glucocorticoid therapy.
- Treatment options include calcium and vitamin D supplementation, bisphosphonates, calcitonin, hormone replacement therapy, parathyroid hormone (PTH) supplementation, and receptor activator of nuclear factor kappa-B ligand (RANKL) inhibition (see Chapter 48, Osteoporosis).

- **Vitamin supplementation**
  - ○ **Calcium carbonate**
    - ▪ **Dosage:** 1000 to 1200 mg PO qday (elemental calcium). This should be taken with food to improve absorption.
    - ▪ **Mechanism:** Supplementation of nutritional element.
    - ▪ **Side effects:** Abdominal pain, nausea, vomiting, diarrhea or constipation, flatulence, hypophosphatemia, hypercalcemia, milk–alkali syndrome, renal failure may occur.
    - ▪ **Contraindications/precautions:** Avoid use in hypoparathyroid patients and those with a history of calcium-containing renal stones.
    - ▪ **Special considerations:** For those on a proton pump inhibitor (PPI) or an H2 blocker for gastroesophageal reflux disease (GERD), use of **calcium citrate** is recommended.
  - ○ **Vitamin D** (D3 = cholecalciferol, D2 = ergocalciferol)
    - ▪ **Dosage:** Cholecalciferol: 800 to 1000 IU/day. Ergocalciferol: 800 to 1000 IU po qday, unless 25(OH) vitamin D levels are low, where doses range from 50,000 IU qweek to qmonth.
    - ▪ **Mechanism:** Supplementation.
    - ▪ **Side effects:** Hypercalcemia, hypercalciuria, and nephrolithiasis may occur.
    - ▪ **Contraindications/precautions:** Use with caution in those with hypercalcemia, sarcoid or malabsorption syndrome.
    - ▪ **Special considerations:** Some data suggests that cholecalciferol increases 25(OH) vitamin D levels more effectively than ergocalciferol. Calcitriol (1,25-dihydroxycholecalciferol) also increases 25(OH) vitamin D levels but frequently causes hypercalcemia and/or hypercalciuria, and its use is not recommended.
  - ○ In November of 2010, the Institute of Medicine has recommended lower daily dietary intake of both calcium (800–1000 mg/day) and vitamin D (400 IU/day). The impact of this on patients with rheumatic diseases is unclear, and updated recommendations for this patient population are pending.
- **Bisphosphonates**
  - ○ **General principles**
    - ▪ **Mechanism:** These drugs inhibit bone resorption by their actions on osteoclasts and osteoclast precursors.
    - ▪ All bisphosphonates should be given on an empty stomach, since absorption of drug is <1% of dose. Patients are advised to remain upright for 30 minutes to minimize risk of reflux.
    - ▪ Caution is advised with patients experiencing upper GI disease or esophagitis, and chronic kidney disease. If creatinine clearance <30 to 35 mL/minute, avoid use.
    - ▪ All patients should limit treatment to 3 to 5 years maximum to reduce risk of **atypical fractures of the femur.**
    - ▪ Oral formulations
      - □ **Class side effects:** Hypocalcemia, hypophosphatemia, headache, GERD, abdominal pain, nausea, diarrhea/constipation, myalgias, and arthralgias.
      - □ **Contraindications/precautions:** Avoid use in those with stage 3 or greater chronic kidney disease, hypocalcemia, esophageal abnormalities which would delay esophageal emptying, and those who cannot remain upright for at least 30 minutes after administration. Use caution in those

who experience musculoskeletal pain, GI irritation, or have had recent oral surgery (risk of osteonecrosis of the jaw).

- □ **Alendronate**
  - **Dosage:** 10 mg PO qday or 70 mg PO qweek. For prophylaxis, 5 mg PO qday or 35 mg PO qweek.
- □ **Risedronate**
  - **Dosage:** 5 mg PO qday, 35 mg PO qweek, or 150 mg PO qmonth.
- □ **Ibandronate**
  - **Dosage:** 2.5 mg PO qday or 150 mg PO qmonth. Also IV formulation (see below).

- ■ IV formulations
  - □ **Class side effects:** A self-limited flu-like reaction lasting 3 to 4 days is common after infusion. Bone pain, edema, hypertension, fatigue, fever, headache, hypocalcemia, renal failure, dyspnea, GERD, abdominal pain, diarrhea/constipation, nausea, myalgias, and arthralgias may occur.
  - □ **Contraindications/precautions:** Avoid use in those with stage 3 or greater chronic kidney disease or hypocalcemia. Use caution in those who experience musculoskeletal pain, GI irritation, and recent oral surgery (risk of osteonecrosis of the jaw). Patients with aspirin-sensitive asthma may develop bronchospasm from taking zoledronic acid.
  - □ **Ibandronate**
    - **Dosage:** 3 mg IV q3 months.
  - □ **Zoledronic acid**
    - **Dosage:** 5 mg IV qyear.
- • Selective estrogen receptor modulators (SERMs)
  - ○ Raloxifene
    - ■ **Dosage:** 60 mg PO qday.
    - ■ **Mechanism:** It binds to estrogen receptors, exhibiting both agonist and antagonist properties, inhibiting bone resorption. It also reduces total and LDL cholesterol (but not the risk of CAD), and reduces risk of breast cancer.
    - ■ **Side effects:** Hot flushes, flu-like syndrome, infections, leg cramps, arthralgias, edema, **venous thromboembolic disease,** and fatal stroke may occur.
    - ■ **Contraindications/precautions:** There is a **boxed warning** for stroke risk and thromboembolic disease. Use with caution in those who have renal or liver impairment, hypertriglyceridemia, concurrent estrogen therapy, and unexplained uterine bleeding.
- • **Estrogen hormone therapy**
  - ○ **Estrogen–progestin**
    - ■ **Dosage:** 0.35 to 0.45 mg conjugated estrogen with 1.5 mg medroxyprogesterone PO qday.
    - ■ **Mechanism:** It inhibits bone resorption through poorly understood mechanisms.
    - ■ **Side effects:** Data from Women's Health Initiative demonstrated increased risk of breast cancer, stroke, venous thromboembolism, biliary tract disease, shorter survival if prior diagnosis of non-small cell lung carcinoma, and perhaps coronary artery disease. Headache, generalized pain, and GI upset also occur.
    - ■ **Contraindications/precautions:** There is a **boxed warning** for risk of invasive breast cancer, dementia, endometrial carcinoma, and cardiovascular

disease. Use with caution in those who have unexplained vaginal bleeding, biliary disease, and SLE. **Because of these concerns, estrogen–progestin is no longer first line therapy.**

- **Parathyroid hormone therapy**
  - ○ **Teriparatide**
    - ▪ **Dosage:** 20 mcg SC qday.
    - ▪ **Mechanism:** This is an "anabolic" agent, which stimulates bone growth and activates bone remodeling. It stimulates preosteoblasts to mature into osteoblasts.
    - ▪ **Side effects:** Hypercalcemia, hypercalcuria, hypotension, tachycardia, muscle cramps, hyperuricemia may occur, and there is a theoretical risk of osteosarcoma.
    - ▪ **Contraindications/precautions:** There is a **boxed warning** for **osteosarcoma risk.** Use with caution in those who have renal or liver impairment, coronary artery disease, and urolithiasis. Limit use to 2 years.
- **RANKL therapy**
  - ○ **Denosumab**
    - ▪ **Dosage:** 60 mg SC q6 months.
    - ▪ **Mechanism:** This is a humanized mAb to RANK which reduces osteoclastogenesis, leading to decreased bone resorption.
    - ▪ **Side effects:** Musculoskeletal pain, dermatitis, eczema, hypercholesterolemia, cystitis, infections, and hypocalcemia may occur.
    - ▪ **Contraindications/precautions:** Do not use in hypocalcemic patients. Use with caution in those with renal impairment.
- **Other therapies**
  - ○ **Calcitonin**
    - ▪ **Dosage:** 200 IU intranasally (one nostril) qday, or 100 IU SC qother day.
    - ▪ **Mechanism:** It binds to osteoclasts and inhibits bone resorption.
    - ▪ **Side effects:** Rhinitis, flushing, nausea, and musculoskeletal pain are fairly common. Nasal mucosal erosion may develop with intranasal administration, particularly in those >65 years old.
    - ▪ **Contraindications/precautions:** Temporarily discontinue if nasal ulcers develops.

REFERENCES

1. Schimmer BP, Parker KL. Adrenocorticotropic hormone; adrenocortical steroids and their synthetic analogs; inhibitors of the synthesis and actions of adrenocortical hormones. In: Brunton LL, Lazo J, Parker K, eds. *The Pharmacological Basis of Therapeutics.* Vol. 11. New York, NY: McGraw Hill; 2005.
2. Buttgereit F, Burmester G-R. Glucocorticoids. In: Klippel JH, Stone JH, Crofford LJ, White PH, eds. *Primer on the Rheumatic Diseases.* New York, NY: Springer Science+Business Media; 2008:644–650.

Rheumatoid Arthritis

Richa Gupta and Prabha Ranganathan

GENERAL PRINCIPLES

Definition

- Rheumatoid arthritis (RA) is **inflammatory symmetric polyarthritis** which untreated can lead to erosions, joint space loss, and destruction of the affected joints.
- RA causes significant morbidity and increased mortality.
- On rare occasions, RA is self-limited but more often is chronic, disabling, and sometimes associated with **systemic manifestations.**

Epidemiology

- RA affects approximately 1% of the population worldwide.
- RA increases in incidence with age. Women are affected approximately three times more often than men. However, after the age of 60, RA affects both genders equally.
- Genetic studies have demonstrated that certain shared epitopes, a group of related epitopes in the DR4 and DR1 alleles of the class II major histocompatibility (MHC) region, increase susceptibility to RA.

Pathophysiology

- Although the etiology of RA is still unknown, there have been major strides in understanding how the inflammatory process leads to joint destruction.
- Evidence supports initial T-cell activation triggered by an unknown antigen, leading to joint inflammation and destruction.
- RA is characterized by **synovial inflammation** with hyperplasia and increased vascularity (**pannus formation**). The synovium shows leukocytic infiltration, increased expression of adhesion molecules, proteolytic enzymes and cytokines including tumor necrosis factor (TNF)-α, and interleukins (IL)-1, 6, and 17. These cytokines provide potential targets for blockade and therapy.
- B lymphocytes act as antigen-presenting cells in the synovium. They also produce antibodies, and secrete pro-inflammatory cytokines. B-cell depletion therapy has been shown to be beneficial in patients with RA.
- The synovial membrane enlarges to become the pannus and begins to invade the cartilage and bone. Finally, proliferation of the pannus leads to more profound cartilage destruction, subchondral bone erosions, and periarticular ligament laxity. Cytokine-stimulated osteoclast activity also contributes to **erosions and periarticular osteoporosis** found in RA.
- Various citrullinated proteins are present in the rheumatoid joint, including fibrinogen, collagen, and fibronectin, and have recently been implicated in the pathophysiology of RA. The process of citrullination involves conversion of

arginine to citrulline by the enzyme peptidylarginine deiminases (PADIs). Of the four isoforms, PADI 2 and PADI 4 are most abundant in the inflamed synovium. In RA, increased citrullination occurs in the inflamed synovium, and antibodies directed against these citrullinated proteins (**anti-cyclic citrullinated peptide [anti-CCP] antibodies**) are produced by resident B cells.

DIAGNOSIS

Clinical Presentation

History

- The presentation and course of RA is variable. Typically, patients present with an insidious onset of **symmetric joint pain, swelling, and morning stiffness** worsening over several weeks. Less common presentations include acute, rapidly progressive polyarthritis and, more rarely, monoarthritis.
- RA commonly involves the **small joints of the hands** (wrists, metacarpophalangeal [MCP] joints, and proximal interphalangeal [PIP] joints) **and feet** (metatarsophalangeal [MTP] joints) (Fig. 10-1). Large joints can also be involved and include the shoulder, knee, ankle, elbow, and hip.
- The severity and duration of morning stiffness often correlate with the overall disease activity.
- Generalized malaise and fatigue can often accompany active inflammation.
- Through the course of RA, patients often experience a waxing and waning pattern of synovitis coupled with progressive structural damage, leading to significant deformities and disabilities with advanced disease. Extensive joint damage can lead to functional limitations in joints as well as neurologic compromise, leading to symptoms of muscle weakness and atrophy.
- Most of the articular destruction occurs in the early years of disease. Hence, it is **important to diagnose and treat RA early.**

Physical Examination

- Physical findings in RA involve the identification of symmetric joint inflammation early in the course of the disease, and manifestations of joint destruction with chronic disease.
- Active **synovitis** is characterized by warmth, swelling, pain, and palpable effusions. **Synovial proliferation** is appreciated on physical examination by the presence of soft or rubbery tissue around the joint margins. **Joint warmth** is frequently appreciated, although redness is uncommon.
- **Range of motion** can be restricted in joints with significant effusions, including deeper joints that may not demonstrate other signs of inflammation. Chronic joint destruction with significant degree of cartilage loss produces **crepitus** on palpation. Specific joint manifestations follow:
  - The **wrists** are involved in most patients and, over time, can lead to radial-ulnar subluxation and subluxation of carpal bones with radial deviation. Synovitis at the wrist can lead to **median nerve entrapment,** resulting in carpal tunnel syndrome (CTS) or, more rarely, **ulnar nerve entrapment,** resulting in Guyon's canal syndrome.
  - In the **hands,** the MCPs are commonly involved and, with extensive damage, may lead to **ulnar deviation** of the hand. The PIP joints are often involved with **sparing of** distal interphalangeal **(DIP) joints.** Chronic inflammation

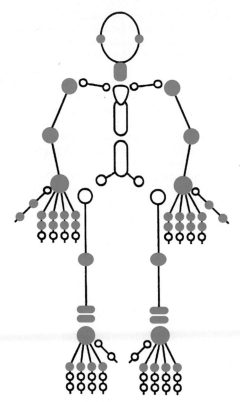

FIGURE 10-1. Distribution of rheumatoid arthritis.

with destruction of surrounding tendons can lead to **Z-shaped thumb** (hyperextension of first interphalangeal joint with palmar subluxation of first MCP), **swan-neck** (hyperextension at PIP, flexion at DIP), and **boutonniere** (flexion at PIP, hyperextension of DIP) deformities. Tenosynovitis of finger tendon sheaths can lead to nodule formation with subsequent catching or tendon rupture.

○ **Elbow** involvement is evident by fullness at the radial-humeral joint with the tendency of patients to maintain the joint in flexion. Over time, this can lead to flexion contractures. In addition, inflammation can lead to **compressive neuropathy of the ulnar nerve** with paresthesias and weakness in the ulnar distribution.

○ Involvement of the **shoulder** usually manifests as loss of range of motion, with decreased abduction and limited rotation. Effusions are difficult to appreciate, because the shoulder joint lies underneath the rotator cuff. Pain in the shoulder can lead to limited range of motion, and adhesive capsulitis, or frozen shoulder, can develop rapidly.

○ **Cervical spine** involvement with RA is common. Inflammation with involvement of the odontoid process, lateral masses, or tenosynovitis of the transverse ligament can lead to **C1–C2 cervical instability.** This may manifest with neck stiffness with decreased range of motion. Compression of cord, nerve roots, or vertebral arteries can occur, leading to neurologic compromise, and may require emergent stabilization. RA involvement of the thoracic and the lumbar spine is rare.

○ **Hip** involvement with RA is also common, but symptoms are often delayed. When present, examination findings include decreased range of motion and pain radiating to the groin, thigh, buttock, low back, or knee.

○ Involvement of the **knee** includes detectable effusions and synovial thickening. Prolonged inflammation can lead to significant instability. Posterior herniation of the synovial capsule can result in a **popliteal (Baker's) cyst,** and rupture can mimic thrombophlebitis.

○ Because of weight-bearing, RA involvement of the **foot and ankle** is often symptomatic. The joints most commonly affected include the MTP, talonavicular, and ankle joints. MTP joints can develop cocking-up deformities with subluxation of the MTP fat pads, causing pain with ambulation. Inflammation of the talonavicular joint and ankle joints results in eversion of the foot and can cause nerve entrapment, resulting in paresthesias of the sole.

○ With the discovery of more effective treatments, extra-articular manifestations of RA occur much less commonly than they did in previous decades. However, severe RA can manifest with sequelae of systemic inflammation, especially in rheumatoid factor (RF)-positive patients. Common extra-articular manifestations follow:

■ **Skin** manifestations include formation of subcutaneous **rheumatoid nodules and vasculitic skin ulcerations.** Rheumatoid nodules typically form during active inflammation over pressure points in bursae and tendon sheaths. Common sites include the olecranon bursa, the extensor surface of the forearm, the Achilles tendon, and the tendons of the fingers.

■ **Ocular** involvement usually involves **sicca symptoms** of dry eyes (and dry mouth in Sjögren's syndrome) but can include **episcleritis** or a more concerning **scleritis** and scleromalacia perforans.

■ **Pulmonary** involvement of RA may include interstitial fibrosis, pulmonary nodules, pleuritis, or bronchiolitis obliterans organizing pneumonia. Interstitial fibrosis generally involves the lower lung fields and is often not clinically symptomatic, but it may be severely debilitating in some cases.

■ **Neurologic** manifestations of RA are usually related to nerve entrapment or cervical spine instability. Vasculitis of vasa vasorum can lead to symptoms of **mononeuritis multiplex.**

■ **Cardiac** involvement may include pericardial effusions, pericarditis, valvular lesions, conduction defects, or cardiomyopathy

■ **Gastrointestinal (GI)** and **renal** manifestations of RA are rare. Amyloidosis can sometimes occur, affecting these organs.

■ Hepatic involvement may include nodular regenerative hyperplasia or portal fibrosis.

■ Hematologic effects of RA include hypochromic-microcytic anemia, **Felty's syndrome** (the triad of leukopenia, lymphadenopathy, and splenomegaly), cryoglobulinemia, and the large granular lymphocyte syndrome.

TABLE 10-1	AMERICAN COLLEGE OF RHEUMATOLOGY CRITERIA FOR THE DIAGNOSIS OF RHEUMATOID ARTHRITIS

1. Morning stiffness. Patients typically have morning stiffness lasting for >1 hour
2. Swelling of ≥3 joints (observed by a physician)
3. Symmetric distribution
4. Involvement of the hand joints, especially the wrist, MCPs, and PIPs, sparing the DIPs
5. Positive RF (found in 80% of patients with RA)
6. Rheumatoid nodules on extensor tendon surfaces, especially the olecranon
7. Radiographic changes (periarticular osteopenia and erosions)

Note: For the diagnosis of RA, a patient should have at least four of the seven criteria. Criteria 1–4 must be present for ≥6 weeks.

MCP, metacarpophalangeal; PIP, proximal interphalangeal; DIP, distal interphalangeal; RF, rheumatoid factor; RA, rheumatoid arthritis.

Diagnostic Criteria

- The diagnosis of RA involves the accumulation of clinical, lab, and radiologic features that develop over the course of the disease. Early RA is often difficult to diagnose definitively, yet it can usually be confirmed as the disease progresses. The American College of Rheumatology (ACR) has provided criteria for the diagnosis of RA (Table 10-1).[1]
  - These criteria were designed for inclusion and monitoring of patients in clinical studies and not for routine clinical diagnosis. However, they can serve as diagnostic guidelines for evaluation of patients with suspected RA.
  - They have 91% to 94% sensitivity and 89% specificity for established RA; the sensitivity of these criteria to diagnose early RA decreases to 40% to 60% with a specificity of 80% to 90%.
  - In practice, a patient with symmetric, inflammatory polyarthritis of the small joints of the hands with positive serologies (RF and anti-CCP antibody described below) most likely has RA.
- The ACR has created a new revised classification criteria for RA, in collaboration with the European League Against Rheumatism (EULAR).[2]
  - This new classification system redefines the preexisting criteria for diagnosis of RA by focusing on features at earlier stages of disease that are associated with persistent and/or erosive disease, rather than defining the disease by its late-stage features.
  - This will focus attention on **the important need for early diagnosis and treatment to prevent or minimize the occurrence of undesirable sequelae** (Table 10-2).[2]

Differential Diagnosis

- The other common causes of **symmetric inflammatory polyarthritis** are systemic connective tissue disorders such as SLE, psoriatic arthritis, and viral (parvovirus B19 and hepatitis B and C associated) arthritis.
- Other causes of **inflammatory arthritis that are less symmetric** and typically oligo- or monoarticular include gout, pseudogout, septic arthritis, HLA-B27 associated spondyloarthropathies, and adult-onset Still's disease.
- Conditions with **noninflammatory polyarthralgias** should not be confused with RA, such as fibromyalgia, osteoarthritis, malignancy, hypo- or hyperthyroidism, or hyperparathyroidism.

TABLE 10-2	THE 2010 AMERICAN COLLEGE OF RHEUMATOLOGY/ EUROPEAN LEAGUE AGAINST RHEUMATISM CLASSIFICATION CRITERIA FOR RHEUMATOID ARTHRITIS

Score

Target population (Who should be tested?): Patients who
1. Have at least 1 joint with definite clinical synovitis (swelling)[a]
2. With the synovitis not better explained by another disease[b]

Classification criteria for RA (score-based algorithm: Add score of categories A–D; a score of ≥6/10 is needed for classification of a patient as having definite RA)[c]

	Score
A. Joint involvement[d]	
1 large joint[e]	0
2–10 large joints	1
1–3 small joints (with or without involvement of large joints)[f]	2
4–10 small joints (with or without involvement of large joints)	3
>10 joints (at least 1 small joint)[g]	5
B. Serology (at least 1 test result is needed for classification)[h]	
Negative RF and negative anti-CCP antibody	0
Low-positive RF or low-positive anti-CCP antibody	2
High-positive RF or high-positive anti-CCP antibody	3
C. Acute-phase reactants (at least 1 test result is needed for classification)[i]	
Normal CRP and normal ESR	0
Abnormal CRP or abnormal ESR	1
D. Duration of symptoms[j]	
<6 weeks	0
≥6 weeks	1

[a]The criteria are aimed at classification of newly presenting patients. In addition, patients with erosive disease typical of rheumatoid arthritis (RA) with a history compatible with prior fulfillment of the 2010 criteria should be classified as having RA. Patients with long-standing disease, including those whose disease is inactive (with or without treatment) who, based on retrospectively available data, have previously fulfilled the 2010 criteria should be classified as having RA.

[b]Differential diagnoses vary among patients with different presentations, but may include conditions such as systemic lupus erythematosus, psoriatic arthritis and gout. If it is unclear about the relevant differential diagnoses to consider, an expert rheumatologist should be consulted.

[c]Although patients with a score of <6/10 are not classifiable as having RA, their status can be reassessed and the criteria might be fulfilled cumulatively over time.

[d]Joint involvement refers to any swollen or tender joint on examination, which may be confirmed by imaging evidence of synovitis. DIP joints, first carpometacarpal joints, and first MTP joints are excluded from assessment. Categories of joint distribution are classified according to the location and number of involved joints, with placement into the highest category possible based on the pattern of joint involvement.

[e]"Large joints" refer to shoulders, elbow, hips, knees, and ankles.

[f]"Small joints" refer to the MCP joints, proximal interphalangeal joints, second through fifth MTP joints, thumb interphalangeal joints, and wrist.

(continued)

TABLE 10-2	THE 2010 AMERICAN COLLEGE OF RHEUMATOLOGY/ EUROPEAN LEAGUE AGAINST RHEUMATISM CLASSIFICATION CRITERIA FOR RHEUMATOID ARTHRITIS (*Continued*)

[g]In this category, at least one of the involved joints must be a small joint; the other joints can include any combination of large and additional small joints, as well as other joints not specifically listed elsewhere (e.g., temporomandibular, acromioclavicular, sternoclavicular, etc.).

[h]Negative refers to IU levels that are less than or equal to the ULN for the laboratory and assay; low positive refers to IU values that are >3 times the ULN for the laboratory and assay. Where RF information is only available as positive or negative, a positive result should be scored as low positive for RF.

[i]Normal and abnormal values are determined by local laboratory standards.

[j]Duration of symptoms refer to patient self-report of the duration of signs or symptoms of synovitis (e.g., pain, swelling, tenderness) of joints that are clinically involved at the time of assessment, regardless of treatment status.

RA, rheumatoid arthritis; RF, rheumatoid factor; CCP, cyclic citrullinated protein; CRP, C-reactive protein; ESR, erythrocyte sedimentation rate; ULN, upper limit of normal; MTP, metatarsophalangeal; DIP, distal interphalangeal; MCP, metacarpophalangeal.

From: Aletaha D, Neogi T, Silman A, et al. Rheumatoid Arthritis Classification Criteria: An American College of Rheumatology/European League Against Rheumatism Collaborative Initiative. *Arthritis Rheum.* 2010;62:2569–2581, with permission.

- **Palindromic rheumatism** is a condition similar to RA in which patients develop recurrent onset of acute, self-limited arthritis.
  - Attacks usually last hours to a few days and may involve any set of joints.
  - Laboratory tests are nonspecific, and synovial fluid analysis reveals an inflammatory reaction.
  - Joint damage and systemic manifestations are rare.
  - Diagnosis is based on the presence of a relapsing and remitting course of arthritis.
  - **Many patients with palindromic rheumatism later progress to develop RA.**
  - Treatment is similar to that for RA. Nonsteroidal anti-inflammatory drugs (NSAIDs) may provide pain relief. Corticosteroids and some disease-modifying anti-rheumatic drugs (DMARDs) may also be beneficial.
- **Relapsing seronegative symmetrical synovitis with pitting edema (RS3PE)** is a condition usually characterized by the sudden onset of polyarthritis associated with pitting edema of the hands and/or feet.
  - Laboratory markers of inflammation are variable, and RF is absent.
  - Synovitis is commonly present but rarely leads to joint destruction.
  - Treatment involves the use of low-dose corticosteroids (prednisone, 5–10 mg), typically with dramatic improvement of symptoms. NSAIDs and hydroxychloroquine may also provide symptomatic relief and may be useful as steroid-sparing agents.
  - RS3PE **may be related to polymyalgia rheumatica and sometimes occur in association with malignancies.**

Diagnostic Testing

Laboratories

- Laboratory evaluation should include a baseline complete blood count (CBC), electrolyte panel, creatinine, hepatic function panel (HFP), urinalysis (UA), and stool occult blood to assess general organ function and comorbidities before initiating medications.

- Serologic markers for RA, including **RF and anti-CCP** antibodies, should be tested. Anti-CCP antibodies have been found in the serum of affected patient's years before the onset of clinically apparent disease, and are more specific for RA than RF.[3]
- RF should be drawn at baseline and repeated 6 to 12 months later if initially negative, as **approximately 50% of RA patients are positive in the first 6 months of illness and 85% become positive over the first 2 years.** Once RF is positive and the diagnosis of RA is made there is no need to repeat this test.
- **A low-titer RF can be associated with other chronic inflammatory conditions** such as bacterial endocarditis, hepatitis C with cryoglobulinemia, and primary biliary cirrhosis. A high-titer RF usually indicates RA.
- The sensitivity and specificity of RF for the diagnosis of RA are roughly 66% and 82%, respectively
- The sensitivity of anti-CCP antibodies for the diagnosis of RA is 70% but specificity is 95%, superior to RF.
- **Up to 35% of patients with a negative RF at presentation will test positive for anti-CCP antibody.**
- A small number of RA patients (10%–15%) will remain seronegative (RF and CCP antibody negative) throughout the course of the disease.
- 20% to 30% of RA patients have a **positive antinuclear antibody (ANA),** but this is at a low titer. **Erythrocyte sedimentation rate (ESR) and C-reactive protein (CRP)** are markers of inflammation and may be useful to monitor disease activity, although they are not specific for RA.
- The synovial fluid in RA patients is inflammatory. Arthrocentesis is useful to rule out infectious and crystalline arthritis, if these are suspected, particularly if one joint is inflamed out of proportion to the others.

Imaging

- **Radiographs** of involved joints may be uninformative early in disease but can be used to monitor disease progression and treatment responses.
- **MRI and ultrasound** have been proven to be more sensitive methods for detecting early joint erosions; synovitis and tenosynovitis (refer to Chapter 6, Radiographic Imaging of Rheumatic Diseases).
- Of note, plain radiographs of feet are more likely to show erosions with early RA than hands.

TREATMENT

- The goals of treatment of RA are to alleviate pain, control inflammation, preserve and improve activities of daily living, and prevent progressive joint destruction.
- **Early recognition of disease and pharmacologic treatment provide the cornerstones for management of RA** and hence early referral to a rheumatologist is imperative.
- Medical treatment includes the use of NSAIDs, DMARDs, and corticosteroids.
- Equally important in the management of RA is non-pharmacologic treatment, including patient education, physical therapy, occupational therapy, orthotics, and surgery.

Medications

Nonsteroidal Anti-inflammatory Drugs

- The use of **NSAIDs** in high doses can help alleviate symptoms from pain and inflammation in most patients with RA.
- Patients should be closely monitored for toxicities, especially GI ulcerations and renal dysfunction.
- Some patients may benefit from selective cyclooxygenase (COX)-2 inhibitors that have documented reduced GI toxicities or addition of GI prophylaxis in the form of misoprostol or proton pump inhibitors.
- **NSAIDs do not prevent progression of bone and cartilage damage;** therefore, current treatment strategies recommend NSAID use in combination with DMARDs for initial therapy.
- For details on dosing, toxicities, and monitoring of specific agents see Chapter 9, Drugs Used for the Treatment of Rheumatic Diseases.

Glucocorticoids

- Corticosteroids in low doses (e.g., prednisone, 5–10 mg) are extremely effective for promptly reducing the symptoms of RA and are useful in helping patients recover their previous functional status.
- Unfortunately, short courses of oral corticosteroids produce only interim benefit, and chronic therapy is often necessary to maintain symptom management.
- Corticosteroids are appropriate in patients with significant limitations in their activities of daily living, particularly early in the course of disease while awaiting the efficacy of slow-acting DMARDs.
- **Every effort should be made to taper to the lowest possible dose and to eliminate steroid therapy when feasible.**
- Toxicities of corticosteroids are well known and include weight gain, cushingoid features, osteoporosis (for details on treatment and prevention of osteoporosis related to corticosteroids, see Chapter 48, Osteoporosis), avascular necrosis (AVN), infection, diabetes mellitus, hypertension, and increases in serum cholesterol levels. Keeping the daily dose of prednisone at ≤5 mg can often reduce toxicities.
- Corticosteroid doses should be slowly tapered over several months to avoid adrenal insufficiency.

Disease-Modifying Anti-Rheumatic Drugs

- **DMARDs can slow or arrest the progression of RA.** DMARDs should be instituted early (within the first few weeks to 3 months of diagnosis). Evidence indicates that **outcomes are improved for patients treated more aggressively at presentation.** Therefore, initiation of therapy with NSAIDs and DMARDs simultaneously is recommended.
- **Many of the DMARDs have significant potential toxicities and may take several months to attain optimal clinical benefit;** therefore, careful monitoring for side effects and symptom relief is required.
- For severe disease flares, the use of oral corticosteroids may also be necessary while waiting for optimal benefit from DMARDs.
- The choice of an initial DMARD is based on disease severity, and the presence of erosive disease and anti-CCP antibodies; the latter are typically associated with a more aggressive disease course. Following is a list of

commonly used DMARDs with associated toxicities and monitoring recommendations.

- For details on dosing, toxicities, and monitoring of specific agents see Chapter 9, Drugs Used for the Treatment of Rheumatic Diseases.
  - ○ **Oral methotrexate is considered to be the DMARD of choice for most patients,** and is imperative in patients with rapid disease progression or functional limitations.
    - ■ From a starting dose of 7.5 to 10 mg once a week, the dose may be increased to 20 mg weekly rapidly.
    - ■ If methotrexate is at least partially effective, it is continued as background therapy while other agents are added.
    - ■ Common side effects include stomatitis, nausea, diarrhea, and hair loss.
    - ■ Supplementation with folic acid, 1 to 2 mg daily, can reduce such side effects without significantly reducing efficacy.
    - ■ Bone marrow suppression is uncommon, but it may occur at low doses in elderly patients.
    - ■ The risk of liver toxicity is increased by alcohol consumption, preexisting liver disease, and possibly by diabetes and obesity.
    - ■ Important contraindications to methotrexate therapy include liver disease, abnormal liver function tests, and regular alcohol consumption.
    - ■ Liver function tests and blood counts are checked every month until the dose is stable and every 2 to 3 months thereafter.
    - ■ A liver biopsy is performed in patients with persistent elevation of liver transaminases or decrease in serum albumin to rule out methotrexate-induced hepatotoxicity.
    - ■ Methotrexate is to be avoided in patients with serum creatinine of greater than 2.0 mg/dL; as such patients are at higher risk of toxicity because of impaired renal clearance of the drug. Women of childbearing age must use appropriate contraceptive measures because of the teratogenic effects of this drug.
  - ○ **Hydroxychloroquine** is effective in mild to moderate, nonerosive RA, at doses of 200 to 400 mg/day, but not to be used in patients with moderate to severe renal or hepatic insufficiency.
    - ■ Macular toxicity is extremely unusual if the dose does not exceed 6 to 7 mg/kg/day, and it rarely occurs before 6 years of treatment.
    - ■ Nonetheless, an ophthalmologist should perform a baseline examination and monitor the patient every 6 to 12 months.
    - ■ Nausea and skin discoloration occur occasionally.
  - ○ **Sulfasalazine** should be started at 500 mg twice daily and gradually increased to 2 to 3 g daily in divided doses.
    - ■ An enteric-coated preparation improves GI tolerability.
    - ■ Monitoring for neutropenia and hepatotoxicity should be performed every 1 to 3 months.
    - ■ GI intolerance due to nausea or abdominal pain may occur.
    - ■ Sulfasalazine should be avoided in patients with sulfa allergies or glucose-6-phosphate dehydrogenase deficiency.
  - ○ **Leflunomide** is a pyrimidine synthesis inhibitor with efficacy comparable to methotrexate in treatment of RA.
    - ■ Diarrhea, nausea, and hair loss are common side effects. Liver functions need to be monitored every 1 to 3 months.

- The effective starting dose is 20 mg/day which can be reduced to 10 mg/day if the medication is not tolerated or if transaminase levels become elevated.
  - **Cyclosporine** is an inhibitor of T-cell activation with known clinical efficacy in treatment of RA.
    - Efficacy is increased when used in combination with methotrexate.
    - Cost and potential for severe renal toxicity, even in low doses, have limited its use to the treatment of severe, refractory RA.
    - Blood pressure and renal function should be monitored closely.
- Other DMARDs less commonly used to treat RA include gold salts, azathioprine, penicillamine, and cyclophosphamide (for rheumatoid vasculitis).

Biologics

- Biologic therapy should be initiated when adequate disease control is not achieved with the oral DMARDs.
- These include **TNF-α antagonists** and other **non–TNF-α mediated biologic agents.**
- **TNF-α antagonists are the initial biologic therapies used in RA patients who fail oral DMARDs. They are often administered in conjunction with methotrexate therapy,** as there is more effective disease control with combination therapy.[4]
- **Serious infections** have occurred rarely.
  - Hence, TNF-α antagonists are **contraindicated in patients with indolent chronic infections** such as osteomyelitis or tuberculosis (TB), and in anyone with an active infection.
  - **Screening for latent TB** should be performed with a tuberculin skin test before beginning therapy with a TNF antagonist, and patients who test positive for latent TB should be treated with isoniazid before beginning therapy. Also, annual skin testing for latent TB is now recommended during treatment with a TNF-α antagonist.
  - Treatment with TNF-α antagonist should be temporarily suspended in patients undergoing surgery.
- **TNF-α antagonists should be used with extreme caution in patients with congestive heart failure or significant coronary artery disease.**
- Rare side effects include demyelinating disorders and lupus-like syndromes, with positive antibodies such as ANA, with or without other features of SLE.
- There is no consensus at the present time regarding the risk of lymphoma and malignancy with use of these drugs, but if their use is warranted in patients with these conditions, these patients need to be monitored closely.
- **Many patients who do not respond to one TNF-α antagonist may respond to a different agent in the same class.**
- Choices for patients with an inadequate response to three or more TNF-α antagonists include **abatacept,** a T-cell costimulation inhibitor, **rituximab,** an anti-CD20 monoclonal antibody, and **tocilizumab,** a monoclonal antibody to the IL-6 receptor.
- For details on dosing, toxicities, and monitoring of specific agents see Chapter 9, Drugs Used for the Treatment of Rheumatic Diseases.
- The five currently available TNF-α antagonists are etanercept, infliximab, adalimumab, golimumab, and certolizumab. Non–TNF antagonizing biologics include anakinra, rituximab, abatacept, and tocilizumab.

- ○ **Etanercept** is a recombinant DNA-derived protein composed of TNF receptor linked to the Fc portion of human IgG1. Etanercept binds TNF and blocks its interaction with cell surface receptors.
- ○ **Infliximab** is a chimeric human/murine monoclonal antibody to TNF.
- ○ **Adalimumab and golimumab** are fully human monoclonal antibodies to TNF.
- ○ **Certolizumab** pegol is made of Fab antigen-binding domain of a humanized anti-TNF antibody, which is pegylated allowing for delayed elimination and an extended half-life.
- ○ **Anakinra** is an IL-1 receptor antagonist.
- ○ **Rituximab** is a monoclonal antibody directed against the CD20 antigen on B lymphocytes.
- ○ **Abatacept** is a selective costimulation modulator which inhibits T-lymphocyte activation by blocking the interaction between antigen-presenting cells and T cells.
- ○ **Tocilizumab** is an antagonist of IL-6.
- Combination regimens of multiple DMARDs or DMARDs plus biologic agents are increasingly popular treatment regimens. If tolerated, methotrexate should be part of every combination.

Other Non-pharmacologic Therapies

- **Ancillary medical services** can augment treatment strategies for patients with RA at any stage of disease.
- **Occupational therapy** usually focuses on the hand and wrist and can help patients with splinting, work simplification, activities of daily living, and assistive devices.
- **Physical therapy** assists in stretching and strengthening exercises for large joints such as the shoulder and knee, gait evaluation, and fitting with crutches and canes. Moderate exercise is appropriate for all patients and can help reduce stiffness and maintain joint range of motion. In general, an exercise program should not produce pain for >2 hours after its completion.

Surgical Management

- **Orthopedic surgery** to correct hand deformities and replace large joints such as the hip, knee, and shoulder may benefit patients with advanced disease.
- The primary indication for reconstructive hand surgery is refractory functional impairment limiting activities of daily living.
- Total joint arthroplasty to replace the knee or hip should also be considered when pain cannot be controlled adequately with medications or when joint instability causes significant fall risk.

COMPLICATIONS

- RA patients are susceptible to **infections** due to the immunosuppressive medications used for treatment.
- RA patients are at increased risk for **lymphoproliferative disorders, particularly lymphomas.**
- **Cervical instability** at the atlantoaxial articulation is a complication of longstanding, severe RA. Evaluation for cervical instability is particularly important

in the perioperative setting, when extension of the neck for intubation may lead to cord compromise with resultant neurologic impairment. Radiographs of the cervical spine, including lateral flexion and extension views, should be taken.

- Rheumatoid **vasculitis** is usually associated with long-standing, severe, erosive RA. Mononeuritis multiplex and skin ulcers are common manifestations of rheumatoid vasculitis.
- There is emerging data on the inflammatory state in RA being an independent risk factor for **cardiovascular disease.**

FOLLOW-UP

- The course of RA differs between patients. Whereas some patients may experience mild disease and have spontaneous remission, others may suffer a chronic course with intermittent disease flares and progressive joint destruction.
- Patients should be monitored on a frequent basis for disease progression or remission, response to therapy, and drug toxicities.
- Drug therapies should be adjusted to attain the minimal effective doses with an emphasis on **limiting use of chronic steroids.**
- **Mortality rates are increased in RA patients due to cardiovascular disease, other comorbidities include infections, pulmonary and renal disease, and GI bleeding and drug toxicities.**

PROGNOSIS

- The presence of erosions at baseline, and high titers of RF and anti-CCP antibodies predict radiographic progression in RA.
- Female sex, smoking, extra-articular disease, functional limitations, a large number of tender and swollen joints, elevated ESR or CRP, HLA-DRB1*0401/*0404 positivity are other poor prognostic factors.

REFERENCES

1. Arnett FC, Edworthy SM, Bloch DA, et al. The American Rheumatism Association 1987 revised criteria for the classification of rheumatoid arthritis. *Arthritis Rheum.* 1988;31:315–324.
2. Aletaha D, Neogi T, Silman A, et al. 2010 Rheumatoid Arthritis Classification Criteria. An American College of Rheumatology/European League against Rheumatism Collaborative Initiative. *Arthritis Rheum.* 2010;62:2569–2581.
3. Nishimura K, Sugiyama D, Kogata Y, et al. Meta-analysis: diagnostic accuracy of anti-cyclic citrullinated peptide antibody and rheumatoid factor for rheumatoid arthritis. *Ann Intern Med.* 2007;146:797–808.
4. Goekoop-Ruiterman YPM, de Vries-Bouwstra JK, Allaart CF, et al. Comparison of treatment strategies in early rheumatoid arthritis: a randomized trial. *Ann Intern Med.* 2007;146:406–415.

Osteoarthritis

11

Hyon Ju Park and Prabha Ranganathan

GENERAL PRINCIPLES

Definition

Osteoarthritis (OA) has evolved from being considered a natural part of the aging process and noninflammatory to now being known as the result of a complex process involving genetic susceptibilities, mechanical forces, and variable inflammation of the synovium, leading to degradation of the articular cartilage.

Classification

- **Primary or idiopathic:** The **localized form** affects one to two joint groups: distal interphalangeal (DIP), proximal interphalangeal (PIP), or carpometacarpal (CMC) joints of hands; cervical or lumbar spine; first metatarsophalangeal (MTP) joints of feet; knees; and hips (Fig. 11-1). The **generalized form** involves three or more joint groups and is frequently associated with Heberden's nodes (bony enlargements of the DIP joints) or Bouchard's nodes (bony enlargements of the PIP joints).
- **Secondary:** This should be considered if a patient develops OA in atypical joints, such as metacarpophalangeal (MCP) joints, wrists, ankles, shoulders, or elbows. Assessment should be made for previous trauma, metabolic disease, blood dyscrasias, or neuropathic joints.
- **Erosive OA:** Also known as inflammatory OA, it affects the DIP and PIP joints of the hand, with negative rheumatoid factor (RF) and anti-cyclic citrullinated protein (CCP) antibodies.

Epidemiology

- OA is the most common articular disease, affecting more than 20 million people in US alone.
- The prevalence of OA increases with age so that, in men and women aged >60 years, the prevalence is 17% and 29.6%, respectively.

Etiology

Cause is unknown although obesity, heredity, biomechanical injuries or overuse, and age are risk factors.

Pathophysiology

- Chondrocytes are responsible for balancing the anabolic and catabolic processes in the joint.
- Biomechanical stressors cause chondrocytes to trigger matrix metalloproteinases and synthesis of matrix proteins including fibrillar type II collagen.

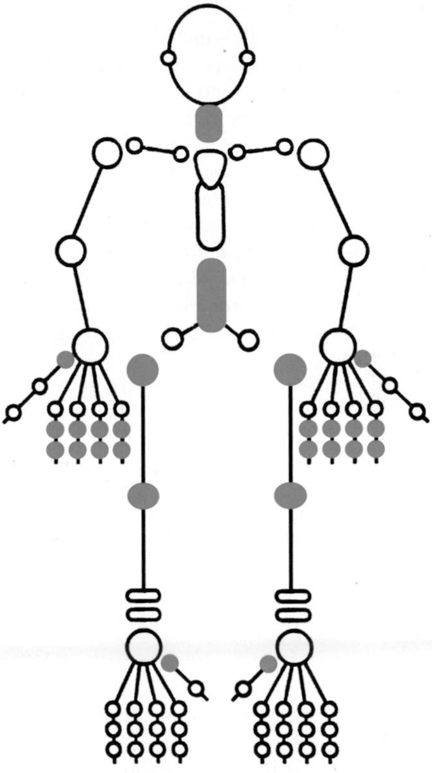

FIGURE 11-1. Distribution of osteoarthritis.

- The triggering of various metalloproteinases lead to cartilage degradation. Synthesis of matrix proteins leads to new bone growth resulting in osteophyte (bony projections at edges of joints) formation.
- Over years, this process of cartilage degradation and osteophyte formation results in the bone-on-bone grinding sensation, and sometimes even instability of the joint with use.

Risk Factors

- Risk factors for primary OA:
  ○ **Age:** The prevalence of OA greatly increases with age.
  ○ **Gender:** Women suffer from OA more often than men.
  ○ **Obesity:** Increased risk in weightbearing joints like knees and hips, as well as the first CMC.
  ○ **High bone mass:** Women with osteoporosis are less likely to have OA.
  ○ **Mechanical factors:** Joints that have been subjected to repetitive use.
  ○ **Genetic:** Although typically thought to be a disease in people over the age of 50, animal models suggest that mutations in genes encoding for extracellular matrix proteins could lead to premature OA.

- Risk factors for secondary OA:
  - **Injured or damaged joints:** This includes mechanical injuries as well as joint damage inflicted by inflammatory arthritides such as rheumatoid arthritis (RA), psoriatic arthritis (PsA), and even septic arthritis.
  - **Metabolic/infiltrative diseases:** Acromegaly, Paget's disease, Cushing's syndrome, crystalline arthropathies, ochronosis, hemochromatosis, Wilson's disease, and amyloidosis increase the risk of OA.
  - **Hemarthrosis:** Whether it be due to trauma, disease states with factor deficiencies or inhibitors, or anticoagulation, persistent or recurrent blood in the synovial fluid leads to cartilage destruction.
  - **Neuropathic joints:** The pattern of joints involved depends on the underlying disease state. Diabetic neuropathy tends to involve foot and ankle; tabes dorsalis involves knees, hips, ankles; and syringomyelia tends to involve shoulders and elbows.

DIAGNOSIS

- Diagnosis is based on history and physical examination.
- If the clinical presentation is confusing, synovial fluid analysis, inflammatory markers, and radiographs can be used to assist in diagnosis.

Clinical Presentation

Unless there is a strong family history, the patient presents with pain usually after the age of 50.

History

- Patients complain of **pain** or "locking" of affected joints that are mechanical in nature and **worsening with activity.**
- As the disease progresses, **stiffness** can become a manifestation but is typically less than 30 minutes, compared to the stiffness in RA lasting more than 60 minutes. Stiffness can occur after a period of inactivity, called a **"gelling" effect.**

Physical Examination

- Examination of the suspected joint may demonstrate **mild tenderness** to palpation, usually without evidence of inflammation. Crepitus, bony enlargement, decreased range of motion, joint effusion, and osteophytes along the periphery of the joint may be found.
- The joints most commonly involved are **DIP, PIP and first CMC joints, knees, hips, and spine.** Secondary OA or another disease process should be considered if other joints are involved.

Diagnostic Criteria

- Listed below are American College of Rheumatology (ACR) criteria for OA involving hands, hips, and knees but it is important to remember that these were created to meet eligibility for clinical trials and should be used more as guidelines rather than absolute criteria:
  - **Hand:** Hand pain or stiffness and at least three of the following: hard tissue enlargement of more than one of the selected joints (second and third DIP or PIP; the first CMC joint of each hand), hard tissue enlargement of more than

one DIP joint, deformity of at least one of ten selected joints, and fewer than three swollen MCP joints.

- ○ **Hip:** Hip pain and at least two of the following: erythrocyte sedimentation rate (ESR) <20 mm/hr, radiographic acetabular or femoral osteophytes, and radiographic joint space narrowing.
- ○ **Knee:** Knee pain plus three of the following: ESR <20 mm/hour, age >50, stiffness <30 minutes, crepitus, no palpable warmth, bony hypertrophy.

Differential Diagnosis

The following diagnoses must be considered when diagnosing OA: RA; seronegative spondyloarthropathies such as PsA, reactive arthritis (ReA), ankylosing spondylitis (AS), and enteropathic arthritis; crystalline arthropathies; infectious arthritis, including bacterial and viral etiologies; paraneoplastic and neoplastic synovitis; hemarthroses, periarticular bursitis and tendonitis; and referred pain from a different joint.

Diagnostic Testing

Laboratories

There are no laboratory tests confirming the diagnosis of OA but if the history is confusing, inflammatory markers can be obtained (ESR should be <20).

Imaging
- Radiographic evidence of OA is very common and does not necessarily correlate with symptomatic disease.
- Typical features seen on radiographs include: **joint space narrowing, subchondral sclerosis, osteophytes** at the periphery of joints, and **subchondral cysts.**

Diagnostic Procedures
- If the patient has an effusion and the clinical picture is confusing, joint aspiration can be performed.
- Synovial fluid has a few WBCs (<2000 WBCs/mL).

TREATMENT

Both the European League Against Rheumatism (EULAR) 2007 guidelines and Osteoarthritis Research Society International (OARSI) 2008 guidelines recommend a combination of nonpharmacologic modalities and the use of pharmacologic agents in a stepwise fashion.

Medications

First Line
- Although the data for using **acetaminophen** up to 4 g/day is not convincing, it is the first line therapy of choice based on its safety profile.
- In practice, most patients require 2 to 3 g/day for pain relief.

Second Line
- No one **nonsteroidal anti-inflammatory drug** (NSAID) has been proven to be more effective than another.
- NSAIDs are often more effective than acetaminophen therapy but long term use has to be balanced with increased cardiovascular, renal, and gastrointestinal (GI) toxicity.

Third Line

Opioid therapy is clearly superior to acetaminophen in terms of pain relief but studies show high drop-out rates secondary to constipation, falls, hypersomnolence, and confusion.

Fourth Line
- Various small trials have demonstrated efficacy of corticosteroid injections in about 60% of patients.
- Trials with hyaluronic acid injections show similar efficacy.[1]
- Current recommendation is to repeat injections at a maximum of every three months.

Topical Therapies
- Although not included in current guidelines, some patients report significant relief with topicals either alone or in conjunction with any of the above therapies.
- 0.025% capsaicin cream applied four times a day over a 6-week period was efficacious in decreasing knee OA pain.
- Topical diclofenac solution (1.5% w/w) at 50 drops four times a day had pain relief equivalent with 150 mg of diclofenac daily but with less GI side effects.
- Randomized controlled studies have not been performed with lidocaine patches for OA pain but they have been shown to be efficacious for neuropathic pain.

Novel Therapies
- **Diacerein** is a novel drug with interleukin (IL)-1 inhibitory activity. In animal models, this drug leads to potent inhibition of metalloproteinases necessary for cartilage destruction. Several large, randomized controlled trials have been performed with conflicting results. Diacerein is currently available in many countries including France and Armenia but is not approved for use in the US due to significant side effect profile without much benefit.[2]
- **Tanezumab** is a humanized monoclonal antibody against nerve growth factor (NGF).[3] Elevated levels of NGF are seen in synovial fluid of patients with inflammatory arthritis and animal models had suggested a benefit in OA. Dramatic response was seen in phase II trials but phase III trials for knee, hip, and shoulder OA were closed by the FDA due to some of the patients developing bone necrosis. Trials for use in metastatic bone disease, endometriosis, and prostatitis are still ongoing.
- **ADAMTS5** is a type II collagen protease thought to be central in cartilage degradation in OA. Research into its role, regulation, and expression in OA is ongoing.[4]

Other Non-Pharmacologic Therapies
- Physical therapy, aerobic, water-based exercises, weight reduction, walking aids, knee braces, footwear, insoles, thermal modalities, transcutaneous electrical nerve stimulation, acupuncture, education, and regular telephone contact to assess for pain have all been shown to improve the functional status of patients both in combination with pharmacologic therapies and by themselves.
- There are no guidelines or data to recommend some of these therapies over others but recommendations should be based on what is readily available to the patient.

Surgical Management

- Arthroscopic irrigations have failed to demonstrate any benefit in knee and hip OA.
- Knee and hip arthroplasty or total joint replacements have demonstrated improvement in function and pain in about 85% of people receiving surgeries.
- Prosthetic joints typically last 15 years.

REFERENCES

1. Leopold SS, Redd BB, Warme WJ, et al. Corticosteroid compared with hyaluronic acid injections for the treatment of osteoarthritis of the knee. A prospective, randomized trial. *J Bone Joint Surg Am.* 2003;85:1197–1203.
2. Fidelix TA, Soares B, Fernandes Moça Trevisani V. Diacerein for osteoarthritis. *Cochrane Database Syst Rev.* 2006, Issue 1. Art. No.: CD005117.
3. Lane NE, Schnitzer TJ, Birbara CA, et al. Tanezumab for the treatment of pain from osteoarthritis of the knee. *N Engl J Med.* 2010;363:1521–1531.
4. Bondeson J, Wainwright S, Huges C, et al. The regulation of the ADAMTS4 and ADAMTS5 aggrecanases in osteoarthritis: a review. *Clin Exp Rheumatol.* 2008;26:139–145.

Systemic Lupus Erythematosus

12

Alfred H.J. Kim and Wayne M. Yokoyama

GENERAL PRINCIPLES

- Systemic lupus erythematosus (SLE) is a **chronic, systemic, inflammatory disease** characterized by **autoantibodies** (particularly antinuclear antibodies [ANAs]) and **immune complex deposition** in multiple target organs.
- Affected organs include skin, musculoskeletal system, nervous system (including psychiatric), serous membranes, hematologic system, reproductive system, heart, lungs, kidneys, and gut.
- Symptoms can range from mild to life-threatening.
- Pattern of symptoms experienced within the first several years of illness tends to predominate throughout the remainder of the disease.
- Mainly affects **women of child-bearing age.**
- Criteria exist to assist in the diagnosis of SLE, but SLE remains a challenging disease to diagnose due to the absence of pathognomonic signs, symptoms, or laboratory findings.

Definition

- The diagnosis of SLE requires the presence of **multiorgan disease** in the setting of immune dysfunction, specifically the presence of **autoantibodies.**
- The American College of Rheumatology has defined diagnostic criteria for SLE (Table 12-1). While helpful for diagnosis, the main role of these criteria is defining SLE for clinical studies. They also fail to highlight common nonspecific manifestations of SLE, such as Raynaud's phenomenon, lymphadenopathy, keratoconjunctivitis sicca (secondary Sjögren's syndrome), elevated erythrocyte sedimentation rate (ESR) and hypocomplementemia.

Classification

- While SLE is the most prevalent form of lupus, there are subsets of lupus that are less severe. These are defined either by the presence of only one aspect of lupus or by a secondary cause.
  - Discoid lupus
  - Subacute cutaneous lupus
  - Drug-induced lupus (DIL)

Epidemiology

- Roughly 20 to 150 cases of SLE per 100,000 patients have been reported.
- Prevalence and severity of the disease depends on **gender and ethnicity.**
  - Gender
    - In children, female-to-male ratio is 3:1. This ratio increases in adults to 7–15:1.

TABLE 12-1	AMERICAN COLLEGE OF RHEUMATOLOGY CRITERIA FOR DIAGNOSIS OF SYSTEMIC LUPUS ERYTHEMATOSUS
Criterion	**Definition**
Malar rash	Fixed erythema, flat or raised, over the malar eminences, tending to spare the nasolabial folds
Discoid rash	Erythematosus raised patches with adherent keratotic scaling and follicular plugging; atrophic scaring may occur in older lesions
Photosensitivity	Skin rash as a result of unusual reaction to sunlight, by patient history or physician observation
Oral ulcers	Oral or nasopharyngeal ulceration, usually painless, observed by a physician
Arthritis	Non-erosive arthritis involving ≥2 peripheral joints, characterized by tenderness, swelling, or effusion
Serositis	Pleuritis: Convincing history of pleuritic pain or rub heard by a physician or evidence of pleural effusion or Pericarditis: Documented by EKG, rub, or evidence of pericardial effusion
Renal disorder	Persistent proteinuria greater than 0.5 g/day or greater than 3+ if quantification not performed or Cellular casts: May be red cell, hemoglobin, granular, tubular, or mixed
Neurologic disorder	Seizures or psychosis: In the absence of offending drugs or known metabolic derangements (uremia, ketoacidosis, or electrolyte imbalance)
Hematologic disorder	Hemolytic anemia: With reticulocytosis or Leukopenia: <4,000/mm^3 total on two or more occasions or Lymphopenia <1,500/mm^3 on two or more occasions or Thrombocytopenia <100,000/mm^3 in the absence of offending drugs
Immunologic disorders	Positive antiphospholipid antibody or Anti-DNA: Antibody to native DNA in abnormal titer or Anti-Sm: Presence of antibody to Smith nuclear antigen or False positive serologic test for syphilis known to be positive for at least six months and confirmed by *Treponema pallidum* immobilization or fluorescent treponemal antibody absorption test
Antinuclear antibody	An abnormal titer of antinuclear antibody by immunofluorescence or an equivalent assay at any point in time in the absence of drugs known to be associated with "drug-induced lupus" syndrome

Four or more of the manifestations must be present, either serially or simultaneously, to establish a diagnosis of SLE. These criteria were developed for classifying SLE patients for study purposes. Virtually all rheumatologists would argue that a negative ANA should exclude an SLE diagnosis.
EKG, electrocardiogram; Sm, Smith.

○ Ethnicity
  ▪ In females, prevalence ranges from 164 (Caucasian) to 406 (African-American) per 100,000.
  ▪ Higher in Asians, African-Americans, Afro-Caribbeans, and Hispanic-Americans compared to Caucasians. Disease is thought to be rare in Africa.

Etiology

- The etiology of SLE is unknown.
- Multiple factors appear to play a role in disease susceptibility, including genetic, hormonal, immune, and environmental.
  ○ Genetic
    ▪ There is a high concordance of SLE between monozygotic twins (14%–57%). In addition, relatives of patients with SLE have a 5% to 12% prevalence rate of SLE.
    ▪ **The genetic factors that confer the highest risk of SLE include the following:**
      □ Deficiencies of the complement component C1q, C4A and B, C2.
      □ Three prime repair exonuclease 1 (TREX1) mutations (enzyme needed to degrade DNA).
    ▪ **The most common genetic factors associated with SLE include the following:**
      □ HLA-DR2 and HLA-DR3.
      □ Genes involved with high levels or enhanced responsiveness to interferon-α (such as STAT4, PTPN22, and IRF5).
      □ Genes involved in lymphocyte signaling or clearance of immune complexes have been also identified, but the significance on disease prevalence remains unclear.
  ○ Hormonal
    ▪ The significant increase in risk seen in women strongly suggests a role of sex hormones in SLE; sex hormones are well-established regulators of the immune system, leading to the hypothesis that they play a role in SLE pathophysiology. Estrogen-containing contraceptives increase the risk of developing SLE (relative risk 1.5).
    ▪ Post-menopausal administration of estrogen and early menarche (age ≤10 years) double the risk of SLE development.
  ○ Immune
    ▪ Numerous abnormalities of the immune system have been observed in SLE patients, but the significance of these abnormalities remains unclear.
    ▪ Currently, it is believed that many of these abnormalities are due to the loss of tolerance to self-antigens.
  ○ Environmental
    ▪ Several environmental factors are associated with triggering disease onset or worsening disease activity in SLE.
      □ Viruses activate the interferon-α pathway, which is an important antiviral immune mechanism. This is the same pathway thought to be critical in promoting SLE activity. Recurrent Epstein–Barr virus infections have been associated with a higher risk of SLE development.
      □ Ultraviolet light exposure commonly triggers cutaneous manifestations of SLE.
      □ Several drugs are associated with DIL (Laboratories below).

Pathophysiology

- Many of the clinical manifestations of SLE are thought to be due to **the presence of autoantibodies and generation of immune complexes.**
- For example, in renal disease, autoantibodies to nuclear antigens either deposit or form within mesangial, subendothelial, or subepithelial regions of the glomerulus. These immune complexes activate the complement system, leading to the inflammation and recruitment of inflammatory cells to the kidney. This cycle eventually leads to fibrinoid necrosis, scarring, and reduction in kidney function.

Risk Factors

Female gender, certain ethnicities, geographical location, ultraviolet exposure, and certain medications (Table 12-2) have been associated with increased SLE prevalence or severity of disease.

TABLE 12-2	DRUGS ASSOCIATED WITH A DEFINITE, PROBABLE, OR POSSIBLE RISK OF DRUG-INDUCED LUPUS	
Definite	**Probable**	**Possible**
Procainamide[a]	Anticonvulsants	Gold salts
Hydralazine[a]	Phenytoin	Penicillin
Minocycline	Ethosuximide	Tetracycline
Diltiazem	Carbamazepine	Reserpine
Penicillamine[a]	Antithyroid drugs	Valproate
Isoniazid	Antimicrobial agents	Statins
Quinidine	Sulfonamides	Griseofulvin
Anti–TNF-α therapies	Rifampin	Gemfibrozil
Interferon-α	Nitrofurantoin	Valproate
Methyldopa	β-blockers	Ophthalmic timolol
Chlorpromazine	Lithium	5-aminosalicylate
Practolol	Captopril	
	Interferon-γ	
	Hydrochlorothiazide	
	Glyburide	
	Sulfasalazine	
	Terbinafine	
	Amiodarone	
	Ticlopidine	
	Docetaxel	

[a]Associated with high risk of inducing DIL.
TNF, tumor necrosis factor.

Prevention

Since the etiology of disease remains unknown, no primary preventative measures are known though patients are routinely advised to avoid sunlight, wear sunscreen, and wide-brimmed hats to prevent disease flares.

Associated Conditions

- As the prototypical connective tissue disease, **SLE can overlap with signs and symptoms from other connective tissue diseases.** For example, SLE can overlap with rheumatoid arthritis ("rupus"), primary Sjögren's syndrome, Raynaud's disease, systemic sclerosis, or polymyositis/dermatomyositis.
- **Mixed connective tissue disease** was initially described as a specific illness consisting of the overlap of SLE, polymyositis, and systemic sclerosis, associated with a positive ANA and very high titers of antiribonucleoprotein (anti-**RNP**) antibody. These patients were thought to have a generally milder disease than those with these diseases separately. The term is often misused by non-rheumatologists to mean an undifferentiated rheumatic illness.
- Non-Hodgkin's lymphoma (particularly diffuse large B cell) is associated with SLE.
- Many other conditions are associated with SLE. These will be covered in the Diagnosis section.

DIAGNOSIS

The diagnosis of SLE remains one of the most challenging diagnoses in medicine. No single sign, symptom, or laboratory value is pathognomonic for SLE.

Clinical Presentation

- SLE presents in a highly variable manner, both in terms of onset and in course.
- Many of the early symptoms are nonspecific (i.e., fatigue, malaise, arthralgias or arthritis, and fever).
- Severe manifestations (i.e., nephritis) usually occur at the onset or early on the course of disease.
- Many of the patient's complaints may be due to SLE, medication side effects, or unrelated intercurrent illnesses.

General Signs and Symptoms

- Virtually all SLE patients present with **fatigue.** This may be due to disease activity but anemia, infections, medications, or fibromyalgia are other causes.
- **Weight loss, lymphadenopathy, and fever** are also common in SLE. Weight loss usually precedes that diagnosis. All fevers must be evaluated for infection.

Musculoskeletal Signs and Symptoms

- **Arthralgias and arthritis** are the most common presenting symptoms in SLE.
  - Arthralgias may involve any joint, but symmetric involvement of hands, wrists, and knees is most typically seen.
  - Arthritis tends to be **symmetric, migratory, and nonerosive.**
  - Although deformities are rare, most deformities associated with SLE are reversible. Both **reversible** "swan-neck" and "boutonniere" deformities (see Chapter 2, Rheumatologic Joint Examination) can be seen. **Jaccoud's**

arthropathy occurs when there is reversible ulnar deviation and subluxation of the second to fifth metacarpophalangeal (MCP) joints.

- Diffuse **myalgias** are also commonly seen, sometimes in association with **fibromyalgia** (see Chapter 36, Fibromyalgia Syndrome). **Myositis** is uncommon but muscle inflammation otherwise typical of primary polymyositis/dermatomyositis may be associated with SLE. Myopathy induced from steroids or hydroxychloroquine (HCQ) can be seen (see Chapter 9, Drugs Used for the Treatment of Rheumatic Diseases).
- **Osteoporosis** is common and worsens from steroids used to treat flares (see Chapter 48, Osteoporosis).

Mucocutaneous Signs and Symptoms
- Approximately 50% of patients have **photosensitivity.**
  - Photosensitivity can take the form of **skin rash or blistering,** but more commonly, **extreme fatigue or malaise** occurs. Usually, symptoms occur **within minutes** of exposure to ultraviolet rays.
- **Malar rash** is seen in 50% of SLE patients.
  - Malar rash (also known as a **butterfly rash**) is a fixed erythema, either flat or raised, over the malar eminences, **sparing the nasolabial folds.**
  - The differential diagnosis for malar rash includes acne rosacea, seborrheic dermatitis, polymorphous light eruption, and contact dermatitis.
- **Discoid rash** starts as erythematous papules or plaques that become infiltrated and have an adherent scale. Follicular plugging is prominent. The lesions expand, leaving **central hypopigmentation, atrophic scarring,** and permanent alopecia. They commonly occur along the hairline and in the ear canals.
  - Some lupus patients only have discoid lesions. This type of lupus is called **discoid lupus. Only 10% of these patients will develop SLE.**
- **Oral and/or nasopharyngeal ulcers** are typically nonpainful. In contrast, herpetic chancre blisters are usually painful.
- 10% of SLE patients have **subacute cutaneous lupus erythematosus (SCLE),** while 50% of SCLE patients have SLE.
  - Erythematous, papulosquamous, or annular lesions commonly occur on sun-exposed skin.
  - Photosensitivity is a prominent feature of SCLE.
  - Most patients with SCLE will have SSA antibody.
- **Nonscarring alopecia,** livedo reticularis, and vasculitis may also be present. Soft tissue swelling and erythema can also occur on the fingers, in between joints (compared to Gottron's papules seen in dermatomyositis, see Chapter 35, Inflammatory Myopathies).

Renal Signs and Symptoms
- Renal involvement is a major cause of morbidity and mortality in SLE patients.
- Clinical involvement of the kidney occurs in **over 50% of SLE patients,** but pathologic abnormalities can be seen in patients with no known renal disease (silent lupus nephritis).
- Findings range from asymptomatic proteinuria to frank nephritic and nephrotic syndrome.
- Classification criteria initially were presented in 1978, but were revised by the International Society of Nephrology/World Health Organization (ISN/WHO) in 2003 (summarized in Tables 12-3 and 12-4).[1,2] The revised criteria are based on glomerular findings on kidney biopsy.

TABLE 12-3	INTERNATIONAL SOCIETY OF NEPHROLOGY/RENAL PATHOLOGY SOCIETY REVISED CLASSIFICATION OF LUPUS NEPHRITIS
Class I	Minimal mesangial lupus nephritis
Class II	Mesangial proliferative lupus nephritis
Class III	Focal lupus nephritis: III (A): Active lesions, focal proliferative lupus nephritis III (A/C): Active and chronic lesions III (C): Chronic inactive lesions with scars, focal sclerosing lupus nephritis
Class IV	Diffuse lupus nephritis IV-S (A): Active lesions, diffuse segmental proliferative lupus nephritis IV-G (A): Active lesions, diffuse global proliferative lupus nephritis IV-S (A/C): Active and chronic diffuse segmental lesions IV-G (A/C): Active and chronic lesions diffuse global lesions IV-S (C): Chronic inactive diffuse segmental lesions with scars IV-G (C): Chronic inactive diffuse global lesions with scars
Class V	Membranous lupus nephritis[a]
Class VI	Advanced sclerotic lupus nephritis

[a]Class V may occur in combination with class II or IV, in which case both will be diagnosed.
Adapted from: Weening JJ, D'Agati VD, Schwarz MM, et al. The classification of glomerulonephritis in systemic lupus erythematosus revisited. *J Am Soc Nephrol.* 2004;15:241–250.

- ○ In general, classes III and IV have more severe nephritis and are associated with poorer prognosis.
- **Kidney biopsies** should be performed when renal functioning is worsening, abnormal urinary sediments are seen, or when the clinical picture is unclear.
  - ○ Other conditions observed in SLE patients and worsening renal function include nonsteroidal antiinflammatory drug (NSAID) toxicity, uncontrolled hypertension, and thrombotic thrombocytopenic purpura (TTP).
- **Vascular disease** occurs in the setting of immune complex deposition within the endothelium of the vessel, immunoglobulin microvascular casts, vasculitis, or a thrombotic microangiopathy similar to TTP.
- **Tubulointerstitial nephritis** is often seen with glomerular disease, and correlates with increased creatinine, hypertension, and advanced clinical course.
- End-stage lupus nephritis requires hemodialysis, and some patients may be suitable for transplantation.
  - ○ Interestingly, many symptoms of SLE become quiescent once dialysis is initiated.
  - ○ Recurrence of nephritis in allograft transplantation occurs in 5% of patients.

Gastrointestinal Signs and Symptoms
- Most symptoms are from **medication side effects,** rather than SLE itself.
  - ○ NSAIDs, azathioprine (AZA), and corticosteroids are associated with **pancreatitis.**

TABLE 12-4 CLINICAL CORRELATES TO LUPUS NEPHRITIS CLASSES

Class	Pattern	Site of Immune Complex Deposition	Urine Sediment	Proteinuria (24 hours)	Clinical Clues[a]			
					Serum Creatinine	Blood Pressure	Anti-dsDNA	C3/C4
I	Normal	None	Bland	<200 mg	Normal	Normal	Absent	Normal
II	Mesangial	Mesangial only	RBC or bland	200–500 mg	Normal	Normal	Absent	Normal
III	Focal and segmental proliferative	Mesangial, subendothelial, ± subepithelial	RBC, WBC	500–3,500 mg	Normal to mild elevation	Normal to elevated	Positive	Decreased
IV	Diffuse proliferative	Mesangial, subendothelial, ± subepithelial	RBC, WBC, RBC casts	1,000–>3,500 mg	Normal to dialysis dependent	High	Positive to high titer	Decreased
V	Membranous	Mesangial, subepithelial	Bland	>3,000 mg	Normal to mild elevation	Normal	Absent to modest titer	Normal

[a]These are only guidelines, and parameters may vary, substantiating the need for biopsy when precise diagnosis is required.
Anti-dsDNA, anti-double stranded DNA; RBC, red blood cell; WBC, white blood cell.
Adapted from: Appel GB, Silva FG, Pirani CL, et al. Renal involvement in systemic lupus erythematosus (SLE): A study of 56 patients emphasizing histologic classification. *Medicine.* 1978;57:371–410.

- ○ Abnormal hepatic function tests can be seen, particularly in the setting of concurrent NSAID use. Frank autoimmune hepatitis is rare in the setting of SLE.
- Most common symptoms include anorexia, nausea, or vomiting.
- Abdominal pain has a wide range of etiologies.
  - ○ Infection, thrombosis (sometimes associated with antiphospholipid antibody syndrome [APLS]), medication side effects, appendicitis, peptic ulcer disease (from steroids or NSAIDs), and gastroenteritis are the most common causes.
    - ■ Cytomegalovirus (CMV) infection should be considered for patients on immunosuppression who have abdominal pain and gastrointestinal bleeding.
  - ○ Abdominal pain due to SLE is usually from **peritoneal inflammation,** though this is much less common than pleural inflammation.
  - ○ Less commonly, mesenteric vasculitis can occur.
    - ■ This can present with lower abdominal pain that can be mild in nature due to the inflammatory blunting associated with immunosuppressive medications.
    - ■ However, these patients can rapidly deteriorate and end up with bowel infarction, perforation, and peritonitis.
  - ○ Consideration for abdominal CT with arteriogram may be necessary to differentiate from more benign causes of abdominal pain. Keep in mind that high-dose steroid use may mask serious abdominal conditions.

Pulmonary Signs and Symptoms

- **Pleuritic chest pain** is the most common pulmonary symptom. This may be due to costochondritis and can be distinguished from pleuritis by palpating the painful areas.
- The most common sign is **pleural effusion,** and is usually associated with **pleuritis.**
  - ○ Most pleural effusions are asymptomatic.
  - ○ Pleural fluid is typically exudative with 3,000 to 5,000 white blood cells (WBC)/ mm^3, normal glucose, decreased complement levels, and positive ANA.
- Less commonly (<10%), pneumonitis, interstitial lung disease, pulmonary hypertension, and alveolar hemorrhage can occur.
  - ○ **Acute pneumonitis** and alveolar hemorrhage both can present identically. Fever, cough, dyspnea, pleurisy along with late inspiratory crackles occur in both settings. CT scanning will demonstrate a ground glass appearance, seen with alveolitis. Pulmonary function testing (PFT) can differentiate the two, as the diffusing capacity of the lung for carbon monoxide (DLCO) is elevated with alveolar hemorrhage. Bronchoscopy may also be useful for directly observing frank blood associated with alveolar hemorrhage.
  - ○ The prevalence of interstitial lung disease is increased in those who were diagnosed with SLE as a child and now are in their 20s to 30s. These patients will have a restrictive pattern in their PFTs.
- **Thromboembolic involvement** occurs in the setting of APLS (see Chapter 39, Antiphospholipid Syndrome).
- A rare complication is **shrinking lung syndrome,** characterized by dyspnea, episodic pleuritis chest pain, and progressive reduction in lung volume in the absence of interstitial fibrosis or pleural disease on CT.

Cardiovascular Signs and Symptoms

- The most frequent cause of symptomatic cardiac disease is **pericardial disease.**
  - ○ Typically presents with positional substernal chest pain that may be associated with an audible rub on auscultation.
    - ■ Often co-presents with other serositis symptoms (pleuritis and pleural effusion).
  - ○ Echocardiogram usually reveals a pericardial effusion that is not hemodynamically compromising.
    - ■ Pericardial effusion is one of the most common echocardiographic findings and may occur in asymptomatic patients.
    - ■ **Pericardial tamponade** most commonly occurs after prolonged periods of uncontrolled pericarditis; it is very unusual to be a presenting manifestation of SLE. When the effusion is severe, pericardiocentesis must be performed. Purulent, neoplastic, or tuberculous causes should be considered.
- **Coronary artery disease (CAD)** is a common cardiac manifestation in SLE patients but is rarely due to coronary artery vasculitis. Most often it is due to **accelerated atherosclerosis.**
  - ○ Young women have up to a 55-fold increase in the risk of CAD compared to their non-lupus cohort.
  - ○ Suspicion for CAD must be high in any SLE patient, even in young females.
- **Systolic murmurs** are common, occurring in up to 40% of SLE patients.
  - ○ Most are functional murmurs, occurring from anemia, fever, tachycardia, or cardiomegaly.
  - ○ **Mitral valve involvement,** particularly mitral valve prolapse, is the most common valvular etiology of systolic murmur.
  - ○ Valvular disease in SLE patient confers an **increased risk** of serious complications from cerebrovascular disease, peripheral embolism, heart failure, and infectious endocarditis.
  - ○ A more extreme example of valvular disease is **Libman–Sacks endocarditis,** developing in 6% to 10% of SLE patients.
    - ■ Nonbacterial verrucous lesions near the edge of the mitral, aortic, or tricuspid valves can lead to **regurgitation** in the most severe cases.
    - ■ While lesions are usually **asymptomatic,** fragments can break off producing **systemic emboli. The risk of infective endocarditis is also increased.**
    - ■ The development of lesions does not correlate with disease activity.
- A common complaint is **Raynaud's phenomenon** of the hands, feet, ears, or nose, which can be induced by cold or emotion. Two color changes (red, white, or blue) must be reported in order to confirm the diagnosis.
- **Myocarditis** is an uncommon, asymptomatic manifestation usually seen concurrently with pericarditis.
  - ○ Most typical presentation is a **resting tachycardia** out of proportion to temperature **with nonspecific EKG findings and cardiomegaly.**
  - ○ Global hypokinesis on echocardiography is a common finding.
- Pediatric considerations
  - ○ In **mothers with positive anti-SSA (Ro) or anti-SSB (La) antibodies,** there is a 3% risk for the fetus of developing **neonatal lupus with congenital heart block.**

Neuropsychiatric Signs and Symptoms

- The range of symptoms is extremely broad, encompassing subtle symptoms such as poor concentration and emotional disturbance to severe symptoms such as stroke, seizures, and psychosis.
- The American College of Rheumatology has defined criteria on the basis of either **central** or **peripheral** manifestations (Table 12-5).
  - ○ Even with these criteria, it can be very difficult to determine whether the symptom is **functional** (i.e., from a psychological basis) or **organic** (i.e., from a central or peripheral source). If organic, one has to determine if the symptom is from SLE or another cause. Some believe that antineuronal antibodies may be able to distinguish SLE-derived disease.
  - ○ From the most to least common, symptoms range from depression, cognitive disturbance, headache, mood disorder, cerebrovascular disease, seizure, polyneuropathy, anxiety, and psychosis.
  - ○ Often, **other signs and symptoms of SLE will accompany the central nervous system (CNS) manifestations.**
  - ○ CNS lupus patients may have **antiribosomal P protein antibody.**
- Many find it easier to separate symptoms into psychiatric or neurologic manifestations.

Psychiatric
- A diagnosis of psychiatric disturbance from SLE is always one of exclusion.
- One must first consider infection, electrolyte abnormalities, renal failure, drug effects, mass lesions, arterial emboli, and primary psychiatric disorders.

TABLE 12-5	ABRIDGED VERSION OF THE AMERICAN COLLEGE OF RHEUMATOLOGY DEFINITIONS FOR NEUROPSYCHIATRIC MANIFESTATIONS OF SYSTEMIC LUPUS ERYTHEMATOSUS

Central	Peripheral
Aseptic meningitis	Guillain–Barré syndrome
Cerebrovascular disease	Autonomic neuropathy
Demyelinating syndrome	Mononeuropathy
Headache	Myasthenia gravis
Movement disorder	Cranial neuropathy
Seizure disorder	Plexopathy
Myelopathy	Polyneuropathy
Acute confusional state	
Anxiety disorder	
Cognitive dysfunction	
Mood disorder	
Psychosis	

Full definitions can be found at: www.rheumatology.org/publications/ar/1999/aprilappendix. asp?aud=mem (last accessed 1/26/12).

- Depression is the most common psychiatric symptom seen in SLE patients, but this is thought to be of functional etiology rather than from SLE itself.
- Most acute psychiatric disturbances occur within the first two years of diagnosis.
- **SLE-associated psychosis is a medical emergency** (see Chapter 7, Rheumatologic Emergencies). Treatment with **antipsychotics and pulse-dose corticosteroids** must be started as soon as possible to prevent permanent brain damage.
  - ○ Corticosteroids are themselves often associated with psychosis. Symptoms often correlate with initiation or dose increase of drug.
  - ○ Nevertheless, given the significant impact SLE-associated psychosis has on long-term brain function, increasing the corticosteroid dose is justified when in doubt.
- **Cognitive defects** range from short- or long-term memory difficulty, impaired judgment and abstract thinking, aphasia, apraxia, agnosia, and personality changes.
  - ○ Cognitive dysfunction has not been directly correlated with disease activity.

Neurologic
- **Stroke syndrome** is seen in 19% of SLE patients, with an age- and sex-adjusted odds ratio of 1:5.
  - ○ Hypertension, hyperlipidemia, and baseline disease activity are established risk factors. Each factor contributes to the vasculopathy seen in SLE patients.
  - ○ Antiphospholipid antibodies are often present in patients with stroke syndrome and SLE (see Chapter 39, Antiphospholipid Syndrome). Transient ischemic attacks and small recurrent strokes are most commonly seen in this cohort.
- **Seizures** are observed in 10% to 20% of SLE patients.
  - ○ Both partial (both complex and focal) and generalized seizures occur.
  - ○ Associated with antiphospholipid and anti-Smith (anti-Sm) antibodies.
- **Headaches,** both tension and migraine, commonly occur in SLE.
- **Neuropathy** occurs in 10% to 15% of patients, usually due to a vasculopathy of the small vessels affecting peripheral nerves.
  - ○ **Sensory nerves** are more affected than motor nerves. Most commonly, bilateral asymmetric paresthesias or numbness occurs and is worse at night. Underdiagnosed is a **small-fiber neuropathy** causing painful symptoms in the absence of nerve conduction study changes.
  - ○ **Generalized sensorimotor peripheral neuropathy** also occurs with electromyographic and nerve conduction abnormalities, suggesting axonal degeneration.
  - ○ Typically, symptoms are worse later in the course of disease.
- Uncommon manifestations include transverse myelitis, CNS vasculitis, reversible posterior leukoencephalopathy syndrome (RPLS), movement disorders (such chorea or ataxia), cranial neuropathies, and aseptic meningitis.
  - ○ **Transverse myelitis** is a medical emergency and requires immediate assessment. It presents with sudden onset of bowel and bladder incontinence and lower extremity weakness that rapidly ascends, possible with sensory loss (see Chapter 7, Rheumatologic Emergencies). Cerebrospinal fluid (CSF) analysis reveals increased protein and pleocytosis. Urgent imaging with MRI is essential.
  - ○ **CNS vasculitis** is an extremely rare manifestation of SLE. This entity distinctly presents with fever, severe headache, and confusion progressing rapidly to psychosis, seizures, and coma.

○ **RPLS** presents with seizures, altered mental status, vision changes, and headache. MRI can help differentiate this from CNS lupus by demonstrating vasogenic cerebral edema predominantly in the posterior cerebral hemisphere.

Hematologic Signs and Symptoms

- **Anemia** is the most common hematologic abnormality in SLE.
  - ○ **Anemia of chronic disease (AOCD) is the most common etiology,** but autoimmune hemolytic anemia (AIHA), microangiopathic hemolytic anemia (MAHA), renal failure, and iron deficiency are also seen.
    - **AIHA** is characterized by elevated reticulocyte count, low haptoglobin levels (which may be obscured by its increase as an acute phase reactant in inflammation), increased indirect bilirubin levels, and a positive Coombs' test. However, a positive Coombs' test can be seen in the absence of AIHA and vice versa.
    - **MAHA** is characterized with a peripheral blood smear demonstrating schistocytes and elevated lactate dehydrogenase (LDH) and bilirubin levels. One must be vigilant to the features of TTP (see below) that requires different therapy.
- **Leukopenia** is also common and correlates with disease activity.
  - ○ **Neutropenia** may result from disease activity, medications (i.e., cyclophosphamide [CYC] or AZA), bone marrow dysfunction, or hypersplenism.
    - Interestingly, CNS lupus has been associated with severe neutropenia.
  - ○ **Lymphopenia,** particularly of T cells, is observed in over 50% of SLE patients, and is also caused by steroid therapy.
  - ○ Depressed eosinophil and basophil counts are typically associated with steroid therapy.
- **Thrombocytopenia** has several potential causes, including iatrogenic (i.e., heparin). Mild thrombocytopenia (platelet counts between 100,000 and 150,000/μL) is seen in up to 50% of patients, with counts of less than 50,000/μL in only 10%.
  - ○ **Idiopathic thrombocytopenic purpura (ITP)** is a major etiology, with antibody binding to platelets, followed by splenic phagocytosis causing immune-mediated destruction. ITP may be the first presenting sign of SLE in some patients.
  - ○ **TTP** leads to platelet consumption, and is a medical emergency (see Chapter 7, Rheumatologic Emergencies).
    - Affected patients will have concurrent renal failure, MAHA, fever, and neurologic involvement.
    - Schistocytes on peripheral blood smear with an elevated LDH, reduced haptoglobin, and elevated bilirubin will be seen.
    - Urgent plasmapheresis should be initiated.
    - Antibodies that function to inhibit ADAMTS13 are typically seen, but therapy should not be delayed until results of this specialized test are reported.
- **Thrombocytosis** is infrequent, and is associated with increased risk of thromboembolic disease, particularly in the setting of APLS or nephrotic syndrome (renal vein thrombosis).
- **Pancytopenia** can be due to peripheral destruction or bone marrow failure.
  - ○ Acute leukemia, large granular lymphocyte leukemia, myelodysplastic syndromes, overwhelming infection and paroxysmal nocturnal hemoglobinuria

(PNH) all can induce bone marrow failure with autoimmune features resembling SLE.

○ **Macrophage activation syndrome (MAS)** is a form of hemophagocytic lymphohistiocytosis (HLH) seen in connective tissue diseases.

■ **Marked cytopenias of two or three cell lines** are seen, with a reduction in ESR, elevations in prothrombin time (PT) and activated partial thromboplastin time (aPTT), hypertriglyceridemia, and hyperferritinemia.

■ Low or absent natural killer cell activity and elevations in soluble CD25 (interleukin [IL]-2 receptor) are typically seen.

■ Fever, weight loss, arthritis, and rash are common symptoms.

■ Bone marrow biopsy will reveal hemophagocytosis.

■ MAS responds well to immunosuppression.

• APLS (see Chapter 39, Antiphospholipid Syndrome) is associated with elevated aPTT, thrombocytopenia, **arterial and venous thrombosis,** and **fetal loss.** The presence of **lupus anticoagulant, anticardiolipin antibodies, or anti–beta-2-glycoprotein-1 antibodies** characterizes this syndrome.

Ophthalmologic Signs and Symptoms

• The most common manifestation of the eye is **conjunctivitis sicca,** also seen in Sjögren's syndrome (see Chapter 37, Sjögren's Syndrome).

• Anterior uveitis, keratitis, and episcleritis present with photophobia and pain. Eye pain in the absence of photophobia is characteristic of scleritis.

• Retinal vasculopathy is characterized by cotton–wool exudates and usually is associated with CNS lupus. Retinal vasculitis can be detected with fluorescein dye angiography where microaneurysms are visible.

• Corticosteroids may worsen or cause glaucoma and cataract formation.

• In addition, retinal detachment associated with a fibrinous exudate can be confused with retinal vasculopathy or vasculitis.

Diagnostic Criteria

• The American College of Rheumatology has defined revised classification criteria in 1997 to establish the diagnosis of SLE for clinical studies (Table 12-1).

• The diagnosis of SLE requires **multiorgan involvement with evidence of autoimmunity.**

○ A patient who likely has SLE may complain of fatigue, joint pain, chest pain, and photosensitivity.

○ Exam reveals malar rash, nontender oral ulcers, and several swollen and tender joints.

○ Laboratory results demonstrate a mild anemia, proteinuria, positive Coombs' test, and ANAs, usually with anti-double stranded DNA (anti-dsDNA) antibodies.

○ Chest radiograph shows small bilateral pleural effusions.

• Symptoms are often vague at initial presentation, and the diagnosis may become more apparent over time.

• A thorough history and physical examination is necessary to confidently diagnose SLE since no single diagnostic test is pathognomonic.

Differential Diagnosis

• The highly variable manifestations of SLE lead to a very broad differential diagnosis.

- Typically, infection, other connective tissue diseases, and other systemic conditions such as sarcoidosis, amyloidosis, and malignancies are considered.

Diagnostic Testing

SLE is one of the diseases where the diagnostic testing only supplements a careful history and physical examination.

Laboratories

- Comprehensive metabolic panel (CMP), complete blood count (CBC) with differential, ESR, C-reactive protein (CRP), and urinalysis (UA) provide diagnostically useful information and should be obtained for every suspected and established SLE patient. **Complement (C3 and C4) levels** can be beneficial in those patients whose complement levels correlate with disease activity (lower complement levels, higher disease activity).
- **Autoantibodies** are characteristic of SLE, and represent autoreactivity to nuclear proteins and nucleic acids. As a result, these are usually the first diagnostic tests ordered (see Chapter 5, Laboratory Evaluation of Rheumatic Diseases).
  - **ANA is present in >99% of SLE patients,** meaning that its absence virtually rules out SLE.
    - Patients with SLE typically have ANA positivity in **significant titers** (>1:160). Suspicion of an autoimmune disorder should be elevated when titers >1:640.
    - **The pattern of ANA reactivity has little diagnostic value** since recognition of patterns is dependent on the experience of the operator and serum dilution.
    - The false positive rate in healthy people varies from 30% with titers of 1:40 (high sensitivity, low specificity) to 3% with titers of 1:320 (low sensitivity, high specificity).[3]
    - Among patients referred to a rheumatologist with a positive ANA (titer ≥1:40), only 19% were diagnosed with SLE.[4] Most of the ANA-positive patients without SLE had no disease whatsoever, or had fibromyalgia-like manifestations.
    - Low-titer ANAs can be found in other autoimmune diseases such as Sjögren's syndrome, scleroderma, juvenile idiopathic arthritis, rheumatoid arthritis, interstitial lung disease, primary autoimmune cholangitis, or autoimmune hepatitis or thyroiditis.
    - Certain medications (Table 12-2) can induce ANA positivity and a condition called **DIL.**
      - DIL presents with mild manifestations of lupus, and typically without internal organ involvement.
      - Symptoms usually cease after stopping the offending medication.
      - **Antihistone antibodies** are characteristic of this condition.
      - Most drug-induced ANAs are not associated with clinical symptoms of SLE.
  - Once a significant titer ANA is obtained, speciation of the autoantibodies should be performed, including assays for **anti-dsDNA, anti-Sm, anti-SSA (Ro), anti-SSB (La), anti-RNP, antiphospholipid antibodies, and anti-ribosomal P protein antibodies.**
    - **Anti-dsDNA** and **anti-Sm** are highly specific for SLE. Anti-dsDNA antibodies may correlate with disease activity and nephritis. Unfortunately,

they have poor sensitivity with only about 30% of SLE patients showing positivity for these tests.

- **Anti-RNP** associates with SLE, mixed connective tissue disease, and scleroderma.
- **Anti-SSA and anti-SSB** are associated with Sjögren's syndrome and neonatal lupus. Anti-SSA is seen with lymphopenia, photosensitivity, C2 deficiency, and subacute cutaneous lupus.
- **Anti-ribosomal P** protein is associated with CNS lupus.

Imaging
- Decision to pursue imaging is dependent on the patient's symptom complex and whether the test will add diagnostic or prognostic value.
  - For chest pain, consider chest radiograph and/or CT, EKG.
  - For joint pain, consider plain radiographs of affected joints.
  - For renal involvement, consider renal ultrasound to assess kidney size and rule out urinary tract obstruction.
  - For abdominal pain, consider abdominal and pelvic CT and/or angiogram if vasculitis is suspected.
  - For CNS manifestations, consider brain MRI.
  - For peripheral neuropathies or weakness, consider nerve conduction studies with electromyography.

Diagnostic Procedures
- As with imaging, decision to obtain fluid or tissue is dependent on the symptoms and the value to diagnosis or prognosis.
  - For rash, consider skin biopsy.
  - For renal involvement, consider kidney biopsy.
  - For fluid associated with serositis (pleural effusion, pericardial effusion, or ascites), consider draining fluid.
  - For cytopenias with suspected bone marrow involvement, consider bone marrow biopsy.
  - For joint effusions, consider arthrocentesis.

TREATMENT

- **Treatment is based on type and severity of clinical manifestations** (see Chapter 9, Drugs Used for the Treatment of Rheumatic Diseases). For example, mild photosensitive rash requires much different treatment than life-threatening lupus nephritis.
- Symptoms that are mild and not organ- or life-threatening are typically treated with less potent immunosuppressive medications or non-pharmacologic therapies in order to minimize side effects.
- Conversely, **organ- or life-threatening disease requires maximal immunosuppression.**
  - A way to think about which immunosuppressant to use in these cases is to divide the medications into **induction** and **maintenance** therapies.
  - Since SLE is a chronic, incurable condition characterized with flares, certain drugs are reserved for quickly resolving lupus flares and some are best for suppression of subsequent flares. Typically, drugs used for flares have side effect profiles preventing their long-term use.

○ The maintenance medications are used for cytotoxic- and steroid-sparing purposes, and to suppress future flares. These medications do not rapidly resolve active flares.

Medications

For Mild Disease

- Usually, mucocutaneous, musculoskeletal, hematologic (excluding hemolytic anemia and MAS), and serositis complaints can be treated with less potent immunosuppressive therapies.
- **NSAIDs/cyclooxygenase (COX)-2 inhibitors**
  ○ Used for the treatment of arthralgias, arthritis, fever, and mild serositis.
- **Aspirin**
  ○ Low-dose aspirin is used for primary prevention of APLS, where it has limited efficacy.
- **HCQ** (antimalarial)
  ○ **Very useful for mucocutaneous disease, arthritis, alopecia, and fatigue.** Because of its beneficial effect on lipid profiles it may also help prevent CAD. **Daily dose of 4 to 6 mg/kg (200–400 mg) after meals is typical.**
  ○ Onset of action is very slow (about 6 weeks) and peak efficacy may not be reached for 4 months.
  ○ GI side effects, especially nausea, are the most common.
  ○ Regular ophthalmologic visits (q6–60 months depending on age, liver and kidney function, and dose) should occur as HCQ can bind to melanin in the retina damaging rods and cones leading to blindness.
  ○ Test for **glucose-6-phosphate deficiency** as these patients are at increased risk for hemolysis.
  ○ If there are no contraindications, most SLE patients are placed on HCQ therapy regardless of type of disease. There is evidence for a reduced frequency of major kidney and CNS damage for those on HCQ therapy.[5]
- **Dapsone**
  ○ **Used in cutaneous lupus** such as bullous lupus, subacute cutaneous lupus, and discoid lupus. Starting dose is 50 mg PO q day, with a typical dose of 100 mg PO q day.
  ○ Test for **glucose-6-phosphate deficiency** as these patients are at increased risk for hemolysis. Hemoglobin and reticulocyte count should be monitored during therapy.
- **Topical steroids**
  ○ Hydrocortisone can be used early in mild skin disease, but most require fluorinated preparations that possess increased potency. Do not use fluorinated steroids on the face.
  ○ Ointments are more effective than creams.
  ○ Scalp lesions should be treated with lotions, gels, or solutions.
- **Low-dose systemic corticosteroids**
  ○ Doses of prednisone ≤15 mg PO daily are effective until a steroid-sparing agent (i.e., HCQ) can take effect.

For Moderate–severe Disease

- **High-dose systemic corticosteroids**
  ○ The most potent and fastest acting class of immunosuppressive medications.
  ○ Used primarily for **induction** therapy.

- ○ **Pulse-dose corticosteroids (methylprednisolone):**
  - Reserved for organ-threatening disease.
  - Dosed 1 g IV q day × 3 days, followed by a taper with oral steroids (prednisone ≤60 mg PO q day).
  - This approach is entirely empiric, with no clinical data supporting this dosing regimen; nevertheless, it is widely used.
- ○ **Oral corticosteroids (prednisone):**
  - Used for moderately severe flares or tapering from pulse-dose steroids.
  - Goal is to change to steroid-sparing therapies as quickly as possible to reduce the risk of the numerous side effects associated with steroids.
  - Every SLE patient on corticosteroids should be considered for a steroid-sparing agent, especially once the acute flare has been controlled, and osteoporosis prevention should be considered.
- **CYC**
  - ○ Reserved for **severe disease manifestations,** such as severe lupus nephritis, CNS lupus, APLS, or vasculitis. **Strongly considered for any life-threatening disease.**
  - ○ Considered **induction therapy,** but onset of action is somewhat longer than that for corticosteroids, so it is often used concomitantly with high-dose steroids in induction therapy.
  - ○ Can be delivered IV (monthly) or PO (daily).
    - In general, **IV CYC** has shown efficacy in inducing the remission of severe SLE manifestations, such as diffuse proliferative nephritis. This approach is advantageous to daily PO CYC since the total dose of drug is less over a fixed period of time. This reduces the risk of severe side effects seen with CYC therapy. Concomitant use of 2-mercaptoethane sulfonate sodium (MESNA) may also reduce the risk of cystitis and bladder cancer. However, oral CYC is considered to be more potent.
    - High-dose IV CYC (National Institutes of Health protocol) has been traditionally used for severe disease. More recently, low-dose IV CYC protocol (Euro-Lupus protocol) has been increasingly used with equal efficacy for proliferative lupus nephritis.[6]
    - Check a CBC 8 to 10 days after IV CYC infusion to monitor for a dose-dependent nadir leukocyte count. The target count should be 2.5 to 3.5/mm^3. Lymphopenia will be common, but **neutropenia should be avoided.**
  - ○ Nausea, vomiting, alopecia, bone marrow suppression, infections, and bladder carcinoma are the most common adverse reactions.
- **Mycophenolate mofetil (MMF)**
  - ○ Typically used to prevent renal allograft rejection, data suggest MMF noninferiority to IV CYC in short-term remission from lupus nephritis with a better safety profile.[7]
  - ○ May also be useful as a steroid-sparing agent.
  - ○ Dosing ranges from 500 to 1,500 mg PO bid.
  - ○ Side effects include GI upset, cytopenias, and increased risk of infections.
- **AZA**
  - ○ Used as a **steroid-sparing agent,** and thus is considered a maintenance mediation.
  - ○ Dosage is 2 to 2.5 mg/kg/day.
  - ○ **Thiopurine methyltransferase** (TPMT) inactivates AZA, so TPMT enzyme activity should be checked prior to use to prevent bone marrow toxicity. Even

low doses of AZA can cause pancytopenia in individuals with low TPMT enzyme activity.

○ **Regularly monitor hepatic and renal function** as it is hepatic metabolized and renal excreted.

○ Be cautious with its use with allopurinol, since acute pancytopenia can occur with concurrent use.

○ Can be used in pregnancy, but does pass into breast milk and breastfeeding is not advised.

- **Methotrexate (MTX)**
  ○ Conflicting results with the use of MTX for SLE exist within the literature.
  ○ It appears that MTX is efficacious for **cutaneous and articular manifestations,** allowing for tapering of steroid. Considered a steroid-sparing agent.
  ○ Usually dosed between 7.5 and 20 mg PO q week.
  ○ Folic acid supplementation (1 mg PO q day) may be needed to abrogate some of the side effects of MTX, including alopecia, gastrointestinal complaints, hepatic function test elevations, and mucositis.
  ○ MTX should be discontinued 6 months prior to pregnancy for both males and females.
- **Cyclosporine**
  ○ Not commonly used for SLE, but has been efficacious for moderate systemic manifestations of lupus as a steroid-sparing agent.
  ○ Dosages range from 2.5 to 5 mg/kg/day.
  ○ Side effects are dose dependent and reversible, including **hypertension,** hepatic function test and **creatinine elevations,** GI complaints, tremor, and infections.
  ○ Although effective for membranous glomerulonephritis, long-term treatment can induce interstitial fibrosis and tubular atrophy.
- **B cell modulating agents**
  ○ **Off-label use of rituximab** has been efficacious in a subset of SLE patients, with or without nephritis. Despite these promising preliminary reports, placebo-controlled randomized trials did not see benefit.[8]
- **Belimumab** has recently been shown to be efficacious in phase III trials.[9]
- **Other therapies** that have been utilized with varying success include intravenous immunoglobulin, plasmapheresis, and immunoablation with or without autologous stem cell transplantation.
- Drug development for SLE is advancing at a very rapid rate with several candidate drugs demonstrating potential.

Other Medications

- **Bisphosphonates** should be started with long-term high-dose prednisone use, or with evidence of osteopenia. Treatment should last for 3 to 5 years.
- **Statins** should be used on the basis of guidelines for the general population.

Lifestyle/Risk Modification

- Sedentary lifestyle is an important feature of SLE. Low impact exercise (i.e., water aerobics) is extremely beneficial for SLE patients. This prevents deconditioning and weight gain.
- For patients with photosensitivity, **avoiding intense sun exposure** with routine sunscreen use and appropriate clothing is necessary.

- **Smoking cessation** is important, as smoking is associated with higher disease activity and can reduce the efficacy of several medications. Strongly advise patients to stop smoking.

SPECIAL CONSIDERATIONS

- While variable, SLE may significantly worsen during **pregnancy.**
- Best outcomes occur when the disease has been quiescent from 6 to 12 months prior to conception.
- Fetal loss is highest when high lupus activity occurs in the first or second trimester or when new onset lupus nephritis occurs in the first trimester.
- Preeclampsia can mimic SLE flares (proteinuria, thrombocytopenia).
- Pregnant SLE patients should be followed closely by a rheumatologist and high-risk obstetrician.

REFERRAL

- It is appropriate to refer to a rheumatologist when you suspect that a patient has symptoms consistent with SLE and has a positive ANA.
- **Any patient with established SLE should see a rheumatologist for disease management and monitoring for side effects from immunosuppressive medications.**
  - For difficult skin manifestations from lupus, dermatology referral is highly recommended.

PATIENT EDUCATION

- At the time of initial diagnosis, patients are unfamiliar with the disease and its complexity. Consequently, education and counseling are important. Several foundations and organizations dedicated to patients with lupus have excellent resources for the newly diagnosed.
- Patients must be informed of the side effects associated with their specific immunosuppression regimen to avoid life-threatening complications.

MONITORING/FOLLOW-UP

- The goal during follow-up is to monitor for drug-induced toxicity, infection, and flares.
- A history and physical examination, along with laboratory testing, should be routinely done during the follow-up period.
  - When relapses occur, the history and physical findings will typically mimic the patient's initial presentation.
  - CMP, CBC, ESR, CRP, and UA should be obtained with each visit. In some patients complement levels and anti-DNA titers parallel disease activity and may be useful in monitoring activity.
  - Lipid profiles and 25-hydroxyvitamin D levels should be checked annually.
  - Dual-emission X-ray absorptiometry (DEXA) scan should be obtained every two years.
  - Routine vaccinations with killed-virus vaccines should be performed.

OUTCOME/PROGNOSIS

- SLE has a variable clinical course.
- Many patients relapse, requiring high-dose steroids or induction treatment with cytotoxic agents.
- Despite this, **the 5-year survival rate is greater than 90%.** Likelihood of survival is highly dependent on organs involved. Best outcomes are associated with skin or musculoskeletal involvement only, while **kidney and CNS involvement confer the poorest prognoses.**
- Early in disease, the major cause of mortality is active disease or infection related to medications. Late in disease, SLE itself (i.e., end-stage renal disease), vascular disease, infections, non-Hodgkin lymphoma, and lung cancer are the leading causes of death.

REFERENCES

1. Weening JJ, D'Agati VD, Schwartz MM, et al. The classification of glomerulonephritis in systemic lupus erythematosus revisited. *J Am Soc Nephrol.* 2004;15:241–250.
2. Buyon JP. Systemic lupus erythematosus: A. Clinical and laboratory features. In: Klippel JH, Stone JH, Crofford LJ, White PH, eds. *Primer on the Rheumatic Diseases.* 13th ed. New York, NY: Springer Science + Business Media; 2008:303–318.
3. Mosca M, Tani C, Bombardieri S. A case of undifferentiated connective tissue disease: Is it a distinct clinical entity? *Nat Clin Pract Rheumatol.* 2008;4:328–332.
4. Shiel WC Jr, Jason M. The diagnostic associations of patients with antinuclear antibodies referred to a community rheumatologist. *J Rheumatol.* 1989;16:782–785.
5. Fessler BJ, Alarcon GS, McGwin G Jr, et al. Systemic lupus erythematosus in three ethnic groups: XVI. Association of hydroxychloroquine use with reduced risk of damage accrual. *Arthritis Rheum.* 2005;52:1473–1480.
6. Houssiau FA, Vasconcelos C, D'Cruz D, et al. Immunosuppressive therapy in lupus nephritis: The Euro-Lupus Nephritis Trial, a randomized trial of low-dose versus high-dose intravenous cyclophosphamide. *Arthritis Rheum.* 2002;46:2121–2131.
7. Ginzler EM, Dooley MA, Aranow C, et al. Mycophenolate mofetil or intravenous cyclophosphamide for lupus nephritis. *N Engl J Med.* 2005;353:2219–2228.
8. Merrill JT, Neuwelt CM, Wallace DJ, et al. Efficacy and safety of rituximab in moderately-to-severely active systemic lupus erythematosus: The randomized, double-blind, phase II/III systemic lupus erythematosus evaluation of rituximab trial. *Arthritis Rheum.* 2010;62: 222–233.
9. A Study of Belimumab in Subjects with Systemic Lupus Erythematosus (SLE) (BLISS-52). 2010; http://clinicaltrials.gov/ct2/show/NCT00424476. Last accessed 1/30/12.

Gout

13

Richa Gupta and Wayne M. Yokoyama

GENERAL PRINCIPLES

Definition

Gout is a disease related to deposition of uric acid, classically in the joints, soft tissues (termed tophi), or kidney interstitium, and/or formation of uric acid nephrolithiasis.

Classification

- The natural history of gout classically has three stages:
  - **Asymptomatic hyperuricemia** usually exists for years before the initial acute attack. It is important to note that most patients with hyperuricemia do not develop gout.
  - **Acute intermittent gout** then develops. Patients have acute attacks of arthritis followed by symptom-free intercritical periods. The attacks become more frequent and severe.
  - **Chronic gouty arthritis** may then ensue. In these patients, the intercritical periods are no longer asymptomatic, and joint pain persists. Tophi (uric acid deposits) are often seen in these patients. Gout may also involve the kidneys (causing gouty nephropathy) and the urinary tract (uric acid stones).

Epidemiology

- Gout is relatively common among the rheumatic diseases.
- Approximately 90% of gout occurs in men between the ages of 30 and 50.
- Gout is very uncommon in premenopausal women.

Pathophysiology

- **Hyperuricemia** may be a primary disorder, i.e., in the absence of conditions or medications that cause hyperuricemia, or secondary.
- Uric acid is normally produced in the liver in the purine metabolism pathway; its immediate precursors are hypoxanthine and xanthine which are converted by xanthine oxidase to uric acid.
- "Normal" uric acid levels reported by clinical laboratories may be misleading with respect to the pathophysiology of gout.
  - In comparison to age-matched controls, two standard deviations above the mean is typically used as the cutoff level to indicate abnormally high levels, frequently >8.5 mg/dL.
  - However, uric acid levels >6.8 mg/dL in men and women are supersaturated in bodily fluids, i.e., they exceed normal soluble concentrations.[1]
- Uric acid levels in children are typically low (<4.0 mg/dL), rising in men at the time of puberty.
- In postmenopausal women, uric acid levels approach those of men because of the loss of the uricosuric effects of estrogen.

- Two-thirds of uric acid excretion is via the kidney, with a small portion of uric acid excretion by the gastrointestinal (GI) tract.
- **Primary hyperuricemia**
  - Patients with a complete deficiency of hypoxanthine–guanine phosphoribosyl transferase (HGPRT) have the X-linked **Lesch–Nyhan syndrome** with hyperuricemia, severe neurologic defects, gout, and uric acid stones.
  - Patients with a partial defect in HGPRT display X-linked, primary hyperuricemia and classically present with early onset gout and/or uric acid nephrolithiasis without neurological problems.
  - However, **most patients with primary hyperuricemia do not have an identifiable cause.**
- **Secondary hyperuricemia**
  - **Many medications, especially thiazide and loop diuretics, can cause hyperuricemia.**
  - Other medications include cyclosporine, tacrolimus, low-dose aspirin, niacin, ethambutol, pyrazinamide, and L-dopa.
  - **Overproduction** of uric acid can occur with psoriasis, myeloproliferative disorders, multiple myeloma, hemoglobinopathies, and cytotoxic drugs.
  - **Underexcretion** of uric acid may occur in chronic renal disease, hypothyroidism, and lead poisoning, leading to hyperuricemia.
- **Acute gout is an inflammatory response to monosodium urate (MSU) crystal deposition in the joint space.** This is more likely to happen in patients with high uric acid levels. It is not clear what initiates the inflammatory process, as crystals can be present in the joint space during asymptomatic periods without inflammation.
- MSU-induced inflammation appears to be a consequence of activation of the nucleotide-binding oligomerization domain (NOD)-like (NLR) family pyrin domain containing 3 (NLRP3, also known as cryopyrin) inflammasome, proteolytic cleavage and activation of caspase 1, proteolytic cleavage and maturation of pro-interleukin-1β, and secretion of mature interleukin (IL)-1β.[2] This process is related to inflammation in diseases associated with gain of function mutations in NLRP3, including familial cold autoinflammatory syndrome, Muckle–Wells syndrome, and neonatal-onset multisystem inflammatory disease.

DIAGNOSIS

Clinical Presentation

- The sudden onset of **severe pain, erythema, swelling, and disability of a single joint** and tenosynovial inflammation characterizes an acute gout attack. The erythema and swelling may be accompanied by pruritus and fever. Inflammation often extends beyond the affected joint. Desquamation of the skin overlying the affected joint frequently occurs after the attack resolves.
- Acute gout initially presents in men between the ages of 40 and 50 and in postmenopausal women. A much earlier age of onset should lead to an investigation for an inborn error of metabolism. Acute gout may be precipitated by alcohol binges, dehydration, recent trauma, surgery, and initiation of drugs that change uric acid levels (either increase, such as cytotoxic drugs, or decrease, such as allopurinol, uricase).

- Early attacks of gout are typically **monoarticular and involve joints in the lower extremities.**
- The initial attack involves the MTP joint of the great toe (**podagra**) in about 50% of cases, with about 90% of patients ultimately experiencing podagra with recurrent attacks. Other common sites are the ankle, knee, and wrist. Gout rarely involves the hips or shoulders.
- An acute attack involves more than one joint in only 20% of cases, but rarely in initial attacks. When it does, it is usually in an asymmetric distribution. A **polyarticular distribution** occurs more frequently with recurrent attacks or gout attributed to secondary causes (e.g., myeloproliferative disease, lymphoproliferative disease, or transplant recipient).
- Acute attacks usually peak within the first 12 hours from onset, typically lasts 5 to 7 days, but a severe attack may last up to 2 weeks. Gouty attacks are self-limited and eventually resolve spontaneously.
- **Acute intermittent gout:** Between acute attacks, patients are asymptomatic for prolonged periods, termed intercritical periods. Without treatment, the typical patient can expect a recurrent attack within 2 years of the initial attack. However, some patients may not experience another attack. Recurrent attacks are usually more severe and more likely to be polyarticular.
- **Chronic gouty arthritis:** Left untreated, the disease may progress to chronic gouty arthritis in approximately 12 years (range, 5–40 years).
- **Chronic tophaceous gout** is characterized by the deposition of MSU in connective tissue as soft tissue masses known as tophi. Smaller tophi may cause joint erosions seen on radiographs, manifested as polyarticular deforming arthritis that particularly involves the hands. In some patients, this arthritis may be difficult to differentiate in clinical appearance from rheumatoid arthritis (RA).
- Tophi occur most commonly at the base of the great toe, fingers, wrists, hands, olecranon bursa, and Achilles tendon. Higher uric acid levels are associated with more tophi. Complications of tophi include pain, deformity, joint destruction, and nerve compression.

Differential Diagnosis

- An acute attack of gout needs to be distinguished from cellulitis, septic arthritis, pseudogout, and RA.
- Gout **mimics cellulitis** in that the affected area is swollen, erythematous, and painful and may be accompanied by fever and leukocytosis.
  - **If cellulitis is suspected, the joint should not be aspirated through the overlying skin infection to avoid seeding a secondary septic arthritis.**
  - In some cases, it may be necessary to treat with antibiotics for 1 to 2 days while awaiting blood cultures and other indications of infection before considering gout as a leading diagnosis.
- **Septic arthritis** must always be considered in a patient with acute monoarticular arthritis, especially with fever and leukocytosis.
  - **Joint aspiration is critical to rule out bacterial infection;** treat suspicious cases with antibiotics as for cellulitis.
  - Gouty joints are more susceptible to bacterial infection, and the two conditions may occur simultaneously.
- **Pseudogout** should always be considered when entertaining the diagnosis of gout. It is most readily distinguished from gout by the presence of calcium pyrophosphate crystals in the joint.

- Chronic gout may **mimic RA** because some chronic gout patients may display a symmetric polyarthritis. They may also develop tophi in sites where rheumatoid nodules typically occur. In contrast to RA, chronic gout typically presents at an older age and is seronegative. Radiographs may show changes typical of gout.

Diagnostic Testing

- The diagnosis is based primarily on history, physical examination, and the presence of **MSU crystals** in joint fluid or tophus.
- **Hyperuricemia alone is not diagnostic for gout**, even with a history of acute arthritis, which could be due to many other possible disorders.

Laboratories

- Patients with gout almost invariably have hyperuricemia, but **uric acid levels may be normal during an attack.**
- Attacks are also associated with an increased erythrocyte sedimentation rate (ESR) and leukocyte count.
- None of these laboratory tests are helpful in making the diagnosis of gout.

Imaging

- **Joint radiographs** early in the course of the disease are normal, but as the disease progresses, **characteristic punched-out joint erosions with overhanging edges** ("rat-bite lesions") in the bone may be evident.
- Significant joint destruction may occur.
- Tophi may be evident on other radiographs.

Diagnostic Procedures

- **Aspiration of the joint is essential for diagnosis and reveals intracellular monosodium urate crystals.**
- Monosodium urate crystals are **needle-shaped** and demonstrate **negative birefringence** with polarized microscopy. Crystals can also be identified during the intercritical period in an asymptomatic patient but are usually not intracellular.
- Leukocyte counts are elevated in the joint fluid, usually 15,000/μL or higher with a predominance of neutrophils. Leukocyte count of greater than 50,000/μL should raise suspicion for a bacterial joint infection.

TREATMENT

First and foremost, one should treat the acute attack; later, consider the need for treating hyperuricemia and also the other components of the metabolic syndrome that are commonly present.

Acute Gouty Attack

- **Nonsteroidal antiinflammatory drugs (NSAIDs) are considered first line therapy,** though contraindications may limit their use because the typical gout patient is somewhat older and has comorbid conditions.
  - ○ Essentially any NSAID may be used but most have not been adequately studied.
  - ○ NSAIDs are typically used at full maximal daily doses with improvement in symptoms expected within a few hours.

- ○ **Contraindications** include peptic ulcer disease, chronic renal insufficiency, and drug allergy.
- ○ Commonly used NSAIDs are ibuprofen in full doses of 800 mg qid, naproxen as 500 mg bid, or indomethacin as 50 mg tid.
- ○ Selective cyclooxygenase (COX)-2 inhibitors may also be used with similar efficacy and lower GI toxicity as compared to indomethacin.
- ○ Aspirin should not be used, as it impairs uric acid secretion.
- **Intraarticular or systemic corticosteroid** therapy is of particular benefit in patients with contraindications to NSAID usage.[3] **Septic arthritis should be ruled out before initiating any corticosteroid therapy.**
  - ○ Intraarticular steroid injections are used frequently as a safe, local treatment in all patients (e.g., methylprednisolone or triamcinolone 10–40 mg).
  - ○ Oral corticosteroid therapy is reserved for patients who have failed or have a contraindication to NSAIDs or colchicine, or are experiencing a polyarticular attack. A typical regimen of prednisone is started at 40 to 60 mg PO qd and tapered over 7 to 10 days. A rebound attack may occur with tapering of corticosteroids.
- **Adrenocorticotropic hormone (ACTH)** is an option in patients who cannot tolerate other recommended therapies.
  - ○ ACTH was believed to exert its main beneficial effect by adrenal corticosteroid release. New evidence shows that, instead, peripheral activation of a melanocortin receptor, melanocortin type 3 receptor (MC3R), could be responsible, at least in part, for ACTH's efficacy in acute gout.[4]
  - ○ The dosage 40 to 80 IU in a single dose or every 12 hours for 1 to 2 days, SC or IM.
- **Colchicine** was once the drug of choice for acute gout but toxicity and delayed effectiveness have diminished enthusiasm for its use in the typical patient. However, it may have a role in a patient with contraindications for other treatment choices.
  - ○ It is most effective if started within the first 12 to 24 hours of the attack. **Oral dosing is limited by GI side effects, most predominately diarrhea with cramping that may be severe.**
  - ○ At the first sign of an attack in patients **with normal renal function,** this agent is usually administered as one or two 0.6-mg tablets, followed by one 0.6-mg tablet 1 hour later. The maximum recommended treatment dosage 1.8 mg over a 1-hour period.[5] The patient should respond within 48 hours.
  - ○ Recommended prophylactic dosage is 0.6 mg once or twice daily.
  - ○ Drug-drug interactions with colchicine occur largely with agents that interfere with the functions of the membrane P-glycoprotein multiple drug resistance transporter and/or the cytochrome P450, as both these are involved in colchicine metabolism.
  - ○ In patients with creatinine clearance of <30 mL/minute, colchicine dose adjustment is not required but redosing within 2 weeks is not recommended. In hemodialysis patients, a maximum dose of 0.6 mg/attack is recommended.
  - ○ **Intravenous colchicine use is associated with the potential for very serious toxicity and in 2008 the United States Food and Drug Administration banned the manufacturing or shipping of IV colchicines in the US.**
- **Experimental antiinflammatory therapy:** IL-1 is a prominent proinflammatory cytokine released as a result of innate immune mechanisms activated by the inflammasome. It is suspected to play a role in inducing the symptoms of

the acute gout flare. Hence, there are currently trials underway examining the recombinant **IL-1 receptor antagonist, anakinra,** in acute gouty arthritis.[6] Although not yet FDA approved for this indication, it may be considered for use in acute gout at a dose of 100 mg subcutaneously daily for 3 days where standard therapy is contraindicated or not effective.

- **Analgesia:** Acute attacks usually resolve spontaneously within 5 to 7 days. Patients with contraindications to the above therapies or complicating factors (e.g., postoperative patients with NPO orders, renal failure, and coagulopathy) **may require opioid analgesics.**

Prophylactic Therapy

- Prophylactic therapy may be given daily to prevent the recurrence of acute attacks.
- It must also be given before the initiation of treatment to lower uric acid levels, as changes in uric acid levels may precipitate acute attacks.
- The dose of **colchicine** is 0.6 mg PO qd or bid or even once every other day, unless the patient has renal or hepatic disease. Possible side effects of long-term colchicine therapy include myositis and mixed peripheral neuropathy.
- **Daily indomethacin or other NSAIDs** are also useful in prophylaxis. Use with caution in the elderly because of the risk of peptic ulcer disease and chronic renal insufficiency. Indomethacin at the dose of 25 mg bid may be effective although the data are very limited.

Treatment of Hyperuricemia

- **Asymptomatic hyperuricemia does not require treatment.**
  - Hyperuricemia is highly prevalent among hypertensive patients.
  - Almost 75% of patients with hypertension and chronic renal insufficiency have increased uric acid levels.
  - Hyperuricemia is independently associated with increased mortality in patients with cardiovascular disease, especially in women, but it is not clear whether treatment of hyperuricemia in these patients is beneficial.
- Treatment of hyperuricemia aims to reduce serum uric acid levels and prevent progression of disease to chronic gouty arthritis.
- **Criteria for initiating treatment of hyperuricemia** in patients with symptomatic gout include:
  - Tophaceous gout.
  - Gouty nephropathy.
  - Uric acid kidney stones
  - Repeated attacks (generally >2/year).
  - It is debatable whether to institute treatment of hyperuricemia after a single acute gout attack.
- The goal of therapy is to achieve a serum uric acid level of approximately 6 mg/dL.[7] When the uric acid level is <6.0 mg/dL, monosodium urate crystals are reabsorbed from the joint and soft-tissue tophi.
- Suppression with chronic therapy eventually leads to alleviation of the arthritis, although bony abnormalities and other structural defects are not affected. Normalization of serum uric acid should prevent further structural damage.
- **Do not start these agents during an acute attack,** rather, start them 4 to 6 weeks after the attack subsides and while the patient has had at least one week of prophylactic therapy.

- **If the patient is on an antihyperuricemic agent, do not discontinue it during an acute attack** because any alteration in serum uric acid levels may precipitate or prolong attacks.
- Continue therapy to lower uric acid levels indefinitely. A common mistake is stopping treatment when uric acid level has normalized, which usually precipitates another attack.

Xanthine Oxidase Inhibitors

- **Allopurinol is currently the preferred agent** for lowering uric acid levels in patients with arthritis and/or kidney involvement. It is useful in patients with overproduction of uric acid and is also beneficial for tophaceous gout.
  - It **decreases urate production** by inhibiting the final step of urate synthesis and, thus, decreases uric acid levels, facilitating tophus mobilization.
  - **Allopurinol may also precipitate acute attacks** when started; therefore, continue prophylactic colchicine or NSAIDs for 2 weeks after initiation of allopurinol or change in allopurinol dose.
  - The initial dose is 100 mg PO qd. After 2 weeks, if the uric acid is still elevated, increase the dose to 300 mg qd. Further titration of allopurinol dose may be necessary depending on the uric acid levels. Because allopurinol is primarily cleared by the kidney, initial **doses must be adjusted in patients with renal insufficiency.**
  - Multiple drug interactions may occur with allopurinol, including azathioprine, probenecid, ampicillin, and cyclosporine.
  - The most common side effects of allopurinol are rash, diarrhea, nausea, liver dysfunction, and pruritus. **If a rash develops, stop the allopurinol immediately.** The rash may herald a more severe but rare (<1 case per 1000 patients treated) reaction especially in patients with renal insufficiency: exfoliative dermatitis, which can be accompanied by vasculitis, fever, liver dysfunction, eosinophilia, and acute interstitial nephritis. This **Stevens–Johnson syndrome** can carry a 25% mortality.
- **Febuxostat** is a newly developed and FDA-approved selective **inhibitor of xanthine oxidase** and is associated with a sharp reduction in serum uric acid levels.
  - Febuxostat produces a dose-dependent decrease in serum urate levels. A daily dose of 40 mg produces a reduction that is roughly equivalent to that seen in patients who are treated with allopurinol at a dose of 300 mg per day.[8] Febuxostat is started at a dose of 40 mg/day and can be increased to 80 mg/day if the goal uric acid is not achieved in 2 weeks on low dose 40 mg daily dose.
  - It has high bioavailability, and less than 5% is excreted as unchanged drug in the urine. No dose reduction of febuxostat is recommended in chronic kidney disease patients.
  - The place for febuxostat within the urate-lowering agents would be for patients showing intolerance to other urate lowering drugs, and those with severe gout in whom the target serum uric acid levels should be lower than usually targeted in order to deplete urate deposits rapidly.

Uricosuric Agents

- **Probenecid and sulfinpyrazone inhibit tubular reabsorption of urate.** These agents are ineffective if the serum creatinine level is >2 mg/dL. Do not use them if the patient has a history of **uric acid kidney stones,** low urinary flow (<1 mL/minute), or high levels of urine uric acid at baseline (>800 mg/24 hours).

- Before initiation of therapy, perform a 24-hour urine collection for creatinine and uric acid to determine if patient fits guidelines for use of uricosuric agents.
- Probenecid is started at 250 mg PO bid, and increments in dose are titrated according to the serum urate concentration. The dose is typically raised every several weeks to a maintenance dose of 500 to 1000 mg two or three times daily; the maximal effective dose is 3 g/day.
- Sulfinpyrazone, where available, is started at a dose of 50 mg twice daily, and increased in increments over several weeks to 100 to 200 mg three or four times daily as needed. The maximum effective dose of sulfinpyrazone is 800 mg/day.
- Advise the patient to maintain a daily urine output >2 L to avoid precipitation of uric acid stones. To decrease this risk, alkalinizing agents (potassium citrate) may be added. Potassium citrate can be used at 10 mEq PO tid. for target urinary citrate >320 mg/day, and urinary pH 6 to 7.
- Less potent uricosuric agents include the angiotensin 1 receptor antagonist **losartan,** and the lipid lowering agents **atorvastatin and fenofibrate.**

Other Urate Lowering Drugs

- **Pegloticase** is a new recombinant porcine PEGylated uricase developed for the treatment of refractory gout.
  - Uricase (urate oxidase) is the enzyme that catalyzes conversion of urate to a more soluble purine degradation product, allantoin. Uricase **is present in most mammals but is absent in humans.** Uricase is indicated as an alternative to xanthine oxidase inhibitors or uricosuric agents in gout patients intolerant of standard therapy.
  - Pegloticase is given as intravenous infusions at a dose of 8 mg every 2 weeks.[9] Gout flare prophylaxis is recommended at least 1 week prior to infusion and continuing for 6 months after the infusion. Side effects may include infusion reactions, development of low titer anti-PEG uricase antibodies, acute gout flares, nausea, and vomiting.
  - **Pegloticase is contraindicated in glucose-6-phosphate dehydrogenase (G6PD) deficiency due to the risk of hemolysis and methemoglobinemia.**
- Brief courses of **non-PEGylated recombinant uricase (rasburicase)** have been used for the prevention of acute uric acid nephropathy due to tumor lysis syndrome in patients with high risk lymphoma and leukemia. Severe hypersensitivity reactions have been reported. Experience with this agent for the treatment of gout is limited largely by the expectation that this unmodified foreign protein is likely to be more immunogenic than PEGylated uricases over the longer term of treatment needed for achieving the aims of gout management.[10]

OTHER NON-PHARMACOLOGICAL THERAPIES

- After the initial attack, educate the patient about weight loss and decreasing alcohol intake. In addition, reevaluate the patient's drug regimen.
- For example, if the patient is being treated with niacin for hypercholesterolemia or diuretics (especially thiazides) for hypertension, consider substitute medications.

REFERENCES

1. Schlesinger N, Norquist JM, Watson DJ. Serum urate during acute gout. *J Rheumatol.* 2009;36:1287–1289.
2. Martinon F, Pétrilli V, Mayor A, et al. Gout-associated uric acid crystals activate the NALP3 inflammasome. *Nature.* 2006;440:237–241.
3. Janssens HJ, Janssen M, van de Lisdonk EH, et al. Use of oral prednisolone or naproxen for the treatment of gout arthritis: a double-blind, randomised equivalence trial. *Lancet.* 2008;371:1854–1860.
4. Getting SJ, Christian HC, Flower RJ, et al. Activation of melanocortin type 3 receptor as a molecular mechanism for adrenocorticotropic hormone efficacy in gouty arthritis. *Arthritis Rheum.* 2002;46:2765–2775.
5. Terkeltaub RA, Furst DE, Bennett K, et al. High versus low dosing of oral colchicine for early acute gout flare: Twenty-four-hour outcome of the first multicenter, randomized, double-blind, placebo-controlled, parallel-group, dose-comparison colchicine study. *Arthritis Rheum.* 2010;62:1060–1068.
6. So A, De Smedt T, Revaz S, et al. A pilot study of IL-1 inhibition by anakinra in acute gout. *Arthritis Res Ther.* 2007;9:R28.
7. Zhang W, Doherty M, Bardin T, et al. EULAR standing committee for international clinical studies including therapeutics. EULAR evidence based recommendations for gout. Part II: Management. Report of a task force of the EULAR standing committee for international clinical studies including therapeutics (ESCISIT). *Ann Rheum Dis.* 2006;65:1312–1324.
8. Becker MA, Schumacher HR, Espinoza LR, et al. The urate-lowering efficacy and safety of febuxostat in the treatment of the hyperuricemia of gout: The CONFIRMS trial. *Arthritis Res Ther.* 2010;12:R63.
9. Sundy JS, Becker MA, Baraf HS, et al. Reduction of plasma urate levels following treatment with multiple doses of pegloticase (polyethylene glycol-conjugated uricase) in patients with treatment-failure gout: Results of a phase II randomized study. *Arthritis Rheum.* 2008; 58:2882–2891.
10. Richette P, Briere C, Hoenen-Clavert V, et al. Rasburicase for tophaceous gout not treatable with allopurinol: An exploratory study. *J Rheumatol.* 2007;34:2093–2098.

Calcium Pyrophosphate Dihydrate Crystal Deposition Disease

14

Amy Archer and Wayne M. Yokoyama

GENERAL PRINCIPLES

Definition

- Calcium pyrophosphate dihydrate (CPPD) crystal deposition disease is characterized by an inflammatory reaction to CPPD crystals in connective tissues.
- CPPD can affect ligaments, tendons, articular cartilage, and the synovium.
- It can have a clinical presentation that mimics other rheumatologic diseases such as gout, rheumatoid arthritis (RA), and osteoarthritis (OA).

Classification

- Asymptomatic
- Acute CPPD
  - "Pseudogout"
- Chronic CPPD
  - "Pseudo-osteoarthritis"
  - "Pseudo-rheumatoid"
  - "Pseudo-neuropathic"
  - Spinal involvement
  - Extra-articular

Epidemiology

- CPPD is **primarily a disease of the elderly.**
  - **Radiographic evidence** of CPPD deposition increases with age, reaching approximately 17% by age 80.
  - There is no predominance among a certain sex although subclassifications may have predilection toward females or males as noted below.

Etiology

- The majority of cases of CPPD are **idiopathic.**
- The occurrence of early onset CPPD is often related to the presence of risk factors or associated conditions.

Pathophysiology

- The pathologic formation of calcium pyrophosphate crystals is believed to be secondary to **high levels of calcium or inorganic pyrophosphate,** which can precipitate to form crystals in a conducive microenvironment.
- The primary components involved in crystal formation are chondrocytes, matrix, and, articular cartilage vesicles (ACVs).
- The crystal formation can be modulated by several factors including transforming growth factor beta (TGF-β), retinoic acid, nitric oxide, thyroid hormone, transglutaminase, and interleukin (IL)-1.

Risk Factors

- **The largest risk factor for CPPD is age.**
- **Joint trauma and/or surgery** have also been associated with an increased risk of developing CPPD.
- **Familial CPPD** has been linked to mutations in ankylosis, progressive homolog (mouse) (ANKH), which has been identified as a pyrophosphate transporter.

Prevention

It has been hypothesized that an increase in dietary calcium could help in the prevention of CPPD.[1]

Associated Conditions

- Hereditary **hemochromatosis, hyperparathyroidism, hypomagnesaemia, and OA** have been shown to be associated with CPPD. In addition, Gitelman's or Bartter's syndromes that cause **hypomagnesaemia** are also associated with CPPD.[2]
- Pseudogout has been reported to be associated with **bisphosphonates, joint injections of hyaluronate, and parathyroidectomy.**[3–5]

DIAGNOSIS

Clinical Presentation

Asymptomatic CPPD

- Identified when calcium pyrophosphate crystals are seen incidentally in cartilage on radiographs.
- This finding is termed **chondrocalcinosis.**

Acute CPPD/Pseudogout

- Acute CPPD is **more common in men.**
- Attacks may be precipitated by severe illness, trauma, or surgery.
- It manifests as severe, **sudden-onset mono- or oligoarthritis with erythema, swelling, and pain.**
- Acute attacks can involve any joint but **most frequently affects the knee** (50% of cases). Subacute attacks can involve more than one joint.
- Acute CPPD can be associated with fever, leukocytosis, and an increased erythrocyte sedimentation rate (ESR).

Chronic CPPD

- **"Pseudo-osteoarthritis" or "pseudo-OA"**
  - Pseudo-OA is **more common in women.**
  - It can present as a **slowly progressive joint pain that may affect multiple joints.**
  - The patient's chronic disease course may be punctuated by acute attacks similar to gout.
  - There is involvement of **joints that are not typically associated with OA** (e.g., wrists, shoulders, and ankles).
- **"Pseudorheumatoid" arthritis**
  - "Pseudorheumatoid" arthritis occurs in less than 5% of patients with CPPD.
  - Patients will typically present with **symmetric joint involvement and prominent systemic complaints** (e.g., morning stiffness and fatigue).

TABLE 14-1	DIAGNOSTIC CRITERIA FOR CALCIUM PYROPHOSPHATE DIHYDRATE DEPOSITION DISEASE (PSEUDOGOUT)

Criteria

I Definitive identification of calcium pyrophosphate crystals in tissue or synovial fluid (by x-ray diffraction or chemical analysis)

IIa Detection of rhomboidal (monoclinic or triclinic) crystals that are either weakly positive or have no birefringence

IIb Demonstration of classic radiographic findings (e.g., chondrocalcinosis, etc.)

IIIa Acute arthritis, especially that which involves large joints

IIIb Chronic arthritis, particularly if the course is punctuated with acute exacerbations and involves the knee, hip, wrist, carpus, elbow, shoulder, or metacarpophalangeal joint

Categories
Definitive: I OR IIa PLUS IIb
Probable: IIa OR IIb
Possible: IIIa OR IIIb

Adapted from: McCarty DJ. Calcium pyrophosphate dihydrate crystal deposition disease: nomenclature and diagnostic criteria. *Ann Intern Med.* 1977;87:241–242.

○ Patients' joints will exhibit **synovial thickening, local edema, flexion contractures, and decreased range of motion.**
- **"Pseudoneuropathic arthritis"**
  ○ Reports describe patients that will present with a **severe destructive and painful monoarthritis,** which is not associated with neurological abnormalities
- **Spinal involvement**
  ○ The presentation may mimic polymyalgia rheumatica (PMR).[6]
  ○ **Cervical spine involvement** is more unusual than the lumbar spine but is believed to be an under-recognized etiology of acute neck pain.[7]
  ○ Cases of cervical cord compression secondary to CPPD have been reported, particularly in older women.
- **Extra-articular CPPD**
  ○ The eye and the spleen have been reported as extra-articular manifestations.

Diagnostic Criteria

Diagnostic criteria for CPPD are presented in Table 14-1.[8]

Differential Diagnosis

- Infection, RA, OA, neuropathic joint disease, trauma, other crystal-associated diseases (e.g., gout, basic calcium phosphate crystal deposition), and malignancy should be considered in the appropriate clinical setting.
- It is important to realize that CPPD is not mutually exclusive to the alternative diagnoses stated above.

Diagnostic Testing

Laboratories

- Screening for the metabolic diseases mentioned above may be appropriate after CPPD diagnosis, particularly in young patients or patients with severe arthritis.
- Check calcium, phosphorus, magnesium, alkaline phosphatase, ferritin, iron, total iron-binding capacity, and thyroid stimulating hormone (TSH) levels.

Imaging

Plain Radiographs

- **Chondrocalcinosis**
  - ○ Chondrocalcinosis represents the accumulation of calcium salt in cartilaginous tissue, but can be found in the articular or periarticular regions. It can be visualized in the absence of an arthropathy.
  - ○ It is classically seen on radiographs in fibrocartilage (knee menisci, triangular ligament of the wrist, symphysis pubis, glenohumeral joint) but may be seen in hyaline and articular cartilage, as well as joint capsules and tendon insertion sites (Achilles, quadriceps).
  - ○ **Fibrocartilage calcification** appears as shaggy and irregular radiodense areas that are typically in the center of the joint. **Hyaline cartilage calcifications** are represented as a parallel thin line in close proximity to the subchondral bone. **Synovial calcification** usually appears as an amorphous opacity in the joint margin. **Tendon calcifications** are thin and linear.
- **Structural Joint Changes**
  - ○ CPPD can be associated with **subchondral sclerosis, subchondral cyst formation, and joint space narrowing.** Although the findings are also seen in osteoarthritis, the location may help differentiate the two diseases.
  - ○ Unlike RA, CPPD **does not have typical bony erosions.**

Ultrasound

- There is increasing utilization of ultrasound to differentiate between CPPD and gout.
- Calcium pyrophosphate crystals can appear as a thin hyperechoic band parallel to the hyaline cartilage, a punctate collection of hyperechoic spots in fibrous cartilage and tendons, or a nodular or oval shape of the hyperechoic densities that are often mobile in the bursa or articular recesses.
- Initial studies suggest a sensitivity and specificity as high as 86.7% and 96.4% respectively.[9]

Alternative Imaging

- Calcifications can be visualized on CT but it is not typically utilized in the assessment of an arthropathy. However, it is the preferred method of identifying calcium deposits in the upper cervical spine and craniovertebral junction.
- Although MRI is often utilized to evaluate a painful joint, it can be difficult to visualize the calcifications.

Diagnostic Procedures

Arthrocentesis

- In an acute attack, the typical synovial **leukocytes** count is 15,000–30,000 cells/mm³, with a neutrophilic predominance.
- CPPD crystals show **positive birefringence** that may vary in intensity (weak to none). They are smaller than urate crystals, frequently intracellular, vary in

shape **from needle to rhomboid** (monoclinic or triclinic crystal structure) and are usually **more difficult to find**. In addition, they can appear in the presence of urate crystals.
- CPPD crystals can be visualized from joints aspirated between acute attacks.
- Even if crystals are seen, it is important to send synovial fluid for culture to **rule out coincident infection.**

Paraffin Embedded Tissue
- CPPD crystals classically appear as amorphous basophilic to amphophilic material that can be surrounded by foreign body giant cell reaction.
- Nonaqueous alcoholic eosin staining allows for the observation of positive birefringence that may not be present on routine hematoxylin and eosin stain slides.

TREATMENT

- Therapeutics are targeted at controlling symptoms.
- The basis for the majority of the treatment options are based on case reports and expert opinion.

Medications

Acute Symptomatic Treatment
- **Nonsteroidal antiinflammatory drugs (NSAIDs)** are frequently utilized if they are tolerated and renal function is normal.
- **Oral or intra-articular corticosteroids** are sometimes needed for severe cases but should be held until infection is ruled out.

Recurrent/Chronic Symptom Treatment
- **Colchicine** (0.6 mg qd or bid) may decrease the frequency of attacks.
- **Methotrexate** (5–20 mg/week) and hydroxychloroquine may be considered in resistant cases.[10,11]
- **Anakinra,** an IL-1 inhibitor, is a novel therapy that may also be utilized in refractory cases at the dosage of 100 mg subcutaneously per day, or three times a week with hemodialysis treatment.[12]

Other Non-pharmacologic Therapies

- Joint aspiration usually provides some pain relief in acute cases.
- Omega-3 polyunsaturated fatty acid (PUFA) supplementation has been reported to improve symptoms in some patients with general inflammatory joint pain.[13]

Surgical Management

In the cases of spinal CPPD disease that are complicated compressive cervical myelopathy, surgical decompression is performed.

REFERENCES

1. Zhang Y, Terkeltaub R, Nevitt M, et al. Lower prevalence of chondrocalcinosis in Chinese subjects in Beijing than in white subjects in the United States: The Beijing Osteoarthritis Study. *Arthritis Rheum.* 2006;54:3508–3512.

2. Richette P, Ayoub G, Lahalle S, et al. Hypomagnesemia associated with chondrocalcinosis: A cross-sectional study. *Arthritis Rheum.* 2007;57:1496–1501.

3. Doshi J, Wheatley H. Pseudogout: An unusual and forgotten metabolic sequela of parathyroidectomy. *Head Neck.* 2008;30:1650–1653.

4. Ali Y, Weinstein M, Jokl P. Acute pseudogout following intra-articular injection of high molecular weight hyaluronic acid. *Am J Med.* 1999;107:641–642.

5. Young-Min SA, Herbert L, Dick M, et al. Weekly alendronate-induced acute pseudogout. *Rheumatology.* 2005;44:131–132.

6. Salaffi F, Carotti M, Guglielmi G, et al. The crowned dens syndrome as a cause of neck pain: Clinical and computed tomography study in patients with calcium pyrophosphate dihydrate deposition disease. *Clin Exp Rheumatol.* 2008;26:1040–1046.

7. Sekijima Y, Yoshida T, Ikeda S. CPPD crystal deposition disease of the cervical spine: A common cause of acute neck pain encountered in the neurology department. *J Neurol Sci.* 2010;296:79–82.

8. McCarty DJ. Calcium pyrophosphate dihydrate crystal deposition disease: nomenclature and diagnostic criteria. *Ann Intern Med.* 1977;87:241–242.

9. Filippou G, Frediani B, Gallo A, et al. A "new" technique for the diagnosis of chondrocalcinosis of the knee: Sensitivity and specificity of high-frequency ultrasonography. *Ann Rheum Dis.* 2007;66:1126–1128.

10. Chollet-Janin A, Finckh A, Dudler J, et al. Methotrexate as an alternative therapy for chronic calcium pyrophosphate deposition disease: An exploratory analysis. *Arthritis Rheum.* 2007;56:688–692.

11. Rothschild B, Yakubov LE. Prospective 6-month, double-blind trial of hydroxychloroquine treatment of CPDD. *Compr Ther.* 1997;23:327–331.

12. McGonagle D, Tan AL, Madden J, et al. Successful treatment of resistant pseudogout with anakinra. *Arthritis Rheum.* 2008;58:631–633.

13. Goldberg RJ, Katz J. A meta-analysis of the analgesic effects of omega-3 polyunsaturated fatty acid supplementation for inflammatory joint pain. *Pain.* 2007;129:210–223.

Undifferentiated Spondyloarthritis

Kristine A. Kuhn and Wayne M. Yokoyama

GENERAL PRINCIPLES

- A group of clinically related disorders were previously known as the **serone-gative spondyloarthropathies,** reflecting the absence of rheumatoid factor and primary involvement of the axial skeleton (spondylopathy) with less prominent involvement of the peripheral joints. These disorders can be contrasted with rheumatoid arthritis (RA) which is typically rheumatoid factor (RF) positive with prominent involvement of the peripheral joints and rare involvement of the axial skeleton. These diseases have recently been renamed **spondyloarthritides** (SpAs) to reflect the inflammatory nature of the disease.[1]
- SpAs are often associated with **HLA-B27.**
- There are five types of SpA: ankylosing spondyloarthritis (AS), psoriatic arthritis (PsA), reactive arthritis (ReA), enteropathic arthritis, and undifferentiated spondyloarthritis (USpA). This chapter focuses on USpA; the other types of SpA are discussed in the following chapters.

Definition

Patients with SpA who do not meet the criteria for AS, PsA, ReA, or enteropathic arthritis but meet criteria for SpA (see below) are considered to have USpA.

Classification

- Common features among the classification criteria for SpA include:
  - Age of onset <45 years old.
  - **Inflammatory back pain** present >3 months, defined as insidious onset, improves with exercise (but not rest), and morning **stiffness. Sacroiliitis** may be a component.
  - **Peripheral arthritis,** usually asymmetric and involving the lower extremities.
  - **Enthesopathy,** which is inflammation of tendon and ligament insertions into bone. This may result in **dactylitis,** or a "sausage-digit."
  - **Family history** of SpA.
  - History of associated diseases such as **psoriasis, inflammatory bowel disease,** or **urethritis, cervicitis,** or **diarrhea** within one month before the onset of arthritis, which would classify the SpA as PsA, enteropathic arthritis, or ReA, respectively.
- Assessment of SpondyloArthritis International Society (ASAS, Table 15-1)[1] have improved sensitivity and specificity over previous criteria sets, particularly for early disease. Separate criteria exist for axial and peripheral SpA.[1,2]

TABLE 15-1	ASAS CLASSIFICATION CRITERIA FOR AXIAL AND PERIPHERAL SPONDYLOARTHRITIS

Axial Spondyloarthritis		Peripheral Spondyloarthritis	
Back pain ≥3 mo. Age at onset <45 years old. AND either column below:		Arthritis, enthesitis, or dactylitis AND either column below:	
HLA-B27 AND ≥2 other SpA features: IBP Arthritis Enthesitis Uveitis Dactylitis Psoriasis IBD Good response to NSAIDs FHx HLA-B27 Elevated CRP	Sacroiliitis on imaging: Active inflammation on MRI OR Radiographic sacroiliitis (grade 2 if bilateral, grade 3 if unilateral) AND ≥ 1 other SpA feature	≥1 SpA feature: Uveitis Psoriasis IBD Preceding infection HLA-B27 Sacroiliitis on imaging	≥2 other SpA features: Arthritis Enthesitis Dactylitis IBP ever FHx of SpA

ASAS, Assessment of SpondyloArthritis international Society; CRP, C-reactive protein; FHx, family history; IBD, inflammatory bowel disease; IBP, inflammatory back pain; nonsteroidal anti-inflammatory drugs, NSAIDs; SpA, spondyloarthritis.

Adapted from: Rudwaleit M, van der Heijde D, Landewé; R, et al. The development of Assessment of SpondyloArthritis international Society classification criteria for axial spondyloarthritis (part II): validation and final selection. *Ann Rheum Dis* 2009;68:777–783.

Epidemiology

- Of the subtypes of SpA, **AS is the most prevalent followed by USpA.**
- The prevalence of HLA-B27 within patient populations with SpA ranges 50% to 95%.
- SpAs occur in about 2% of the general population and in just over 10% of HLA-B27 positive individuals.
- The frequency of HLA-B27 in the general Western European population is about 10%, but the rate fluctuates based on the population studied.

Etiology

- At present, the etiology of SpA is not known but several observations suggest it likely results from a combination of genetic risk factors and an environmental trigger.
  - The most studied genetic risk factor for SpA is HLA-B27. HLA-B27 positivity carries a 20-fold increased risk for SpA but only explains about one-third of the genetic risk for disease.
  - Other genes associated with USpA include the genes for chemokine receptor type 4 (CXCR4), interleukin (IL)-1β, IL-8, and integrin-1. Other genes are being identified and risk assessed in genome-wide association scans.

- Specific environmental triggers have not been identified, but SpA is associated with prior enteropathic illnesses (reactive SpA) and IBD, suggesting possible links to gastrointestinal (GI) flora. Moreover, animal models that have suggested enterobacterial infections may elicit disease in a favorable genetic setting.

Pathophysiology

- Two major observations support the concept that SpAs are immune-mediated diseases.
- SpAs associated with HLA-B27 possibly result from the presentation of "**arithrogenic**" **peptides** to T cells. Alternatively, **enterobacterial antigens** may carry sequence homology with HLA-B27 subtypes, suggesting that HLA-B27 itself may be recognized.
  - Either possibility is supported by animal studies: Mice transgenic for HLA-B27 can develop enthesopathy and ankylosis similar to human AS; however, in germ-free environments, these mice do not develop disease.
- Tumor necrosis factor (TNF)-α appears central to the pathology of SpA because TNF blockade ameliorates disease activity of most forms of SpA. TNF may act through several mechanisms because it:
  - Stimulates production of adhesion molecules and recruitment of inflammatory cells.
  - Activates T cells and production of other inflammatory cytokines.
  - Induces expression of vascular endothelial growth factor and matrix metalloproteinases that lead to angiogenesis and bone erosions.
  - Stimulates production of receptor activator of nuclear factor kappa-B ligand (RANKL) resulting in osteoclast maturation.

DIAGNOSIS

- Diagnosis of SpA relies upon clinical presentation and imaging.
- Classification criteria (Table 15-1) provide a guide to the diagnosis of SpA but it should be emphasized that they were developed for purposes of unifying clinical studies. They may be less helpful in an individual patient, particularly when seen just once early in the disease.

Clinical Presentation

- Clinical manifestations include **inflammatory back pain, sacroiliitis, peripheral arthritis, enthesitis,** and **anterior uveitis. Cardiovascular** involvement is a relatively rare, late manifestation.
- The majority of patients present **before the age of** 45.
- The highest likelihood ratios for disease include inflammatory back pain lasting longer than 3 months, positive MRI findings, and positive HLA-B27 status.

History

- A thorough history will elicit symptoms of inflammatory back pain such as **morning stiffness,** improvement of pain with activity and worsening with rest, and insidious onset. **Alternating buttock pain** may be present.
- Additional articular symptoms include:
  - **Peripheral, asymmetric inflammatory arthritis,** usually in the lower limbs and usually oligoarticular.
  - **Enthesitis,** which can lead to dactylitis, plantar fasciitis, and Achilles' tendinitis.

- Extra-articular symptoms may identify the type of SpA:
  - **Psoriasis** (PsA).
  - **Symptoms of inflammatory bowel disease or infectious diarrhea** (enteropathic arthritis or ReA, respectively).
  - **Urethritis or cervicitis** (ReA), often asymptomatic in women.
  - **Uveitis** typically causing eye pain with exposure to bright lights.
- A family history of SpA or related disease such as psoriasis or inflammatory bowel disease may suggest SpA.

Physical Examination
- The musculoskeletal examination can be divided into the axial skeleton and peripheral joints.
  - Within the **axial skeleton,** early findings are **reduced lateral spinal flexion, chest expansion, and cervical rotation.** Restriction of spinal mobility and kyphosis are more advanced findings.
  - **Peripheral joint findings** include swelling, effusions, erythema, reduced range of motion, and dactylitis.
- The **skin** should be thoroughly assessed for evidence of psoriasis, including small patches in the umbilicus or gluteal fold. Dermatology referral and skin biopsy may need to be considered.
- Referral to an ophthalmologist may be required for evaluation for uveitis.

Diagnostic Criteria
- Many refer to the classification criteria to aid in diagnosis of SpA.
- Strictly, a diagnosis of USpA is given when a patient meets the classification criteria for SpA but not specific criteria for AS, PsA, ReA, or enteropathic arthritis.

Differential Diagnosis
- **Mechanical back pain** is the most common cause of lower back pain. Typically, its symptoms are **acute onset,** often with an inciting event, and pain that is **worse with exercise** and relieved by rest. Contrast these symptoms with the classical symptoms of SpA. Only 5% of patients seen in a primary care setting with chronic low back pain are ultimately diagnosed with SpA.
- For inflammatory back pain, the differential diagnosis includes the five types of SpA.
- Peripheral inflammatory arthritis may be infectious arthritis, seronegative RA, systemic lupus erythematosus (SLE), or undifferentiated connective tissue disease (CTD).

Diagnostic Testing
Laboratories
- The serum acute phase reactants such as erythrocyte sedimentation rate (ESR) and C-reactive protein (CRP) are of limited use to follow disease activity as they have poor sensitivity and specificity.
- HLA-B27 testing is included in the ASAS classification criteria. However, given that SpA occurs in only approximately 10% of HLA-B27 individuals, the positive predictive value for disease is relatively low. Thus, **HLA-B27 testing is generally not clinically useful by itself.**

Imaging

- **Plain radiography** of the sacroiliac joints is included in the classification criteria for SpA.
  - Definite sacroiliitis can be difficult to evaluate and requires expertise.
  - When present it carries nearly 80% specificity.
  - However, structural damage appears late in disease.
  - Only 30% of patients with early disease have radiographic changes; thus, it has a poor sensitivity in early disease.
- **MRI** has emerged as a valuable tool for the assessment of early SpA.
  - **Bone marrow edema and fat infiltration** on MRI are signs of inflammation with about 60% sensitivity for early sacroiliitis.[3]
  - However, over 20% of patients with mechanical low back pain and healthy individuals have inflammatory features on MRI as well.[4]
  - Further, not all patients with evidence of sacroiliitis on MRI will develop radiographic evidence. The positive predictive value of MRI for the development of sacroiliitis on radiographs several years later is less than 20%.
  - Therefore, the patient's history and examination remain critical in interpreting the results from MRI.

TREATMENT

Medications

- Pharmacologic treatment of SpA varies on the type. For USpA, treatment is based on whether symptoms are predominantly axial, in which therapy will be most similar to that for AS, or peripheral, in which therapy is similar to PsA.
- Most clinical trials evaluating the efficacy of medications for the treatment of SpA have focused on either AS or PsA; little data exist to support specific treatments for USpA.

Nonsteroidal Antiinflammatory Drugs

- First line treatment of SpA is **nonsteroidal antiinflammatory drugs (NSAIDs) for either axial or peripheral disease.**
- These agents decrease inflammation and control pain but do not alter the underlying course of disease.
- Initially indomethacin was the preferred agent, but any NSAID can be effective.
- NSAIDs work quickly, with improvement in morning stiffness and pain within 48 hours. Conversely, stiffness and pain return quickly, within 48 hours, after discontinuation of the NSAID.
- In the case of inefficacy, trial of an alternate NSAID is indicated before changing class of agents.
- Use of NSAIDs is limited by side effects of GI intolerance and increased risk of cardiovascular events.

Oral Disease-Modifying Antirheumatic Drugs

- Oral disease-modifying antirheumatic drugs (DMARDs) have limited efficacy in axial SpA, although **methotrexate, sulfasalazine, leflunomide, and azathioprine** have been used. There are conflicting data on the efficacy of these agents.[5]
- Sulfasalazine and methotrexate are commonly used for the treatment of peripheral SpAs; again the data regarding efficacy of these agents in USpA are lacking.

TABLE 15-2	BATH ANKYLOSING SPONDYLITIS DISEASE ACTIVITY INDEX (BASDAI)

The following questions are rated on a scale of 0 (none)–10 (very severe):

1. How would you describe the overall level of fatigue/tiredness you have experienced?
2. How would you describe the overall level of inflammatory neck, back, or hip pain you have had?
3. How would you describe the overall level of pain/swelling in joints other than neck, back or hips you have had?
4. How would you describe the overall level of discomfort you have had from any areas tender to touch or pressure?
5. How would you describe the overall level of morning stiffness you have had from the time you wake up?
6. How long does your morning stiffness last from the time you wake up? (0 minute = 0 score, 1 hour = 5, 2 hours = 10)

Scoring:

1. Add the scores for questions 1–4.
2. Add the scores for questions 5 & 6 and divide by 2.
3. Add the results from steps 1 & 2 and divide by 5 for the final BASDAI score.

Interpretation:

Score >4 suggests suboptimal control of disease.

—

Adapted from: Garrett S, Jenkinson T, Kennedy LG, et al. A new approach to defining disease status in ankylosing spondylitis: the Bath Ankylosing Spondylitis Disease Activity Index. *J Rheumatol* 1994;21:2286–2291.

Antitumor Necrosis Factor Agents

- **Etanercept, infliximab, and adalimumab** have been demonstrated to be effective in the treatment of SpA. Few patients with USpA have been evaluated in trials utilizing these agents for SpA and thus the long-term efficacy is unknown. Nevertheless, of the few patients evaluated, antitumor necrosis factor (anti-TNF) agents have been demonstrated to improve in axial and peripheral symptoms. However, **they do not alter the potential for progression of radiographic disease,** as they do in RA.
- Anti-TNF agents have also been demonstrated to have good efficacy in controlling extra-articular manifestations.
- International ASAS and US consensus guidelines for the use of anti-TNF agents in AS suggest use of these agents when patients have severe disease (Bath Ankylosing Spondylitis Disease Activity Index score >4, see Monitoring/Follow-Up and Table 15-2) and have failed NSAIDs. As a significant number of patients with USpA progress to AS the same guidelines are appropriate for use of anti-TNF agents in USpA.

Analgesics and Glucocorticoids

- **Analgesic** medications are often needed for pain control. Opiates carry high risk of addiction in these patients with a chronic disease.

- Systemic glucocorticoids have historically been felt to be ineffective for the treatment of SpA; however, **intra-articular and systemic corticosteroids** may be useful in cases of peripheral joint involvement. They have minimal efficacy in axial disease.

Other Non-Pharmacologic Therapies

- **Physical therapy and exercise** are mainstays for all SpAs.
- A combination of an exercise program with pharmacologic agents has been shown to be more effective than pharmacologic treatment alone.
- Extension exercises are preferred.[6]

Surgical Management

- **Surgical intervention** may be required to treat late manifestations of axial disease such as deformities, traumatic fractures, and radiculopathy.[7]
  - Corrective surgery for kyphosis of the lumbar spine and cervicothoracic junction can improve field-of-vision, swallowing function, gait stability, axial pain, and radiculopathy symptoms.
  - Decompression surgery such as laminectomy is warranted in some cases of symptomatic spinal stenosis and cauda equina syndrome.
  - Three column fractures are stabilized with instrumentation.
- Peripheral joint arthroplasty, fusion, or soft tissue release for contractures is indicated when there is significant joint pain unresolved by medical treatment or loss of function.

COMPLICATIONS

- Complications of SpA result from long-standing inflammation affecting the target joint(s).
  - In the case of axial USpA, 30% to 60% of patients will ultimately develop AS. As a result, these patients may develop **ankylosis** of the spine and major joints (hips, shoulders) and **decreased chest wall expansion,** which may cause restrictive lung disease.
  - **Radiculopathies** can also result from ankylosis of the spine.
  - Inflammatory arthritis and enthesitis of peripheral joints may lead to joint erosions and/or ankylosis of the affected joint.
- **Extra-articular manifestations** may result in other complications.
  - **Uveitis** can lead to vision loss.
  - Late **cardiac complications** include aortic dilation, aortic and mitral regurgitation, atrioventricular conduction blocks, and arrhythmias.
  - **Restrictive lung disease** may develop due to late stage stenosis of costovertebral and costosternal joints in AS but typically not in other SpA.
  - Bilateral **apical pulmonary fibrosis** may develop
  - **Renal amyloidosis** may develop
- Pharmacologic treatments also have side effects that may lead to other complications. See Chap. 9, Drugs Used for the Treatment of Rheumatic Diseases for further discussion.

REFERRAL

- Patients with chronic back pain lasting longer than three months and one or more of the following should be referred to a rheumatologist:
  - Inflammatory back pain.
  - HLA-B27 positivity.
  - Sacroiliitis on imaging.
  - Refractory peripheral arthritis.

PATIENT EDUCATION

- Patients should be educated on the manifestations, complications, and therapeutic options of their disease.
- Additionally the benefits of exercise and physical therapy for improving functional status and limiting pain should be emphasized.

MONITORING/FOLLOW-UP

- As noted above, monitoring serum acute phase reactants is of limited value for assessing disease activity.
- Rather, disease activity should be monitored based on clinical features of morning stiffness, pain, physical examination, and imaging when indicated.
  - The Bath Ankylosing Spondylitis Disease Activity Index (BASDAI, Table 15-2) was developed for assessment of symptoms for clinical trials; however, it can serve as a guide for monitoring disease activity in a clinical setting.[8]
- Monitoring for development of late cardiovascular, pulmonary and renal complications is warranted.
- Monitoring of pharmacologic agents is discussed in Chapter 9.

OUTCOME/PROGNOSIS

- Prospective studies over a duration of 10 years have shown that, in patients classified as USpA, up to 40% will go into remission and 30–60% will meet criteria for AS.
- The outcome and prognosis of AS is discussed in Chap. 16, Ankylosing Spondylitis.

REFERENCES

1. Rudwaleit M, van der Heijde D, Landewé R, et al. The development of Assessment of SpondyloArthritis international Society classification criteria for axial spondyloarthritis (part II): validation and final selection. *Ann Rheum Dis.* 2009;68:777–783.
2. Rudwaleit M, van der Heijde D, Landewé R, et al. The Assessment of SpondyloArthritis international Society classification criteria for peripheral spondyloarthritis and for spondyloarthritis in general. *Ann Rheum Dis.* 2011;70:25–31.
3. Heuft-Dorenbosch L, Landewé R, Weijers R, et al. Combining information obtained from magnetic resonance imaging and conventional radiographs to detect sacroiliitis in patients with recent onset inflammatory back pain. *Ann Rheum Dis.* 2006;65:804–808.

4. Weber U, Hodler J, Kubik RA, et al. Sensitivity and specificity of spinal inflammatory lesions assessed by whole-body magnetic resonance imaging in patients with ankylosing spondylitis or recent-onset inflammatory back pain. *Arthritis Rheum.* 2009;61:900–908.

5. Kabasakal Y, Kitapcioglu G, Yargucu F, et al. Efficacy of SLZ and MTX (alone or combination) on the treatment of active sacroiliitis in early AS. *Rheumatol Int.* 2009;29:1523–1527.

6. Ortancil O, Sarikaya S, Sapmaz P, et al. The effect(s) of a six-week home-based exercise program on the respiratory muscle and functional status in ankylosing spondylitis. *J Clin Rheumatol.* 2009;15:68–70.

7. Etame AB, Than KD, Wang AC, et al. Surgical management of symptomatic cervical or cervicothoracic kyphosis due to ankylosing spondylitis. *Spine.* 2008;33:E559–E564.

8. Garrett S, Jenkinson T, Kennedy LG, et al. A new approach to defining disease status in ankylosing spondylitis: the Bath Ankylosing Spondylitis Disease Activity Index. *J Rheumatol.* 1994;21:2286–2291.

Ankylosing Spondylitis

16

Lesley Davila and Wayne M. Yokoyama

GENERAL PRINCIPLES

Ankylosing spondylitis (AS) belongs to a group of clinical disorders characterized by prominent involvement of the axial skeleton, known as the spondyloarthritides (SpAs).

Definition
- AS is an inflammatory arthritis causing back pain and progressive stiffness of the spine.
- It involves the sacroiliac (SI) joints and the articular joints of the spine.
- Additionally, AS may be associated with peripheral arthritis of the knees, hips, and shoulders as well as extra-articular manifestations involving the eyes, heart, and lungs.
- AS may be difficult to distinguish from the other SpAs.
  - If the patient has psoriasis, a recent history of enteric or genitourinary infection, or inflammatory bowel disease, the patient is considered to have psoriatic arthritis, reactive arthritis, or enteropathic arthritis, respectively, rather than AS.
  - Some patients do not meet the classification criteria for AS (see below), in which case they are considered to have undifferentiated spondyloarthritis. These disorders are discussed separately in their respective chapters.

Epidemiology
- AS occurs with a male to female ratio of approximately 2 to 3:1. The age of onset is most often <40 years, with peak incidence between the ages of 20 and 30. The prevalence of AS ranges from 0% to 1.4% with a wide variation noted in different ethnic populations.
- **HLA-B27** is well known to be associated with AS; the primary reason for ethnic variation relates to the expression of HLA-B27.
  - In the United States, HLA-B27 is more common in whites of Northern European descent and less common in blacks.
  - In white males, 80% to 95% of AS patients express HLA-B27.
  - The prevalence of AS in HLA-B27-positive individuals is estimated to be 10% to 20%.
  - Like all of the seronegative spondyloarthropathies, AS has a strong familial aggregation; however, HLA-B27 confers only about 30% of the genetic risk, suggesting other genes may also predispose to AS.

Pathophysiology
- The etiology of AS is unknown. However, the strong association with HLA-B27 suggests an immune-dependent component. Other evidence, particularly response to therapy with antitumor necrosis factor (anti-TNF) agents, supports

a role for inflammatory cytokines in disease pathogenesis. Chapter 15, Undifferentiated Spondyloarthritis discusses this in more detail.

- Pathologically the differentiating feature of AS from rheumatoid arthritis (RA) is its predominant involvement of the **entheses** (where ligaments, tendons, and joint capsules attach to bone) instead of the synovium. Histologically, synovitis and enthesitis in AS are difficult to distinguish from that of RA.

DIAGNOSIS

Clinical Presentation

- The key to diagnosing AS is having a high index of suspicion in young to middle-aged patients who complain of inflammatory-type back pain.
- Direct further history and physical examination at pursuing this diagnosis.
- Family history of similar complaints or rheumatologic diseases is important.

History

- Patients typically complain of **low back pain and stiffness.** The pain is inflammatory in nature (e.g., insidious onset without trauma, exacerbation of pain with rest, and improvement with activity). The pain may wake the patient at night. A warm shower, exercise, and antiinflammatory drugs usually provide some relief.
- **Sacroiliitis,** a common initial feature, can present with pain in the buttock, typically alternating sides, and radiating down the thigh posteriorly.
- Occasionally **uveitis, enthesitis, or oligoarticular arthritis** may be the presenting symptom.
- Symptoms progress gradually over a period of months to years and, over time, may lead to significant spinal deformities and loss of range of motion of the neck and/or lower back.

Physical Examination

- Significant morbidity and physical disability result from flattening of the lumbar lordosis, kyphosis of the thoracic spine, flexion of the cervical spine, and flexion contractures in the pelvis and knee joints.
- The physical examination should include **evaluation of range of motion** of the spine.
  - One measure is the modified **Schober's test:** Make marks 10 cm above and 5 cm below the level of the sacral dimples (approximately L5). Next, have the patient maximally reach for the floor without bending his or her knees. The distance between these two marks should increase from 15 cm to ≥20 cm if normal spinal motion is present.
  - **Evaluate lateral rotation and lateral flexion** of the spine in both directions as well. Lateral rotation can be measured by the examiner standing behind the patient and placing examiner's hands on the patient's iliac crest then having the patient laterally rotate the shoulders. The plane of the shoulders should normally reach a 45-degree angle with respect to the plane of the pelvis. For lateral flexion, ask the patient to stand upright and laterally flex to the floor. The distance from fingertip of the middle finger to the floor can be measured and followed.
  - The **occiput to wall distance** can be measured by having the patient stand with both heels and buttocks against the wall, and measuring the gap between the occiput and the wall. The normal distance is zero, and increasing distance indicates loss of lumbar and cervical lordosis.

○ Evaluate **chest expansion** by measuring the circumference of the chest at the level of T4 at the end of both maximal inspiration and maximal expiration. Expansion should be >2.5 cm.

• Clinical examination for **sacroiliitis** is variable and generally does not contribute to the diagnosis.

• **Extra-articular manifestations** of AS include anterior uveitis, increased risk of fracture of the fused spine, C1–2 subluxation, and restrictive lung disease (mostly from stiffness of the chest wall, but these patients can also develop pulmonary fibrosis). Less common manifestations include cardiac abnormalities (including conduction abnormalities, myocardial dysfunction, or aortitis leading to aortic regurgitation), renal disease from nonsteroidal antiinflammatory drugs (NSAIDs) or amyloid deposition, and bowel mucosa ulcerations.

Diagnostic Criteria

• The New York criteria for AS, last revised in 1984, are commonly used to diagnose AS.[1] The criteria rely on both clinical and radiologic components.
  ○ The **clinical criteria** consist of the following three components:
    ■ **Low back pain and stiffness** of >3 months duration, improving with exercise but not relieved with rest.
    ■ **Limitation of motion** of the lumbar spine in both the sagittal and frontal planes.
    ■ Limitation of chest expansion relative to normal values corrected for age and gender.
  ○ The **radiographic criteria** consist of the following two components:
    ■ **Sacroiliitis** with more than minimum abnormality bilaterally.
    ■ Sacroiliitis of unequivocal abnormality unilaterally.
  ○ A patient is designated as having definite AS if at least one radiologic criterion and one clinical criterion are present. A patient is designated as having probable AS if three clinical criteria are present or if one of the radiologic criteria is present without any signs or symptoms of the clinical criteria.
  ○ In practice, these criteria are highly specific for AS, but they **lack sensitivity to serve as a reliable screening tool.** Therefore, AS is likely to be underdiagnosed if these criteria are strictly followed. Furthermore, these criteria fail to address the presence of familial associations, HLA-B27, or extra-articular manifestations of AS.

• The Assessment of SpondyloArthritis international Society (ASAS) classification criteria for axial spondyloarthritis are **useful for diagnosing early AS** and are described in Table 15-1.[2]

Differential Diagnosis

The differential diagnosis of AS includes noninflammatory causes of low back pain, other seronegative spondyloarthropathies (see Chapter 15, Undifferentiated Spondyloarthritis), other peripheral inflammatory arthritides, and diffuse idiopathic skeletal hyperostosis (DISH).

Diagnostic Testing

Laboratories

• Most laboratory tests for AS are nonspecific. Indicators of inflammation (e.g., elevated erythrocyte sedimentation rate [ESR] or C-reactive protein [CRP]) support the diagnosis but may not correlate with disease severity.

- Measurement of HLA-B27 may support the diagnosis and provide evidence of heritability, but in clinical practice it is only useful for ruling out the diagnosis if absent in white males.

Imaging
- **Radiographs** play an important role in the diagnosis of AS.
  - Anterior–posterior radiographs of the SI joints and other affected joints, including the spine or peripheral joints, are usually adequate and should be performed initially.
  - The modified Ferguson view of the SI joints may be useful (a posterior–anterior radiograph taken of the SI joints with the patient in the prone position and the x-ray tube angled 30 degrees obliquely).
  - Standardization of scoring systems for sacroiliitis has increased the reliability of x-rays for diagnosis. However, radiographs are less sensitive in early disease.
- **MRI** has a higher sensitivity and specificity for sacroiliitis, but is limited by cost. If the clinical suspicion for AS is high and plain radiographs are negative or unequivocal for sacroiliitis, an MRI of the SI joints is recommended.
  - CT is also sensitive for detection of sacroiliitis while offering the same degree of specificity. However, it does involve more radiation than MRI so it should probably be reserved for patients unable to undergo an MRI.
- **Sacroiliitis** in AS is typically bilateral and symmetric, as is the sacroiliitis associated with inflammatory bowel disease. By contrast, sacroiliitis in psoriatic and reactive arthritis is often asymmetric.
- In severe AS, radiographs of the spine may demonstrate ankylosis of the spine with **syndesmophytes** (osseous formations that attach to ligaments) and a **"bamboo spine"** appearance. Spinal involvement in AS is typically ascending without "skip" areas whereas discontinuous spinal involvement is more typical of psoriatic and reactive arthritis.
- MRI of the spine can provide an image of the amount of inflammation in the spine. Specialized techniques, such as STIR and T1 images obtained after contrast administration can detect inflammation with a high degree of specificity. Abnormalities on MRI include vertebral corner erosions and bone marrow edema. It is unclear if areas of inflammation on MRI correlate to ankylosis of the spine over time.

TREATMENT

- Treatment of AS is focused on providing symptomatic relief and returning the patient to best functional capacity, as well as preventing (as much as possible) the long-term consequences such as spinal fusion, peripheral joint destruction, and extra-articular manifestations.
- Combinations of medications, stretching, physical therapy, and/or surgical management are tailored to the individual patient to achieve these goals.

Medications
Nonsteroidal Antiinflammatory Drugs
- The first-line therapy for patients with AS is NSAIDs to limit symptoms of inflammatory arthritis and back pain.
- Classically, AS is treated with either indomethacin or naproxen but patient satisfaction should ultimately dictate which NSAID works best.

- Maximum doses of NSAIDs are generally required.
- Monitor NSAID-associated toxicities closely (see Chapter 9, Drugs Used in the Treatment of Rheumatic Diseases).
- One study showed a decrease in radiographic progression of spinal disease with the continuous use of NSAIDs, although these results have yet to be replicated.[3]

Oral Disease-Modifying Antirheumatic Drugs

- Peripheral joint symptoms have been successfully treated with escalating doses of **sulfasalazine.**
  ○ Sulfasalazine is initiated at a dose of 500 mg PO bid and is increased until a daily dose of 3 g is reached or toxicities prevent escalation.
  ○ At maximum tolerated doses, sulfasalazine has been shown to improve peripheral joint symptoms but has limited effects on axial symptoms.
  ○ Discontinue sulfasalazine if no response has been attained by 4 months or if severe toxicities occur.
  ○ Monitor patients periodically (at least every 3 months) for leukopenia and neutropenia.
- Traditional disease-modifying antirheumatic drugs (DMARDs) for RA such as oral **methotrexate and leflunomide** have been used for peripheral joint symptoms associated with AS.
  ○ Methotrexate has conflicting data regarding its efficacy and is not used frequently.
  ○ Leflunomide also has not been shown to be effective in treatment of AS.

Antitumor Necrosis Factor Agents and Other Biologics

- Recent studies have demonstrated significant symptomatic improvement with the use of **antitumor necrosis factor (anti-TNF) agents** in AS. Specifically, the anti-TNF agents **infliximab, etanercept, adalimumab, and golimumab** are approved by the FDA for AS and have been shown to significantly limit disease activity and signs of inflammation in early AS.
  ○ These are the only agents that significantly improve the axial symptoms (inflammatory back pain and morning stiffness).
  ○ They are commonly used as first line DMARD therapy for patients who do not respond to NSAIDs alone.
  ○ Although they significantly improve quality of life, the anti-TNF agents have not been shown to prevent or slow down spinal fusion although research in this area is ongoing.[4]
- Recent data have shown that **rituximab** may be efficacious in reducing disease activity in TNF-inhibitor naive patients, but not in those previously exposed to anti-TNF agents.[5] Randomized control studies have not yet been published.
- **Pamidronate** (an IV bisphosphonate) has also been studied in patients with AS and in a small study has shown to decrease disease activity in a dose-dependent fashion.[6]

Analgesics and Glucocorticoids

- Systemic corticosteroids are not routinely used in treatment of AS, unlike other inflammatory rheumatic disorders. However, **local injections of steroids** may provide symptomatic relief to patients with otherwise poorly controlled joint pain. Either blind injections of SI joints or radiographically guided injections can be used.

- Analgesics such as opiates are commonly needed to alleviate the pain caused by damaged joints and spinal fusion that occurs with prolonged disease.

Other Non-Pharmacologic Therapies

- All patients diagnosed with AS should be referred for **physical therapy** to initiate treatment with range of motion exercises and postural training.
  - Physical therapy can limit pain and improve functional status in most patients with AS.
  - Patients should be taught motion and flexibility exercises of the cervical, thoracic, and lumbar spine; stretching exercises for shortened muscles; and chest expansion exercises. Patients should be instructed to perform these exercises regularly at home.
- **Smoking cessation** should be encouraged in all patients with AS, as smoking is a predictor of worse outcome.

Surgical Management

- Surgery may be beneficial for AS patients with significant morbidity from skeletal deformities.
  - **Total hip arthroplasty** can improve pain and decreased mobility resulting from damaged hip joints. This surgery may be performed at a younger age (40–60 years) than in osteoarthritis patients to improve mobility and quality of life in patients with AS.
  - **Spinal fusion** can be considered in patients with unstable vertebral articulations (including atlanto-axial subluxation).
  - **Wedge osteotomies** can be performed for patients with severe flexion deformities, restoring their ability to look forward.
- Anesthesiologists should be made aware of the AS diagnosis in an AS patient undergoing general anesthesia because intubation may be difficult.

COMPLICATIONS

Complications of AS are identical to those discussed in Chapter 15, Undifferentiated Spondyloarthritis.

MONITORING/FOLLOW-UP

- Patients should be followed for development of worsened symptoms, physical deformity, and late complications (cardiovascular, pulmonary and medication related complications).
- Two **functional indexes** shown to be sensitive in detecting improvement or deterioration in clinical disease include the Bath Ankylosing Spondylitis Functional Index and the Dougados Functional Index.[7] While initially designed for assessment of symptoms in clinical trials, they can be used to monitor disease activity in a clinical setting.

OUTCOME/PROGNOSIS

- AS has not been associated with an increase in mortality but can produce significant morbidity if not recognized and treated appropriately.

- AS may progress to fusion of the entire axial skeleton at which point pain from spondyloarthritis itself frequently subsides. A complication of spinal fusion is **pseudoarthrosis** where a false "joint" is formed, frequently as a result of minor trauma. Clinical clues to pseudoarthrosis are increased local pain and enhanced spinal mobility. **Surgical referral is immediately recommended** because of possible spinal cord encroachment.
- Most patients with AS have mild to moderately severe disease, usually characterized by a chronic relapsing and remitting course.
  - ○ Severe AS occurs less commonly but produces significant morbidity related to axial skeletal fusion.
  - ○ One study has correlated seven **prognostic factors** with more severe disease.[8] The presence of hip arthritis was the most prognostic of a severe outcome. The other factors included ESR >30 mm/hour, dactylitis, oligoarthritis, decreased range of motion of the lumbar spine, limited efficacy of NSAIDs, and onset before age 16.

REFERENCES

1. Van der Linden S, Valkenburg HA, Cats A. Evaluation of diagnostic criteria for ankylosing spondylitis. A proposal for modification of the New York criteria. *Arthritis Rheum.* 1984;27:361–368.
2. Rudwaleit M, van der Heijde D, Landewé R, et al. The development of Assessment of SpondyloArthritis international Society classification criteria for axial spondyloarthritis (part II): Validation and final selection. *Ann Rheum Dis.* 2009;68:777–783.
3. Wanders A, Heijde D, Landewe R, et al. Nonsteroidal anti-inflammatory drugs reduce radiographic progression in patients with ankylosing spondylitis: A randomized clinical trial. *Arthritis Rheum.* 2005;52:1756–1765.
4. Van der Heijde D, Landewe R, Baraliakos X, et al. Radiographic findings following two years of infliximab therapy in patients with ankylosing spondylitis. *Arthritis Rheum.* 2008;58:3063–3070.
5. Song IH, Heldmann F, Rudwaleit M, et al. Different response to rituximab in tumor necrosis factor blocker-naive patients with active ankylosing spondylitis and in patients in whom tumor necrosis factor blockers have failed: A twenty-four-week clinical trial. *Arthritis Rheum.* 2010;62:1290–1297.
6. Maksymowych WP, Jhangri GS, Fitzgerald AA, et al. A six-month randomized, controlled, double-blind, dose-response comparison of intravenous pamidronate (60 mg versus 10 mg) in the treatment of nonsteroidal anti-inflammatory drug-refractory ankylosing spondylitis. *Arthritis Rheum.* 2002;46:766–773.
7. Ruof J, Sangha O, Stucki G. Comparative responsiveness of 3 functional indices in ankylosing spondylitis. *J Rheumatol.* 1999;26:1959–1963.
8. Spoorenberg A, van der Heijde D, de Klerk E, et al. A comparative study of the usefulness of the Bath Ankylosing Spondylitis Functional Index and the Dougados Functional Index in the assessment of ankylosing spondylitis. *J Rheumatol.* 1999;26:961–965.

Psoriatic Arthritis

17

Amy Archer and Wayne M. Yokoyama

GENERAL PRINCIPLES

Definition

- Psoriatic arthritis (PsA) is an inflammatory arthritis that is associated with psoriasis. It is one of the five types of **spondyloarthropathies** (SpA).
- The disease can range from asymptomatic to severely debilitating.

Classification

- PsA can be classified on the basis of the pattern of arthritis (numbers in parentheses represent relative occurrence of each pattern).
  - **Asymmetric oligoarthritis:** Maximum of five joints affected in an asymmetric distribution (30%–50%).
  - **Symmetric polyarthritis:** Involvement of multiple joints in a symmetric pattern (30%–50%).
  - **Spondyloarthropathy:** Includes sacroiliitis and spondylitis (5%–30%). This form may be difficult to distinguish from the other spondyloarthritides, especially reactive arthritis, which can also cause asymmetric sacroiliitis and discontinuous spondylitis.
  - **Distal arthritis:** Involves the distal interphalangeal (DIP) joints (10%).
  - **Arthritis mutilans:** Severe destructive arthritis leading to significant joint deformities (rare).
  - Some patients will have more than one pattern of arthritis.

Epidemiology

- Consistent with the age of onset of SpA, PsA has a mean age of onset between 35 and 45 years.
- The overall prevalence of PsA in the United States is 0.25% and among patients with psoriasis is 11%. The prevalence appears to be increasing.

Pathophysiology

- As a member of the family of SpA, genetic, immunologic, and environmental factors are believed to have important roles in the development of the disease.
  - PsA has a **familial association** and has been linked to several human major histocompatibility complex (HLA) class I and II loci.
    - Like the other spondyloarthritides, PsA is associated with **HLA-B27.** However, the association is primarily with the spondyloarthropathy form of PsA.
  - The **immune system** appears to play an active role in the pathogenesis of the disease.

- There is an accumulation of immune cells at sites of disease as well as the production inflammatory cytokines. T cells and monocytes have a central role in this process.[1]
  ○ Treatments aimed at blocking **tumor necrosis factor** (TNF) have improved symptomatic disease activity, implicating TNF in disease pathogenesis, but do not alter the radiographic progression of disease.
  ○ **Bacterial infections, viral infections, and localized trauma** have all been implicated in contributing to the disease.

Associated Conditions

PsA, like rheumatoid arthritis (RA) and other chronic inflammatory arthritides, is associated with increased risk of cardiovascular disease.[2]

DIAGNOSIS

Clinical Presentation

History
- Typical of SpA, patients with PsA classically present with **inflammatory arthritis** (symptoms of pain and stiffness in affected joints that is worsened with immobility and improved with activity and nonsteroidal anti-inflammatory drugs [NSAIDs]). The pattern of arthritis can be variable as mentioned above.
- **Most patients already have psoriasis when arthritis develops;** however, a small percentage of patients develop arthritis before manifestations in the skin appear. Hence, it is important to search thoroughly for psoriatic skin lesions in a patient with rheumatic symptoms reminiscent of PsA, even if the patient does not complain of a rash. For example, the skin lesions may be present only in the gluteal fold or the periumbilical area.
- The severity and activity of skin and arthritic disease are independent of each other.

Physical Examination
- The physical examination should evaluate for musculoskeletal system, integumentary system, and ocular manifestations of disease.
- **Musculoskeletal:**
  ○ **Joint pain and effusions** are identified in one of the five distribution patterns noted above.
  ○ **Enthesitis** can be present and is typically manifested as pain in the heel and/or sole of the foot.
  ○ **Dactylitis** can be identified as inflammation at tendon insertions, along the tendon sheaths and in the joint spaces of the fingers and toes. It commonly causes the appearance of "**sausage digits.**"
- **Integumentary:**
  ○ The skin changes of psoriasis include salmon-colored hyperkeratotic scaling plaques commonly located on extensor surfaces. However, occult psoriasis can be present in the external auditory canal, umbilicus, intergluteal cleft, and axilla.
  ○ Typical **nail changes** include pitting, onycholysis, leukonychia, nail plate crumbling, oil-drop discoloration, nail bed hyperkeratosis, splinter hemorrhages, and red spots in the lunula.

TABLE 17-1	CLASSIFICATION OF PSORIATIC ARTHRITIS (CASPAR) CRITERIA

The presence of an inflammatory articular disease (joint, spine, or entheseal) plus ≥3 points from the following:
Evidence of psoriasis (one of the following)
Current psoriasis (2 points)
Personal history of psoriasis (1 point)
Family history of psoriasis (1point)
Psoriatic nail dystrophy (1 point)
Negative test for rheumatoid factor (1 point)
Dactylitis (one of the following)
Current dactylitis (1 point)
History of dactylitis by a rheumatologist (1 point)
Radiological evidence of juxtaarticular new bone formation

Adapted from: Taylor W, Gladman D, Helliwell P, et al. Classification criteria for PsA: Development of new criteria from a large international study. *Arthritis Rheum.* 2006;54:2665–2673.

- ○ Onycholysis is commonly mistaken for onychomycosis; therefore, it is important to examine nail scrapings for fungal elements and culture. **Nail changes can occur in up to 90% of patients with PsA.**
- • **Ocular:**
  - ○ As in other SpA, ocular inflammation may be present.

Diagnostic Criteria

Although the Amor criteria for spondyloarthropathy and European Spondyloarthropathy Study Group have provided diagnostic criteria for the broad group of SpA, newer criteria have focused on delineating the classification of individual types of SpA, including the Assessment of SpondyloArthritis International Society (ASAS) (Table 15-1) and Classification of PsA (CASPAR) (Table 17-1).[3] Axial disease diagnosis is based on ASAS criteria.

Differential Diagnosis

The differential diagnosis includes reactive arthritis, RA, ankylosing spondyloarthropathy, and gout.

Diagnostic Testing

Laboratories
- • As with SpA in general, laboratory tests are not routinely useful in the diagnosis of PsA.
- • Erythrocyte sedimentation rate (ESR) and C-reactive protein (CRP) are variably elevated and nonspecific.
- • Anemia associated with chronic inflammation can occur but is also not specific.
- • PsA usually occurs in the absence of rheumatoid factor (RF) or antinuclear antibodies (ANA), but these tests may be positive in a small percentage of cases.

- Anti-cyclic citrullinated protein (anti-CCP) antibody can be present in patients with PsA and tends to be associated with a greater number of involved joints, with deformities and functional impairment of peripheral joints and with radiographic changes.[4]

Imaging
- **Joint radiographs:** Classic findings include erosive changes and new bone growth in the distal joints, "pencil-in-cup" erosion, lysis of terminal phalanges, periostitis, and new bone growth at sites of enthesitis.
- **MRI:** As discussed in Chapter 15, MRI may be useful to identify early signs of disease: subclinical enthesitis, arthritis, and periarthritis. However, cost can preclude its routine use in diagnosis.

TREATMENT

- The goals of treatment are to provide symptomatic relief of arthritis and skin disease and **limit disease progression.** The choice of agent depends on the severity/presentation of disease. For more aggressive disease or refractory symptoms steroid-sparing anti-rheumatic drugs are utilized.
- Group for Research and Assessment of Psoriasis and PsA (GRAPPA) treatment guidelines suggest the approach for selected manifestations of PsA presented in Table 17-2.[5]
- Composite measures are being developed by GRAPPA to assess disease activity in PsA, similar to the Bath Ankylosing Spondylitis Disease Activity Index (BASDAI) for ankylosing spondylitis in Table 15-2.[6]

Medications
Nonsteroidal Antiinflammatory Drugs
- Symptomatic joint relief can often be attained with the use of NSAIDS or selective cyclooxygenase (COX)-2 inhibitors if the patient is at risk for gastrointestinal toxicities.
- NSAIDs are not beneficial for skin manifestations.

Intra-Articular Corticosteroids
Intra-articular injections of steroids may also provide symptomatic relief, but are contraindicated if psoriatic skin lesions overlie access to joint spaces due to risk of intra-articular seeding with Gram-positive bacteria.

Disease-Modifying Anti-Rheumatic Drugs
- **Sulfasalazine** has been shown to be efficacious in the treatment of peripheral PsA.
- **Methotrexate**
  ○ Can be an effective treatment option for peripheral PsA.
  ○ American College of Rheumatology (ACR) guidelines for monitoring **liver toxicity** in RA are often followed with patients who have PsA.
    ■ Obtain baseline aspartate aminotransferase (AST), alanine aminotransferase (ALT), albumin, bilirubin, hepatitis serologies, complete blood count (CBC), and creatinine.
    ■ Baseline liver biopsy should be considered in patients with a history of previous or current excessive alcohol consumption, persistently elevated AST or chronic hepatitis infection.

TABLE 17-2	GROUP FOR RESEARCH AND ASSESSMENT OF PSORIASIS AND PsA (GRAPPA) TREATMENT GUIDELINES

Recommended treatments are listed in the order of intervention. Therapies are not mutually exclusive.

Peripheral arthritis
NSAIDs
Intra-articular steroids
DMARDs (e.g., methotrexate, cyclosporine, sulfasalazine, leflunomide)
Biologics (e.g., anti-TNF agents)

Skin and nail disease
Topical agents
PUVA/UVB
Systemic agents (e.g., methotrexate, cyclosporine, etc.)
Biologics (e.g., anti-TNF agents)

Axial disease
NSAIDs
Physical therapy
Biologics (e.g., anti-TNF agents)

Dactylitis
NSAIDs
Steroid injections
Biologics (e.g., anti-TNF agents)

Enthesitis
NSAIDs
Physical therapy
Biologics (e.g., anti-TNF agents)

NSAID, nonsteroidal antiinflammatory drug; DMARD, disease-modifying anti-rheumatic drug; TNF, tumor necrosis factor; PUVA, psoralen and ultraviolet A photochemotherapy; UVB, ultraviolet B.

Adapted from: Ritchlin CT, Kavanaugh A, Gladman DD, et al. Treatment recommendations for PsA. *Ann Rheum Dis*. 2009;68:1387–1394.

- Every 4 to 8 weeks AST, ALT, and albumin should be monitored and only if there is an increase in AST/ALT or a decrease in albumin should biopsy be considered.
  ○ Folic acid should be administered concomitantly with methotrexate.
- **Azathioprine** may be effective in the treatment of PsA.

Biologic Agents

TNF Inhibitors
- TNF inhibitors are considered for use in patients who have failed to respond to disease-modifying anti-rheumatic drug (DMARD) therapy, and may also be considered first line in patients with poor prognosis.
- Failure to respond is defined as a lack of improvement after treatment for more than three months, of which two months need to be at the standard target dose.
- **Etanercept, infliximab, and adalimumab are equally effective in both treatment and stopping disease progression.** Moreover, it may be possible to tailor

therapy within this class of medications as data suggests that **etanercept may be better for articular disease whereas adalimumab and infliximab may be more effective for cutaneous disease.**[5,7,8]

- Appropriate dosing can depend on the predominant symptom that is being treated, with twice-weekly dosing sometimes needed for refractory skin disease.[9]
- The use of TNF-blockers in RA patients highlights the concern for higher rates of malignancy and serious infection as well as the need for further long-term studies.
- All patients should be tested for tuberculosis prior to the initiation of anti-TNF therapy.

T-cell Modulators

When **alefacept** is used in combination with methotrexate, patients had more improvement in both arthritis and psoriasis when compared to methotrexate alone.[10]

Interleukin-12/23 Antagonists

Studies with **ustekinumab** reveal improvement in signs and symptoms of arthritis and psoriasis as well as quality of life.[11]

Other Systemic Treatments

- **Systemic corticosteroid** treatment is not recommended for long-term treatment of PsA but may provide symptomatic relief until the delayed action of steroid-sparing anti-rheumatic drugs takes effect. However, a post-steroid psoriasis flare can occur.
- **Cyclosporine**
  - This treatment can be used when both skin and joint symptoms are present, as it will decrease signs of inflammation and psoriasis when used in combination with methotrexate.
  - This approach can take several months to attain a response and has significant potential for renal toxicity, although dosages for PsA are less than those utilized in transplantation.
  - Therapy should be limited to no more than 12 months.

Topical Agents

- **Retinoids such as acitretin** can be useful for skin involvement.
- Psoralen and ultraviolet A photochemotherapy/ultraviolet B (**PUVA/UVB**) can be used when both skin and joint symptoms are present.
- The scalp, groin, and axilla are areas that should not be treated with phototherapy.
- Aggressive immunosuppression should not be utilized after phototherapy due to the higher risk of melanoma and non-melanoma skin cancers.

Surgical Management

In severely disabled patients with significant joint deformities, surgery with joint replacements or arthroplasties may provide functional benefit and symptomatic relief.

REFERRAL

- As with all seronegative SpA, therapy should include consultation with physical and occupational therapists.

- Consultation with dermatologist is recommended to coordinate treatment and is especially useful in patients with severe skin involvement.

OUTCOME/PROGNOSIS

- A poor prognosis is associated with an increased number of actively inflamed joints, elevated ESR, treatment failure, evidence of joint damage, decreased function as per the Health Assessment Questionnaire (HAQ) and reduced quality of life.
- Particular HLA antigens have been associated with disease progression; these include HLA-B39, B27, and Dqw3.

REFERENCES

1. Ritchlin CT, Proulx S, Schwarz ES. Translational perspectives on PsA. *J Rheumatol.* 2009; 83:30–34.
2. Ahlehoff O, Gislason GH, Charlot M, et al. Psoriasis is associated with clinically significant cardiovascular risk: A Danish nationwide cohort study. *J Intern Med.* 2011;270:147–157.
3. Taylor W, Gladman D, Helliwell P, et al. Classification criteria for PsA: Development of new criteria from a large international study. *Arthritis Rheum.* 2006;54:2665–2673.
4. Abdel Fattah NS, Hassan HE, Galal ZA, et al. Assessment of anti-cyclic citrullinated peptide in PsA. *BMC Res Notes.* 2009;2:44.
5. Ritchlin CT, Kavanaugh A, Gladman DD, et al. Treatment recommendations for psoriatic arthritis. *Ann Rheum Dis.* 2009;68:1387–1394.
6. Gladman DD, Landewe R, McHugh NJ, et al. Composite measures in PsA: GRAPPA 2008. *J Rheumatol.* 2010;37:453–461.
7. Atteno M, Peluso R, Costa L, et al. Comparison of effectiveness and safety of infliximab, etanercept, and adalimumab in PsA patients who experienced an inadequate response to previous disease-modifying antirheumatic drugs. *Clin Rheumatol.* 2010;29:399–403.
8. Mease PJ, Woolley JM, Singh A, et al. Patient-reported outcomes in a randomized trial of etanercept in psoriatic arthritis. *J Rheumatol.* 2010;37:1221–1227.
9. Sterry W, Ortonne JP, Kirkham B, et al. Comparison of two etanercept regimens for treatment of psoriasis and PsA: PRESTA randomised double blind multicentre trial. *BMJ.* 2010;340:c147.
10. Mease PJ, Gladman DD, Keystone EC. Alefacept in combination with methotrexate for the treatment of PsA: Results of a randomized, double-blind, placebo-controlled study. *Arthritis Rheum.* 2006;54:1638–1645.
11. Gottlieb A, Menter A, Mendelsohn A, et al. Ustekinumab, a human interleukin 12/23 monoclonal antibody, for PsA: Randomised, double-blind, placebo-controlled, crossover trial. *Lancet.* 2009;373:633–640.

Reactive Arthritis

18

Reeti Joshi and Wayne M. Yokoyama

GENERAL PRINCIPLES

Definition

- Reactive arthritis (ReA) is a term for disorders that include the disease previously known as Reiter's syndrome (arthritis, uveitis, and conjunctivitis). Hans Reiter was revealed to be a Nazi war criminal who designed studies on internees in concentration camps.[1] For this reason and because ReA is a broader term, usage of the descriptor "Reiter's syndrome" is declining, even though there is no consensus on defining ReA.[2–4]
- ReA belongs to the group of disorders known as spondyloarthropathies (SpA, Chapter 15), differentiated from other types of SpA as a syndrome of sterile, **inflammatory arthritis** occurring in patients after a **genitourinary (GU) or gastrointestinal (GI) infection.** However, the arthritis in ReA is classically sterile and occurs after a latent period rather than during acute GU or GI infection, thereby distinguishing it from septic arthritis due to direct infection.
- **Extra-articular manifestations** include urethritis, uveitis, oral ulcers, skin rashes, and nail changes.

Epidemiology

- The precise prevalence and incidence of ReA are not well known in part due to the absence of well-accepted diagnostic criteria and study of different populations.[3,4] For example, among a military personnel cohort, the incidence was 4.1 cases per 100,000 persons for ReA after GI infections,[5] but other estimates were much higher (28/100,000) in a Swedish population.[6] Nonetheless, ReA appears to be **less common than the other SpA.**
- Typically, ReA affects the young and middle aged, probably influenced by infectious exposures.
- **ReA occurring after GU infections is generally much more common in men,** while **ReA occurring after GI infections affects men and women equally.**[7]
- ReA tends to have a familial association, but appears to be less strongly **associated with HLA-B27** than ankylosing spondylitis.[8] Nevertheless, the risk of developing ReA after an infection is about 1% to 4% whereas in HLA-B27+ individuals, the risk increases to more than 20%.[3]

Etiology

- While the arthritis in ReA is classically sterile (no organisms isolated), ReA follows GU or GI infections due to only selected bacterial species, such as *Chlamydia, Salmonella, Shigella* (especially *S. flexneri*), *Yersinia,* and *Campylobacter,* suggesting that they are causative agents.

○ However, systematic epidemiologic studies have only been performed after *Salmonella* and *Shigella* enteric outbreaks, primarily for the older, more restrictive definition of Reiter's syndrome.[4]

○ Koch's postulates for a causative role of these organisms have not been satisfied. With the possible exception of *Chlamydia,* it has been difficult to reliably isolate live organisms from affected areas, including joints, although there have been reports of bacterial DNA identified by sensitive techniques, such as polymerase chain reaction (PCR).[9]

• In addition to the classic triggers for ReA, numerous case reports also implicate other organisms but they have not been studied systematically.

Pathophysiology

The pathogenesis of ReA is still poorly understood. However, the **strong clinical associations with certain bacterial infections and HLA-B27** implicate the immune system in pathogenesis as discussed in Chapter 15.

DIAGNOSIS

Clinical Presentation

Clinical features of ReA after GI and GU infections are quite similar.

History

• Acute onset of asymmetric inflammatory oligoarthritis (<4 joints) within 2 to 4 weeks of the initial infection is a common presentation.

• As the preceding infection may be clinically mild or occult, relying on symptoms of a triggering infection often results in underdiagnosis.

Physical Examination

• The joints most commonly affected include **knees, ankles, sacroiliac (SI) joints, lower lumbar spine, and feet.**

• **Enthesitis** (inflammation at the site of insertion of a tendon or muscle into a bone) is a hallmark feature, the commonest being **Achilles tendonitis and plantar fasciitis,** often causing heel pain.

• **Dactylitis** ("sausage digits") may be seen.

• **Inflammatory low back pain** occurs, with symptoms consistent with sacroiliitis or spondylitis.

• Other symptoms associated with ReA include **conjunctivitis** and, in more severe instances, **anterior uveitis.**

• Mucosal features include **painless oral ulcers and sterile pyuria/dysuria** (seen in ReA following either GI or GU infections).

• Skin manifestations occur later and may include **circinate balanitis,** skin inflammation on the glans penis, and **keratoderma blennorrhagicum,** hyperkeratotic pustular lesions found on the palms and soles that are histologically identical to pustular psoriasis.

• **Nail changes including pitting and onycholysis** can mimic psoriatic changes.

• On rare occasions, ReA can lead to **cardiac involvement,** including aortic insufficiency.

Diagnostic Criteria

• ReA is essentially a clinical diagnosis. Unlike other rheumatic disorders such as RA and SLE, there are no validated diagnostic criteria for ReA.[3,4] However, ReA is classified as one of the SpA and there are now classification criteria for the SpA, including ReA, as discussed in Chapter 15 (Table 15-1).

- Except for the history of a preceding GI or GU infection, there are no clear clinical features that differentiate ReA from the other seronegative SpA. ReA can be distinguished from septic arthritis which occurs in the setting of obvious, acute infection and/or when organisms are cultured from the joint. ReA typically occurs some time after the acute GI or GU infection has passed.
- When symptoms persist for more than 6 months, ReA is considered chronic.[10] It may have all of the features described in the acute phase, as well as chronic arthritis and enthesitis producing radiographic features described below.
- Other disorders involving arthritis and GI and/or GU tract should be considered. These include SpA associated with inflammatory bowel disease, gonococcal infection, Behçet's syndrome, and Whipple's disease.

Diagnostic Testing

Laboratories

- General makers of inflammation such as erythrocyte sedimentation rate (ESR) and C-reactive protein (CRP) may be elevated in ReA but are not useful diagnostically.
- **HLA-B27 has a limited positive predictive value and testing should not be used as diagnostic tool** as discussed in Chapter 15.
- Serologic tests may sometimes substantiate prior infections with typical organisms but are usually not clinically useful because they have a high false-negative rate and if positive, usually do not indicate if the infection was recent. Joint aspirations for microbiologic culture should be negative; positive results indicate septic arthritis.
- PCR for microorganisms may be helpful for research studies but is generally not useful clinically.

Imaging

- Imaging studies may help exclude other diagnoses such as rheumatoid arthritis.
- Features including **sacroiliitis, syndesmophytes, periosteal new bone formation,** and **erosions** are often evident in chronic disease.
- Additional findings such as fluffy erosions at the calcaneus or pencil-in-cup erosions at the proximal interphalangeal (PIP) joints support the diagnosis.
- **MRI or ultrasound of SI** or other joints to detect earlier changes may be helpful but has not been studied in patients with ReA.

TREATMENT

- Treatment should be guided by the generally good prognosis for ReA which is usually self-limited and abates spontaneously after several months. For example, the prognosis is generally better for ReA, as defined by ability to perform full work capacity, than other inflammatory arthritides.[11]
- Nonetheless, recurrent or chronic ReA can lead to significant joint destruction and disability.
- Disease activity is typically monitored primarily by clinical signs and symptoms. There are no set criteria for disease activity but elevated ESR may respond to therapeutic intervention.

Medications

First Line

- In most cases of ReA, **nonsteroidal antiinflammatory drugs (NSAIDs)** provide symptomatic relief for arthritis, but they are not efficacious for extra-articular manifestations.
- For limited joint involvement, and for circinate balanitis and keratoderma blennorrhagicum, **intra-articular and topical steroids,** respectively, provide symptomatic short-term relief.

Second Line

- **Corticosteroids generally should be avoided since they appear to be of limited benefit** and carry significant morbidity and toxicity.
- For more severe or relapsing and chronic disease states, use of steroid-sparing **disease-modifying antirheumatic drugs (DMARDs)** may be helpful.
- **Sulfasalazine (SSZ)** is the best studied DMARD for ReA with a modest, though significant, response rate of 62% for patients on 2,000 mg of SSZ per day versus 48% on placebo at 36 weeks in a Veterans Affairs Cooperative study.[12] Similar responses were reported by others.[13] SSZ is generally considered to be helpful for peripheral arthritis but not axial disease.[14]
- Several **tumor necrosis factor (TNF)-α receptor antagonists** have been FDA approved for use in ankylosing spondylitis. For ReA specifically, two open label studies show benefit of etanercept[15,16] and other TNF blockers.[16]
- The use of **methotrexate, azathioprine, cyclosporine** and other agents in ReA has been used but not formally studied.
- Antibiotic therapy is controversial. With regard to acute GI and GU infections, antibiotic usage should follow standard infectious disease guidelines for the specific organism. For chronic ReA, it remains unclear if antibiotic therapy affects the outcomes of patients. Consequently, **routine antibiotic therapy is not generally recommended for chronic ReA.**

Other Non-Pharmacologic Therapies

Physical therapy may be beneficial, especially to prevent contractures and muscle atrophy in patients with spinal involvement.

REFERENCES

1. Wallace DJ, Weisman MH. The physician Hans Reiter as prisoner of war in Nuremberg: A contextual review of his interrogations (1945–1947). *Semin Arthritis Rheum.* 2003;32: 208–230.
2. Lu DW, Katz KA. Declining use of the eponym "Reiter's syndrome" in the medical literature, 1998–2003. *J Am Acad Dermatol.* 2005;53:720–723.
3. Rohekar S, Pope J. Epidemiologic approaches to infection and immunity: The case of reactive arthritis. *Curr Opin Rheumatol.* 2009;21:386–390.
4. Townes JM. Reactive arthritis after enteric infections in the United States: The problem of definition. *Clin Infect Dis.* 2010;50:247–254.
5. Curry JA, Riddle MS, Gormley RP, et al. The epidemiology of infectious gastroenteritis related reactive arthritis in U.S. military personnel: A case-control study. *BMC Infect Dis.* 2010;10:266.
6. Soderlin MK, Borjesson O, Kautiainen H, et al. Annual incidence of inflammatory joint diseases in a population based study in southern Sweden. *Ann Rheum Dis.* 2002;61: 911–915.

7. Leirisalo M, Skylv G, Kousa M, et al. Follow up study on patients with Reiter's disease and reactive arthritis, with special reference to HLA-B27. *Arthritis Rheum.* 1982;25:249–259.

8. Kaarela K, Jantti JK, Kotaniemi KM. Similarity between chronic reactive arthritis and ankylosing spondylitis. A 32–35-year follow-up study. *Clin Exp Rheumatol.* 2009;27: 325–328.

9. Carter JD. Bacterial agents in spondyloarthritis: A destiny from diversity? *Best Pract Res Clin Rheumatol.* 2010;24:701–714.

10. Braun J, Kingsley G, van der Heijde D, et al. On the difficulties of establishing a consensus on the definition of and diagnostic investigations for reactive arthritis. Results and discussion of a questionnaire prepared for the 4th International Workshop on Reactive Arthritis, Berlin, Germany, July 3–6, 1999. *J Rheumatol.* 2000;27:2185–2192.

11. Kaarela K, Lehtinen K, Luukkainen R. Work capacity of patients with inflammatory joint diseases. An eight-year follow-up study. *Scand J Rheumatol.* 1987;16:403–406.

12. Clegg DO, Reda DJ, Weisman MH, et al. Comparison of sulfasalazine and placebo in the treatment of reactive arthritis (Reiter's syndrome). A Department of Veterans Affairs Cooperative Study. *Arthritis Rheum.* 1996;39:2021–2027.

13. Egsmose C, Hansen TM, Andersen LS, et al. Limited effect of sulphasalazine treatment in reactive arthritis. A randomised double blind placebo controlled trial. *Ann Rheum Dis.* 1997;56:32–36.

14. Clegg DO, Reda DJ, Abdellatif M. Comparison of sulfasalazine and placebo for the treatment of axial and peripheral articular manifestations of the seronegative spondyloarthropathies: A Department of Veterans Affairs cooperative study. *Arthritis Rheum.* 1999;42: 2325–2329.

15. Flagg SD, Meador R, Hsia E, et al. Decreased pain and synovial inflammation after etanercept therapy in patients with reactive and undifferentiated arthritis: An open-label trial. *Arthritis Rheum.* 2005;53:613–617.

16. Meyer A, Chatelus E, Wendling D, et al. Safety and efficacy of anti-tumor necrosis factor alpha therapy in ten patients with recent-onset refractory reactive arthritis. *Arthritis Rheum.* 2011;63:1274–1280.

Enteropathic Arthritis

19

Kristine A. Kuhn and Wayne M. Yokoyama

GENERAL PRINCIPLES

- Enteropathic arthritis is one of the five types of spondyloarthropathies (SpA). It is distinguished from the other types by its association with the **inflammatory bowel diseases** (IBD): **Crohn's disease** (CD) and **ulcerative colitis** (UC).
- This chapter will discuss the features of enteropathic arthritis that are shared with other SpAs and distinguish enteropathic arthritis from the other forms of SpA.

Definition

Patients with enteropathic arthritis meet the criteria for SpA as described in Chapter 15, in association with IBD.

Classification

- Three types of arthritis are associated with IBD:[1]
  - **Type I is a peripheral, pauciarticular arthritis,** usually asymmetric, that occurs during active bowel disease. The inflammation typically is transient, migratory, and non-deforming. It may precede a diagnosis of IBD.
  - **Type II is a peripheral, polyarticular arthritis** that occurs independently of the activity of bowel disease.
  - **Type III is axial disease,** which occurs independently of the activity of bowel disease. Features of type III arthritis can range from inflammatory back pain and sacroiliitis to a disease mimicking ankylosing spondylitis (AS).
  - **Enthesitis** can occur with all types.
- **Arthralgias** (non-inflammatory joint pain) also commonly occur in patients with IBD; however, these are not part of the spectrum of enteropathic arthritis.

Epidemiology

- Overall, arthritis occurs in about 20% of patients with IBD.[1] In these patients:
  - Type 1 arthritis will occur in 10% to 20%;
  - Type II arthritis in 2% to 4%; and
  - Type III inflammatory back pain and/or sacroiliitis in 20% to 30%, while about 2% to 10% will develop AS.

Etiology

- As in other diseases, enteropathic arthritis likely occurs as a result of an environmental trigger in a genetically appropriate setting. One hypothesis links chronic gut inflammation to the loss of tolerance to gut pathogens and the development of arthritis.[2]

- Several candidate genes for IBD have been linked to the development of SpA.[1]
  - Mice transgenic for HLA-B27 and human β2-microglobulin develop sacroiliitis, peripheral arthritis, colitis, and psoriasiform skin lesions.[3] Disease, however, does not develop when mice are housed in germ-free conditions.
  - Specific interleukin (IL)-23 receptor polymorphisms have been demonstrated to be protective against CD, AS, and psoriasis.[4,5]
  - Nucleotide-binding oligomerization domain containing 2 (NOD 2), also known as caspase recruitment domain family member 15 (CARD15), polymorphisms are genetically associated with CD.[6] Although no association is found with SpA, SpA patients with certain CARD15 polymorphisms have an increased risk for chronic gut inflammation.
  - Genome-wide association studies are demonstrating other genetic susceptibility loci that associate with IBD, SpA, and chronic gut inflammation.

Pathophysiology

Like other SpA, enteropathic arthritis appears to be immune mediated, with tumor necrosis factor (TNF)-α central to the pathogenesis of disease. See Chapter 15 for further review.

Risk Factors

- No specific risk factors have been identified for the development of enteropathic arthritis, other than the presence of IBD.
- There is suggestion of a genetic risk with the presence of **HLA-B27**. However, the frequency of HLA-B27 in patients with IBD is 30%, compared to up to 95% of patients with AS.[1]

DIAGNOSIS

- Diagnosis is based on a clinical presentation of SpA and a history of IBD.
- Classification criteria for SpA (Table 15-1) guide which clinical features and testing suggest a diagnosis of SpA.

Clinical Presentation

- Bowel pathology usually occurs before extra-intestinal manifestations develop; however, **arthritis can sometimes be the presenting symptom of IBD.**[1]
- The peripheral arthritis associated with IBD is typically **oligoarticular, migratory, and asymmetric, and it generally affects the lower limbs.** The inflammatory arthritis may lead to large joint effusions, especially in the knees.
- Other associated conditions include **uveitis, aortic regurgitation,** and skin manifestations. **Erythema nodosum and pyoderma gangrenosum** are associated with CD and UC, respectively.

History

- The patient may describe symptoms of inflammatory arthritis (morning stiffness lasting longer than 60 minutes, improvement of stiffness with activity, and/or joint swelling and warmth).
  - Peripheral joint involvement is usually asymmetric and affecting the lower extremity joints.
  - Axial skeletal involvement may cause alternating buttock pain.

- One should assess for signs and symptoms of IBD in patients presenting with SpA who do not have a prior history of IBD. In those patients with an established diagnosis of IBD, activity of disease should be assessed. Signs and symptoms include the following:
  - Frequent **diarrhea**, with or without hematochezia, mucous, steatorrhea, and malabsorption.
  - **Crampy abdominal pain.**
  - **Fistulas, abscesses, and aphthous ulcers.**
  - Extra-intestinal manifestations including **uveitis, pyoderma gangrenosum, and erythema nodosum.**

Physical Examination

- The physical examination should evaluate for musculoskeletal as well as other extra-intestinal manifestations of IBD.
- The musculoskeletal exam can be divided into the axial and peripheral findings:
  - Examination of the axial skeleton may demonstrate **decreased spinal mobility.**
  - Peripheral joint findings include **swelling, effusions, erythema, reduced range of motion, dactylitis, and enthesitis.**
- **Scleral injection** raises suspicion for eye involvement. Referral to an ophthalmologist and evaluation for uveitis may be required.
- Evaluation of the **skin** may reveal enterocutaneous fistulae, erythematous nodules, or ulcers. Dermatology referral and skin biopsy may need to be considered.
- Findings upon examination of the gastrointestinal system may reveal aphthous ulcers, abdominal tenderness, rectal ulcers, and guaiac-positive stool.

Diagnostic Criteria

- No specific diagnostic criteria exist. Diagnosis is based on clinical suspicion and excluding other causes for symptoms.
- The criteria for SpA, as proposed by the Assessment of SpondyloArthritis International Society (ASAS), (Table 15-1) are useful as general diagnostic guidelines.[7,8]
- Patients with enteropathic arthritis obviously would be expected to meet the criteria for diagnosis of SpA and have active IBD or a history compatible with IBD. **Some patients may develop IBD after a diagnosis of undifferentiated SpA is made.**

Differential Diagnosis

- **Mechanical back pain** is the most common cause of lower back pain. Only 5% of patients seen in a primary care setting with chronic low back pain are diagnosed with SpA.
- In those without a prior diagnosis of IBD who present with inflammatory back pain, the differential diagnosis includes the five types of SpA. Peripheral arthritis may be infectious or rheumatoid arthritis (RA).
- In patients with established IBD presenting with monoarticular arthritis, **infectious arthritis** must be considered.
- **Arthralgias,** joint pain without inflammatory symptoms, may be found in patients with IBD. These are not part of the spectrum of enteropathic arthritis.

Diagnostic Testing

- Few diagnostic tests are of use for establishing a diagnosis of enteropathic arthritis.

- Laboratory testing of erythrocyte sedimentation rate (ESR) and C-reactive protein (CRP) may suggest systemic inflammation, but are nonspecific.
- Imaging may demonstrate sacroiliitis or other inflammatory changes in the joint.

Laboratories
- ESR and CRP may indicate a systemic inflammatory process. Unfortunately, these tests **rarely correlate with disease activity.**
- **HLA-B27 is only positive in about 30% of patients** with enteropathic arthritis. Furthermore, only 1% to 2% of people who carry HLA-B27 develop SpA. Therefore, **HLA-B27 testing is not clinically useful.**[1]

Imaging
- **Plain radiography of the sacroiliac joints and spine** may demonstrate sacroiliitis, syndesmophytes, or ankylosis consistent with AS (see Chapter 16).[2]
- **MRI of the spine** may demonstrate early inflammatory changes including bone marrow edema and fat infiltration (see Chapter 15).
- For peripheral joints, three modalities are used for imaging. Plain radiography may demonstrate **enthesitis and periosteal reaction.** Ultrasound and MRI may also be helpful in identifying subtle inflammatory changes within the joint and surrounding structures.

Diagnostic Procedures
- Gastroenterology referral and **endoscopy** should be considered in patients with a clinical presentation of SpA and bowel symptoms to evaluate for IBD if not already established.
- An **arthrocentesis** should be performed in any patient presenting with peripheral monoarticular arthritis with synovial fluid submitted for cell count and culture to evaluate for infectious arthritis.

TREATMENT

- Pharmacologic treatment of enteropathic arthritis depends upon the type of arthritis.
- Regardless of the type of enteropathic arthritis, all patients benefit from exercise and/or physical therapy.

Medications
- **Often, control of IBD will result in control of arthritis** and, therefore, should be the goal of therapy. However, when the arthritis is independent of bowel inflammation additional therapy should be considered.
- The pharmacologic therapy of axial and peripheral enteropathic arthritis is similar to that for AS and psoriatic arthritis (PsA), respectively. Many statements about treatment of undifferentiated SpA apply to axial enteropathic arthritis.

Nonsteroidal Antiinflammatory Drugs
- **Nonsteroidal antiinflammatory drugs (NSAIDs)** are first-line therapy for the treatment of SpA and are used in enteropathic arthritis.
  - They are used with caution in enteropathic arthritis as NSAIDs **have been shown to worsen IBD in some patients.**[9]
- Brief courses (up to two weeks) of cyclooxygenase (COX)-2 inhibitors appear to be safe, but long-term data are lacking.

Oral Disease-Modifying Antirheumatic Drugs
- Second-line agents include oral disease-modifying antirheumatic drugs (DMARDs) such as **sulfasalazine, methotrexate, and azathioprine.**[10]
  - **Sulfasalazine** is the preferred oral DMARD given its use in controlling IBD. Although no clinical trials have demonstrated its value in enteropathic arthritis, clinical experience suggests efficacy in early disease and in peripheral disease. It does not alter the course of axial disease or peripheral enthesopathy.
  - Similarly, there is little trial evidence for the use of methotrexate and azathioprine; but anecdotally, these agents appear to have greater benefit in treating peripheral compared to axial disease.

Antitumor Necrosis Factor Agents
- Biologic therapy with **antitumor necrosis factor (anti-TNF) agents** has emerged as a mainstay for treatment of IBD and SpA.
  - Several small trials have demonstrated good results with **infliximab** in specifically treating enteropathic arthritis. Patients' gastrointestinal disease and arthritis, both peripheral and axial manifestations, rapidly improved after infusion of the drug.
  - Other anti-TNF agents have demonstrated efficacy in the treatment of SpA.
  - Etanercept, however, has less efficacy than monoclonal anti-TNF antibody therapies for the treatment of IBD.[11]

Analgesics and Glucocorticoids
- Pain control may require use of analgesics.
- **Glucocorticoids, oral or intra-articular,** are useful in controlling bowel inflammation and may be useful for peripheral joint involvement. They are ineffective for the treatment of axial disease.

Other Non-Pharmacologic Therapies
- **Physical therapy and exercise** are mainstays for all SpAs. An exercise program in combination with pharmacologic agents has been shown to be more effective than pharmacologic treatment alone.
- **Surgical management** is discussed in Chapter 15.

COMPLICATIONS

- Complications of SpA depend upon the type of arthritis.
- Type I arthritis is usually non-deforming.
- Type II arthritis can lead to joint erosions and/or ankylosis of an affected joint, similar to that found in PsA. See Chapter 17.
- Those with type III arthritis may develop complications related to spinal involvement, similar to AS. See Chapter 16.

REFERRAL

- IBD patients with one or more of the following should be referred to a rheumatologist:
  - Inflammatory back pain.
  - Sacroiliitis on imaging.
  - Peripheral arthritis, enthesitis, or dactylitis.

- Those patients who have inflammatory back pain or peripheral arthritis, enthesitis, or dactylitis with signs and symptoms suggestive of IBD should be referred to a gastroenterologist for further diagnostic testing.

PATIENT EDUCATION

- Patients should be educated on the manifestations, complications, and therapeutic options of their disease.
- In addition, the benefits of exercise and physical therapy for improving functional status and limiting pain should be emphasized.

MONITORING/FOLLOW-UP

- Disease activity should be monitored on the basis of clinical features of bowel disease, morning stiffness, pain, physical exam, and imaging when indicated.
- The Bath Ankylosing Spondylitis Disease Activity Index (BASDAI) (Table 15-2) can be used as a guide for assessment of articular disease activity.[12]

REFERENCES

1. De Vos M. Joint involvement associated with inflammatory bowel disease. *Dig Dis.* 2009;27:511–515.
2. Davis JC Jr, Mease PJ. Insights into the pathology and treatment of spondyloarthritis: From the bench to the clinic. *Semin Arthritis Rheum.* 2008;38:83–100.
3. Khare SD, Luthra HS, David CS. Spontaneous inflammatory arthritis in HLA-B27 transgenic mice lacking beta 2-microglobulin: A model of human spondyloarthropathies. *J Exp Med.* 1995;182:1153–1158.
4. Duerr RH, Taylor KD, Brant SR, et al. A genome-wide association study identifies IL23R as an inflammatory bowel disease gene. *Science.* 2006;314:1461–1463.
5. Capon F, Di Meglio P, Szaub J, et al. Sequence variants in the genes for the interleukin-23 receptor (IL23R) and its ligand (IL12B) confer protection against psoriasis. *Hum Genet.* 2007;122:201–206.
6. Hugot JP, Chamaillard M, Zouali H, et al. Association of NOD2 leucine-rich repeat variants with susceptibility to Crohn's disease. *Nature.* 2001;411:599–603.
7. Rudwaleit M, van der Heijde D, Landewé R, et al. The development of Assessment of SpondyloArthritis international Society classification criteria for axial spondyloarthritis (part II): Validation and final selection. *Ann Rheum Dis.* 2009;68:777–783.
8. Rudwaleit M, van der Heijde D, Landewé R, et al. The Assessment of SpondyloArthritis international Society classification criteria for peripheral spondyloarthritis and for spondyloarthritis in general. *Ann Rheum Dis.* 2011;70:25–31.
9. Takeuchi K, Smale S, Premchand P, et al. Prevalence and mechanism of nonsteroidal anti-inflammatory drug-induced clinical relapse in patients with inflammatory bowel disease. *Clin Gastroenterol Hepatol.* 2006;4:196–202.
10. Kabasakal Y, Kitapcioglu G, Yargucu F, et al. Efficacy of SLZ and MTX (alone or combination) on the treatment of active sacroiliitis in early AS. *Rheumatol Int.* 2009;29:1523–1527.
11. Braun J, Baraliakos X, Listing J, et al. Differences in the incidence of flares or new onset of inflammatory bowel diseases in patients with ankylosing spondylitis exposed to therapy with anti-tumor necrosis factor alpha agents. *Arthritis Rheum.* 2007;57:639–647.
12. Garrett S, Jenkinson T, Kennedy LG, et al. A new approach to defining disease status in ankylosing spondylitis: The Bath Ankylosing Spondylitis Disease Activity Index. *J Rheumatol.* 1994;21:2286–2291.

Vasculitis

20

Alfred H.J. Kim and John P. Atkinson

GENERAL PRINCIPLES

- Vasculitis is **inflammation of the vessel wall.** It is an uncommon manifestation of a wide variety of autoimmune, infectious, malignant, and iatrogenic conditions.
- It is characterized by nonspecific signs and symptoms due to systemic inflammatory disease, but specific signs and symptoms depend on which vessels are involved.
- Damage to tissues occurs via ischemia or infarction secondary to a reduction in perfusion to tissue distal to the vasculitic lesion.
- The severity of symptoms ranges from self-limiting rash to life-threatening disease.

Definition

- Vasculitis is defined as inflammatory infiltration of vessel walls with damage to mural structures.
- **Vasculitis is a pathologic finding, not a diagnosis.** Efforts must be made to determine the cause.

Classification

Vasculitis can be divided into primary or secondary, on the basis of etiologies.

Primary Vasculitis

- This typically refers to autoimmune causes.
- Several classification schemes exist, but the most commonly used scheme was derived from the 1993 Chapel Hill Consensus Conference presented in Table 20-1.[1]
- The Chapel Hill Consensus stratified the vasculitides into the size of vessel affected:
  - Large
  - Medium
  - Small
  - Often, a vasculitis will affect vessels of more than one size. These are classified on the basis of which sized vessel the condition *primarily* affects.

Large Vessel Vasculitides

- **Takayasu's arteritis** (see Chapter 21, Takayasu's Arteritis).
  - **Granulomatous inflammation** affects primarily the **aorta and its main branches** and may involve all or just a portion of these vessels.
  - Separate classification criteria exist to aid diagnosis. Typically, in **young women from Far East Asia** (Japan) with pulseless disease in the upper extremities.

TABLE 20-1   CLASSIFICATION OF VASCULITIS

Large vessel
Takayasu's arteritis
Giant cell arteritis

Medium vessel
Polyarteritis nodosa
Kawasaki disease
Primary angiitis of the central nervous system

Small vessel

Immune complex related
Hypersensitivity vasculitis[a]
Henoch–Schönlein purpura
Cryoglobulinemic vasculitis[b]
Connective tissue disease–associated vasculitis[c]

Pauci-immune
ANCA-associated granulomatous vasculitis[d]
Churg-Strauss syndrome
Microscopic polyangiitis

---

[a]Most often caused by medications, infections, and malignancies.
[b]Most often associated with hepatitis B and C, Epstein–Barr virus, plasma cell dyscrasias, chronic inflammatory/autoimmune disorders, and lymphoproliferative malignancies.
[c]Most often associated with rheumatoid arthritis, SLE, and Sjögren's syndrome.
[d]Also known as Wegener's granulomatosis.
ANCA, antineutrophil cytoplasmic antibody.
Adapted from:Jennette JC, Falk RJ, Andrassy K, et al. Nomenclature of systemic vasculitides. Proposal of an international consensus conference. *Arthritis Rheum.* 1994;37:187–192.

- **Giant cell arteritis** (see Chapter 22, Giant Cell Arteritis and Polymyalgia Rheumatica).
  ○ **Granulomatous arteritis** occurs primarily in the **cranial branches of arteries arising from the aortic arch,** also affecting medium-sized vessels. Classically involves the **temporal artery.**
  ○ Associated with **polymyalgia rheumatica.**
  ○ Separate classification criteria exist to aid diagnosis. Usually seen in patients **>50 years old, erythrocyte sedimentation rate (ESR) >50,** and is associated with headache and less commonly jaw or tongue claudication.

Medium Vessel Vasculitides
- **Polyarteritis nodosa** (PAN) (see Chapter 23, Polyarteritis Nodosa)
  ○ A **necrotizing systemic vasculitis** affecting both medium and **small muscular arteries,** without glomerulonephritis or vasculitis of the arterioles, capillaries or venules.
  ○ Separate classification criteria exist to aid diagnosis. Although accounting for <10% of cases due to increased vaccinations, PAN is typically associated with hepatitis B. Clinically, **skin nodules, mononeuritis multiplex, orchitis, and mesenteric artery involvement are most common.**

- **Kawasaki disease**
  - ○ Primarily a medium vessel vasculitis, but can affect large and small vessels.
  - ○ Separate classification criteria exist to aid diagnosis. Mostly seen in **children**. Predilection for **coronary arteries**. Occasionally associated with a **mucocutaneous lymph node syndrome**.
- **Primary angiitis of the central nervous system**
  - ○ A rare granulomatous vasculitis isolated to the medium and small arteries in the leptomeninges.

Small Vessel Vasculitides

- The small vessel vasculitides are further **subdivided into the presence or absence of immunoglobulin within the vessels.**
- **Presence of immune complexes in vessels** (immune complex related).
  - ○ **Henoch–Schönlein purpura** (see Chapter 27, Henoch–Schönlein Purpura)
    - ▪ **Systemic** vasculitis where **IgA-containing immune complexes** deposit within tissues, such as the renal glomerulus, skin and gut.
    - ▪ Most common form of systemic vasculitis in children.
    - ▪ Associated with arthralgias or arthritis, myalgias, and subcutaneous edema.
    - ▪ Post-capillary venules are most affected.
  - ○ **Cryoglobulinemic vasculitis** (see Chapter 28, Cryoglobulinemia and Cryoglobulinemic Vasculitis)
    - ▪ Characterized by the presence of **cryoglobulins,** serum proteins that precipitate in the cold.
    - ▪ Associated with **hepatitis B and C infection. Skin** (extremities) and **glomeruli** often involved.
    - ▪ Affects arterioles, capillaries, and venules.
  - ○ **Connective tissue disease–associated vasculitis**
    - ▪ Seen in small muscular arteries, arterioles, and venules.
    - ▪ Typically associated with rheumatoid arthritis (see Chapter 10, Rheumatoid Arthritis), systemic lupus erythematosus (SLE) (see Chapter 12, Systemic Lupus Erythematosus), and Sjögren's syndrome (see Chapter 37, Sjögren's Syndrome).
    - ▪ Behçet's syndrome (see Chapter 31, Behçet's Syndrome), relapsing polychondritis (see Chapter 43, Relapsing Polychondritis), and inflammatory bowel disease also may present with a vasculitis in a similar vessel distribution to connective tissue diseases.
- **Absence of immune complexes in vessels** (pauci-immune); these conditions are usually associated with antineutrophil cytoplasmic antibodies (ANCAs).
  - ○ **Wegener's granulomatosis,** also known as ANCA-associated granulomatous vasculitis (see Chapter 24, Wegener's Granulomatosis)
    - ▪ Systemic vasculitis affecting small and medium arteries, along with arterioles and venules.
    - ▪ **Lower respiratory tract chronic granulomatous vasculitic inflammation** is characteristic. Upper airways have chronic inflammation, but typically in the absence of granulomatous inflammation.
    - ▪ Typically, patients start with sinus and upper airway symptoms, then lower airway and next kidney disease. Systemic vasculitis can occur at anytime during the disease process.
    - ▪ **Necrotizing, pauci-immune glomerulonephritis** in the kidneys.
    - ▪ Associated with **anti-proteinase 3 (anti-PR3) antibody,** with a **cytoplasmic ANCA** staining pattern (c-ANCA).

○ **Churg–Strauss syndrome** (see Chapter 25, Churg–Strauss Syndrome)
  ▪ Also known as allergic granulomatosis and angiitis.
  ▪ Also affects medium-sized vessels.
  ▪ Classically affects **lung and skin arteries,** but can be systemic.
  ▪ **Extravascular granulomatosis** is characteristic.
  ▪ Associated in approximately 50% of cases with **anti-myeloperoxidase (anti-MPO)** antibodies, yielding a **perinuclear ANCA** staining pattern (p-ANCA).
  ▪ Separate classification criteria exist to aid diagnosis. Classic presentation is **older person with new onset, relatively refractory, and progressive asthma with eosinophilia.**
○ **Microscopic Polyangiitis** (see Chapter 26, Microscopic Polyangiitis)
  ▪ Systemic vasculitis similar to Wegener's granulomatosis with the exception of absence of upper airway involvement, granulomatous inflammation, and serologic specificity.
  ▪ Associated with **anti-MPO** antibodies, yielding a positive p-**ANCA.**

Secondary Vasculitis
- Usually refers to non-autoimmune causes of vasculitis.
- **Medications, infections, and malignancies are the most common etiologies for secondary vasculitis.**
- **Medications** typically cause hypersensitivity vasculitis manifested by skin findings, specifically **leukocytoclastic vasculitis** (see Chapter 29, Cutaneous Vasculitis). Separate classification criteria exist to aid diagnosis of hypersensitivity vasculitis.
- **Viruses** associated with medium and small vessel vasculitis include hepatitis B, human immunodeficiency virus, cytomegalovirus, Epstein–Barr virus, and parvovirus B19.
  ○ Viral vasculitides often present similarly to PAN or microscopic polyangiitis.
  ○ It is important to differentiate between non-viral and viral vasculitis since treatment options differ significantly.
- **Hematologic,** more so than solid, malignancies can be associated with vasculitis.
  ○ Typically presents with palpable purpura.
  ○ Hairy cell leukemia presents with a PAN-like picture or as a cutaneous vasculitis.
  ○ Lymphoproliferative disorders including myelodysplastic syndromes, Waldenström's macroglobulinemia, lymphocytic lymphoma, and chronic lymphocytic leukemia all can have associated vasculitis, with or without cryoglobulins.

Etiology
Multiple factors appear to play a role is disease susceptibility, including genetic, immune, and environmental. Much is yet to be learned about each.

Pathophysiology
- The mechanisms underlying the vasculitides remain poorly understood.
- Currently, it is believed that while immune complexes themselves are not innately pathogenic, their inflammatory potential can be augmented in the setting of increased antigen load, decreased clearance efficiency by the reticulo-endothelial system (RES), or decreased solubility. The pathogenic immune complexes fix complement, leading to intense inflammation.

- ○ Regarding immune complex solubility, when there are equal parts of antigen and antibody, large immune complexes form that are cleared by the RES without tissue damage.
- ○ When an excess of antibody is present, small immune complexes are generated but remain soluble, and are not pathogenic.
- ○ **When there is an excess of antigen, the immune complexes precipitate,** and get trapped in capillaries or vessels damaged by turbulent blood flow. This leads to immune complex–mediated inflammation.
- Activating Fcγ receptors and the alternative pathway of complement are critical for ANCA-associated pauci-immune vasculitis induction. Activation of neutrophils and macrophages ensues, leading to endothelial injury.
- In giant cell arteritis, dendritic cells, T cells and macrophages are strongly implicated in arterial wall destruction.
- Several models have been proposed to describe why vasculitic syndromes have a predilection for certain vessels[2]:
  - ○ Antigens distribute preferentially to tissues, thus inducing vasculitis in those vessels.
  - ○ Endothelial cells control the severity of inflammation at the vessel through expression of adhesion molecules and secretion of proteins, peptides, and hormones. This will control how the immune cell interacts with the vasculature.
  - ○ Nonendothelial cells modulate immune cell and/or endothelial cell behavior, modulating the level of inflammation.

DIAGNOSIS

- The diagnosis of vasculitis should be entertained whenever a patient with systemic symptoms has organ dysfunction.
- Characteristic symptoms are associated with the involvement of certain sized vessels. Thus, it is best to try to **assign the patient's signs and symptoms to a particular vessel size category,** then **determine what features of each disease within the category best fit the patient.**
- Use laboratory testing and diagnostic procedures to define the extent of disease or better elucidate any other characteristic features, particularly **biopsy of affected organs** as this typically yields the diagnosis.

Clinical Presentation
- Most common constitutional symptoms are fatigue, malaise, fever, and arthralgias.
- Several clinical features strongly suggest the presence of vasculitis:
  - ○ **Purpura**
    - ■ These are nonblanching skin lesions due to bleeding in the skin.
    - ■ Those with isolated skin lesions are considered to have cutaneous leukocytoclastic vasculitis.
    - ■ If the purpura is palpable and systemic involvement is seen, Henoch–Schönlein purpura or microscopic polyangiitis should be suspected.
  - ○ **Mononeuritis multiplex**
    - ■ This occurs when two or more nerves in separate parts of the body are damaged.

- **"Foot-drop"** occurs due to damage to the sciatic or peroneal nerve; **"wrist-drop"** occurs due to damage to the radial nerve.
- Of all the neurologic symptoms seen in vasculitis, mononeuritis multiplex is the most specific.
  - **Pulmonary–renal involvement**
    - Alveolar hemorrhage from capillaritis can cause **hemoptysis**. Hemoptysis can also be associated with a medium-sized vessel vasculitis due to a ruptured bronchial artery aneurysm.
    - Glomerulonephritis will be associated with **red blood cell casts or dysmorphic red blood cells** in the urine.
    - While the ANCA-associated vasculitides can cause pulmonary–renal syndrome, anti-glomerular basement membrane syndrome, embolic disease, infection, and SLE should also be considered.

History
- Detailed history significantly helps differentiate between primary and secondary causes of vasculitis.
- Ask about past history of:
  - Medications (hypersensitivity vasculitis).
  - Hepatitis B or C (PAN or cryoglobulinemia, respectively).
  - Connective tissue disease.
  - Sexual history (HIV infection).
  - Illicit drug use (ergots, cocaine, or amphetamines).
- Certain age groups and gender are associated with specific vasculitides.
  - Wegener's granulomatosis and PAN have mean age of onset between 45 and 50, while HSP and Takayasu's arteritis between 17 and 26 within the adult population.
  - Giant cell arteritis affects an older population, with a mean age of onset of 69.
  - Takayasu's and giant cell arteritis occur predominantly in females.

Physical Examination
Certain clues are seen depending on vessel size, see Table 20-2.

Diagnostic Criteria
- The American College of Rheumatology has defined classification criteria for several of the vasculitides, including:
  - Takayasu's arteritis (see Chapter 21, Takayasu's Arteritis).
  - Giant cell arteritis (see Chapter 22, Giant Cell Arteritis and Polymyalgia Rheumatica).
  - PAN (see Chapter 23, Polyarteritis Nodosa).
  - Kawasaki disease.
  - Churg–Strauss syndrome (see Chapter 25, Churg–Strauss Syndrome).
  - Hypersensitivity vasculitis (see Chapter 29, Cutaneous Vasculitis).
- The remainder of the vasculitides do not have set criteria for diagnosis, but are diagnosed clinically with the help of laboratory testing.

Differential Diagnosis
- Look for secondary causes of vasculitis when the patient does not appear to fit within any of the primary vasculitides.

TABLE 20-2	PHYSICAL EXAMINATION FEATURES OF VASCULITIS

Large vessel
Pulse deficits
Bruits

Medium vessel
Cutaneous nodules
Livedo reticularis
Digital infarction

Small vessel
Palpable purpura
Superficial ulcerations
Mononeuritis multiplex
Papulonecrotic lesions

- **Embolic disorders** (endocarditis, left atrial myxoma, cholesterol emboli) can mimic a small vessel vasculitis.
- **Infections** such as sepsis, fungal infections (especially mycotic aneurysm with embolization), mycobacterial infections, Rickettsial infections, and syphilis may mimic a small vessel vasculitis.
- **SLE and amyloidosis,** in the absence of vasculitis, can present with vasculitis-type symptoms.
- **Ergots, cocaine, and amphetamines** can mimic medium or small vessel vasculitis.
- **Malignancies** seen with vasculitis-like symptoms include lymphomatoid granulomatosis, intravascular lymphoma, and angioimmunoblastic T-cell lymphoma.
- **Thrombocytopenia and myelodysplastic syndromes** can present with non-vasculitic purpura.

Diagnostic Testing

Laboratories
- Basic laboratory analysis should include:
  - Complete blood count with differential.
  - Comprehensive metabolic panel (elevated creatinine).
  - Muscle enzymes (creatine kinase, aldolase).
  - ESR and C-reactive protein (CRP).
  - Hepatitis and HIV serologies.
  - Urinalysis and urine toxicology screen.
- More specific laboratory testing can include (see Chapter 5, Laboratory Evaluation of Rheumatic Diseases):
  - **Antinuclear antibodies** (ANA) if suspecting a connective tissue disease.
  - **Complement** (low levels are seen in cryoglobulinemia, hypocomplementemic urticarial vasculitis, and the vasculitis associated with SLE).
  - Although not diagnostic, when **ANCA** is directed to PR3 by ELISA, strongly consider Wegener's granulomatosis. When directed to MPO, consider microscopic polyangiitis or Churg–Strauss syndrome.

Imaging
- Decision to pursue imaging is dependent on the patient's symptom complex.
- Chest radiography may reveal pulmonary infiltration including alveolar hemorrhage.
- Sinus CT may reveal sinusitis in Wegener's granulomatosis.
- Echocardiogram to rule out vegetations and atrial myxoma.
- Angiogram may reveal characteristic alternating dilatations and strictures in large or medium-sized vasculitides—especially in PAN and temporal arteritis.

Diagnostic Procedures
- Usually, biopsy of affected tissue (e.g., skin, nerve, kidney, lungs) can reveal the pathologic findings of vasculitis.
- Delay in obtaining material from affected tissue is a common mistake in establishing a diagnosis in these conditions.

TREATMENT

- The goal of treatment is to first induce remission of disease, then maintain the patient on a less toxic immunosuppressant to prevent relapses.
- Treatment is based on type and severity of clinical manifestations (see Chapter 9, Drugs Used for the Treatment of Rheumatic Diseases).
- In general, **immunosuppression** is the mainstay for treatment.

Medications
- **Glucocorticoids** are used in virtually all systemic vasculitis patients.
  - Giant cell arteritis and Churg–Strauss Syndrome often undergo remission with glucocorticoids alone.
- **Cyclophosphamide** is combined with corticosteroids for rapidly progressive vasculitides, such as the ANCA-associated conditions. **Mycophenolate mofetil** has been used with efficacy for treatment of relapses in these patients.
- **Methotrexate, azathioprine,** and **mycophenolate mofetil** have been used for less severe forms of vasculitis and also for maintenance therapy following cyclophosphamide.
- **Rituximab** is a B-cell depleting agent and is non-inferior to cyclophosphamide for ANCA-associated vasculitis.[3] Rituximab may replace cyclophosphamide due to the potential reduction in long-term side effects.

COMPLICATIONS

- Inadequately treated or aggressive forms of vasculitis can lead to permanent end-organ damage and death.
- Relapse after induction treatment is unfortunately common, but re-treatment usually leads to a good response.

REFERRAL

- Referral to a rheumatologist should occur once a vasculitis is suspected to help confirm the diagnosis and direct the management of immunosuppression.

- Other specialists may be necessary depending on severity of disease in a particular organ (such as nephrologists).

PATIENT EDUCATION

- Due to the relative infrequency of these syndromes, patient education is important to help the patient understand their disease and also to dispel inaccuracies found on the internet.
- Patients must be informed of the side effects associated with their specific immunosuppressive regimen.

MONITORING/FOLLOW-UP

- The goal during follow-up is to slowly wean the level of immunosuppression to reduce potential drug-induced toxicity and monitor for flares and infections.
- Commonly, the procedures used to diagnose the patient are employed for monitoring, except for biopsy.
- A history and physical examination, along with laboratory testing, should be routinely done during the follow-up period.
  - When relapses occur, the history and physical findings will typically mimic the patient's initial presentation.
  - Routine vaccinations with killed vaccines should be done with every immunosuppressed patient.

OUTCOME/PROGNOSIS

- There is limited amount of data regarding outcome.
- Most patients who are treated early and respond appropriately to treatment do not have significant reduction in survival.

REFERENCES

1. Jennette JC, Falk RJ, Andrassy K, et al. Nomenclature of systemic vasculitides. Proposal of an international consensus conference. *Arthritis Rheum.* 1994;37(2):187–192.
2. Deng J, Ma-Krupa W, Gewirtz AT, et al. Toll-like receptors 4 and 5 induce distinct types of vasculitis. *Circ Res.* 2009;104:488–495.
3. Stone JH, Merkel PA, Spiera R, et al. Rituximab versus cyclophosphamide for ANCA-associated vasculitis. *N Engl J Med.* 2010;363:221–232.

Takayasu's Arteritis

21

Michael L. Sams and John P. Atkinson

GENERAL PRINCIPLES

Definition

- The Chapel Hill Consensus Conference defined Takayasu's arteritis (TA) as a rare **granulomatous inflammation of the aorta and its major branches.**[1]
- TA may also affect the pulmonary and coronary arteries.
- It is a chronic vasculitis characterized primarily by **stenotic,** but also, less frequently, by aneurysmal lesions of the large arteries.

Epidemiology

- TA is most common in **Asians.** The incidence is highest in Japan, with 100 to 200 new cases documented in this country per year. In the United States, the incidence is approximately 2.5 cases per million per year.
- TA characteristically affects **women** more than men, approximately 10:1.
- Peak onset is in the **third decade.** Onset of the disease after age 40 is rare.

Pathophysiology

- The cause of TA is unknown.
- TA is a focal **panarteritis affecting large vessels and their major branches,** with subsequent stenosis and aneurysm formation. Approximately 98% of patients develop **stenoses. Aneurysms** are less common but may occur.
- On gross examination, the affected vessels are thick and rigid. The lumen is affected in a characteristic "skipped" fashion, with normal lumen alternating with stenoses or aneurysms.
- Microscopic examination of acute aortic inflammation reveals:
  - **Infiltration around the vasa vasorum** by lymphocytes and plasma cells.
  - Thickening of the adventitia is present along with leukocytic infiltration of the tunica media and intimal hyperplasia.[2]
  - **Granuloma formation and giant cells** are typically located in the media. Destruction and fibrosis of the media can lead to aneurysm formation.
  - **Intimal hyperplasia** due to myofibroblast proliferation leads to characteristic stenotic lesions.
- **Chronic inflammation** in TA is characterized by **fibrosis** of all the three vessel layers. Both acute and chronic inflammations are typically seen in the same patient at the same time, implying a **recurrent process.**
- The manifestations of TA are related either to the systemic effects of chronic inflammation or the effects of localized occlusion or aneurysm formation on organ function.

DIAGNOSIS

Clinical Presentation

History

- The clinical features of TA have been divided into **three monophasic stages.**
  - **Phase one** is the "prepulseless" inflammatory phase characterized by nonspecific **constitutional symptoms** such as fever, malaise, arthralgias, and weight loss.
  - **Phase two** is characterized by **vessel inflammation manifesting as vessel pain and tenderness.** This most commonly results in carotidynia (i.e., pain on palpation of the carotid artery).
  - **Phase three** is called the "burnt-out" or **fibrotic stage** and is characterized by arterial stenoses leading to **ischemic symptoms.**
- Disease presentation is variable. Only about half of the patients have constitutional symptoms, and many patients have both inflammatory and fibrotic manifestations at the same time. Monophasic disease may also occur.
- The classic presentation of TA is that of a young woman with signs and symptoms of abnormal cerebral or upper extremity blood flow.
- **Diagnosis prior to this stenotic phase of the disease is unlikely, given the nonspecific constitutional symptoms.**
- The signs and symptoms are dependent upon the vessels affected.
  - **Subclavian** involvement occurs in over 90% of patients, resulting in arm claudication and pulselessness in about two-thirds.
  - **Aortic** involvement occurs in more than half of the patients, and may result in signs and symptoms of aortic insufficiency, hypertension, and abdominal angina. **Hypertension** in this case is believed to be due to aortic stenosis resulting in decreased blood flow to the kidneys.
  - **Common carotid** involvement is also frequent, and poses at risk for visual defects, strokes and transient ischemic attack (TIA).
  - The **renal arteries** are diseased in about one-third of the patients, typically leading to renovascular hypertension.
  - **Vertebral artery** involvement occurs at a similar rate and may trigger for dizziness and visual impairment.
- Other signs and symptoms include arrhythmia, ischemic chest pain, syncope, and visual loss. Lastly, congestive heart failure may occur and is typically related to the presence of hypertension.
- The average time between onset of symptoms and diagnosis is about 10 months.

Physical Examination

- Common findings on physical examination include **pulselessness, unequal brachial blood pressures, subclavian/carotid bruits and carotidynia.** These manifestations are attributed to ascending aorta and aortic arch involvement with resultant stenoses of their major branches and distal organ hypoperfusion.
- **Hypertension** may be noted as well and is often due to aortic or renal artery stenosis.

Diagnostic Criteria

- The American College of Rheumatology 1990 classification criteria for TA require that at least three of the following six criteria be met for diagnosis (sensitivity 90.5% and specificity 97.8%)[3]:

○ Age of disease onset <40 years.

○ Claudication of the extremities, especially the upper extremities.

○ Decreased pulses in one or both brachial arteries.

○ Systolic blood pressure difference of >10 mm Hg between arms.

○ Bruit over one or both subclavian arteries or abdominal aorta.

○ Arteriogram showing narrowing or occlusion, usually focal or segmental, of the aorta, its primary branches, or large arteries in the proximal upper or lower extremities not due to arteriosclerosis or fibromuscular dysplasia.

Differential Diagnosis

The differential diagnosis of TA includes the **infectious aortitis** (e.g., tuberculous, mycotic, and syphilitic aortitis), **Ehlers–Danlos syndrome, Marfan syndrome, sero-negative spondyloarthropathies** with aortic root involvement, **giant cell arteritis, sarcoid vasculopathy,** and **fibromuscular dysplasia.**

Diagnostic Testing

Laboratories

- Lab data in TA are nonspecific. Anemia of chronic disease, mild to moderate thrombocytosis, hypergammaglobulinemia, and elevated erythrocyte sedimentation rate (ESR) are common.
- Elevations in C-reactive protein (CRP) and/or ESR may correlate with active disease, but are not reliable in all patients.

Imaging

- Intra-arterial angiography has been the gold standard for detecting diseased vessels. However, it does not provide detail of the vessel wall, only the diameter of the lumen and pressure differences across stenotic lesions.
- MR and CT angiography are now available and can provide details about the vessel wall itself. Both modalities identify wall edema and vessel thickness. However, correlation between these wall changes and disease activity is not clear.
- Ultrasound can be used to evaluate for carotid and abdominal arterial disease.
- 18F-fluorodeoxyglucose PET scanning can detect glucose uptake in inflamed tissue and is being investigated as a technique to detect active arteritis. Also being studied is combining PET with CT scanning to help improve location of the inflammation.[2]

TREATMENT

Medications

- Medical treatment is used to treat the active inflammation in hopes of preventing the end-stage stenotic and aneurysmal arterial changes.
- Active inflammatory TA is treated initially with **oral corticosteroids.**
  ○ The typical starting dose is 1 mg/kg/day or a maximum of 60 mg of prednisone per day.
  ○ This dose may be continued for 1 to 3 months until improvement.
  ○ If the disease continued to respond, steroids may be tapered to an alternate day regimen.

- If disease fails to improve or if the patient displays intolerance of the steroid dose a **cytotoxic agent** is typically started.
  - ○ **Methotrexate** 0.3 mg/kg/week is the first choice, with an initial maximum dose of 15 mg/week that can be titrated up to 25 mg/week.
  - ○ Steroids are continued in addition to a cytotoxic agent.
  - ○ Approximately half of the patients will require a cytotoxic agent due to relapse or insufficient initial response to steroids.[1]
  - ○ If steroids cannot be tapered to an alternate day regimen within 6 months or cannot be discontinued within 12 months of initiating a cytotoxic agent, the agent is considered a failure and is stopped.
  - ○ While results of methotrexate promoting remission have been promising, limited conclusions can be drawn because of the lack of randomized controlled studies. In addition, given the extremely low prevalence of the disease, it is difficult to enroll enough subjects to provide sufficient statistical power to perform a randomized study.
- **Other cytotoxic agents** that have been used include **azathioprine and mycophenolate mofetil.** Cyclophosphamide is avoided given the long-term risk of cystitis, as well as bladder and other malignancies.
- **Tumor necrosis factor** (TNF)-α **antagonists (infliximab and etanercept)** have been studied in an open label investigation in patients with relapsing disease and steroid toxicity with promising results.[4] However, given the lack of controlled studies, further investigation is needed.
- **Hypertension** is difficult to treat as ischemia may occur in vascular beds distal to stenotic lesions when blood pressure is lowered.
  - ○ The risks of ischemia must be weighed against that of prolonged hypertension.
  - ○ Furthermore, although limb blood pressure readings are useful in detecting occlusive disease and in monitoring the progression of stenoses and limb ischemia, they are inadequate in monitoring the treatment of hypertension.
  - ○ Stenotic lesions may make peripheral blood pressure readings lower than that of central pressures.
  - ○ β-blockers and angiotensin-converting enzyme (ACE) inhibitors are not contraindicated in TA.

Surgical Management

- **Bypass surgery** and **angioplasty** are used to treat the permanent arterial damage that results.
- The indications for surgery may include:
  - ○ Hypertension associated with renal artery stenosis.
  - ○ Extremity ischemia that limits activities of daily living.
  - ○ Severe (>70%) stenosis of at least three cerebral vessels.
  - ○ Symptoms of cerebral ischemia.
  - ○ Moderate aortic regurgitation.
  - ○ Cardiac ischemia with proven coronary artery stenosis.
  - ○ An expanding aneurysm at risk of rupture also warrants surgical intervention.
- Angioplasty and endovascular stenting may also be used for stenosis. Most commonly it is used for renal artery stenosis, although there is increasing experience with angioplasty and stenting of subclavian, coronary, and aortic stenoses.
- In one long-term cohort of 60 patients, 23 required 50 bypass procedures, while 11 required angioplasty. Autologous grafts fared better than synthetic bypass grafts.[5]

- Angioplasty appears to be complicated by restenosis much more frequently than bypass surgery.
- Success rates for revascularization procedures are highest in those patients who have inactive disease by histology at the time of operation.
- It is often very difficult to determine clinically whether disease is active, but systemic features (e.g., fever, myalgias, or arthralgias), elevated ESR, features of vascular ischemia (e.g., claudication, pulse deficits, bruits, vascular pain, or asymmetric blood pressure readings), and typical angiographic features are usually used as indicators. Unfortunately, patients often fail to meet these criteria of active disease despite pathologic specimens that demonstrate active inflammation. As mentioned previously, newer imaging modalities, such as CT and MR angiography, may give information about the vessel wall that correlates with active inflammation, but further study is needed.

MONITORING/FOLLOW-UP

- For most patients, TA is a chronic disease; few patients experience a monophasic course.
- The follow-up of patients who are in clinical remission has yet to be defined.
- Current markers of active disease are recognized as inadequate indicators of inflammation. Thus, when to start or taper treatment is a difficult decision.
- Monitoring disease via serial aortography is expensive and associated with risks and the role of other imaging modalities has yet to be defined.
- Unfortunately, pathologic tissue is difficult to obtain and cannot be used for following disease activity.
- Reevaluate patients with recurring or relapsing signs and symptoms of systemic vascular inflammation as described above.

REFERENCES

1. Jennette JC, Falk RJ, Andrassy K, et al. Nomenclature of systemic vasculitides. Proposal of an international consensus conference. *Arthritis Rheum.* 1994;37:187–192.
2. Mason JC. Takayasu arteritis—advances in diagnosis and management. *Nat Rev Rheumatol.* 2010;6:406–415.
3. Arend WP, Michel BA, Bloch DA, et al. The American college of rheumatology 1990 criteria for the classification of Takayasu arteritis. *Arthritis Rheum.* 1990;33:1129–1132.
4. Molloy ES, Langford CA, Clark TM, et al. Anti-tumour necrosis factor therapy in patients with refractory Takayasu arteritis: long-term follow-up. *Ann Rheum Dis.* 2008;67: 1567–1569.
5. Kerr GS, Hallahan CW, Giordano J, et al. Takayasu arteritis. *Ann Intern Med.* 1994;120: 919–929.

Giant Cell Arteritis and Polymyalgia Rheumatica

22

Alfred H.J. Kim and John P. Atkinson

GIANT CELL ARTERITIS

GENERAL PRINCIPLES

- Giant cell arteritis (GCA, also known as temporal arteritis) is a **large- and medium-vessel vasculitis** affecting the **second- to fifth-order aortic branches,** often in the **extracranial vessels.**
  - It is characterized by **granulomatous inflammation** in vessel walls.
  - GCA is the **most common primary form of vasculitis among adults** in the United States and Europe, and occurs almost exclusively in older adults (>50 years).
- GCA presents with two major symptom complexes:
  - **Vascular insufficiency** leading to impaired blood flow.
    - **Vision loss** from ischemic optic neuropathy is the most feared complication.
    - **Headache,** scalp tenderness, jaw claudication, or central nervous system (CNS) ischemia due to **cranial arteritis** can be seen.
    - **Large-vessel GCA** can lead to **arm claudication,** pulselessness, Raynaud's phenomenon, aortic aneurysm or aortic insufficiency. All patients suspected of GCA should be screened for large vessel involvement.
  - Signs of **systemic inflammation,** including malaise, fever, and weight loss are common.
- Patients with a reasonable suspicion of GCA should be **immediately started on high-dose oral or intravenous glucocorticoid therapy** to suppress the onset of GCA-related blindness. This will not interfere with temporal artery biopsy results if the biopsy is done within 10 to 14 days of glucocorticoid initiation.
  - **Once visual compromise has started, recovery in the affected eye rarely occurs even with aggressive treatment.**

Definition

- GCA is defined by the Chapel Hill Consensus Conference as **granulomatous arteritis** of the aorta and its major branches, particularly the **extracranial branches of the carotid artery.**[1]
- Two forms of GCA have been identified, which are differentiated by the vascular bed involved:
  - **Cranial arteritis** occurs when the extracranial branches of the carotid artery are involved. This manifests as headache, **jaw claudication,** and visual changes.
  - **Large-vessel GCA** occurs when the carotid, subclavian, axillary, and other large vessels branching off the aorta are affected. Aortic arch syndrome (especially arm claudication) and aortitis can be seen.
  - Typically, cranial arteritis and large-vessel GCA do not occur in the same patient.

Epidemiology

- GCA is seen almost exclusively in older individuals. **Mean age at diagnosis is >70 years.**
- Incidence is estimated to be 1:500 individuals >50 years of age.
- Women are affected two to three times more often than men.
- 40% to 50% of GCA patients have polymyalgia rheumatica (PMR).

Etiology

- The pathogenesis of GCA is unknown.
- Genetic factors have been correlated with GCA.
  - The presence of HLA-DR4 has been significantly associated with GCA.
  - A polymorphism in the second hypervariable region of HLA-DRB1 (the region of HLA that binds to antigen) has been associated with both GCA and PMR. This polymorphism is not seen in RA patients.[2]
- Infections may play an influential role in GCA development.
  - Cyclic (every 5–7 years) peaks of the incidence of GCA suggest that some triggering event such as infection may be important.[3]
  - Gamma-herpes virus infections in interferon-γ receptor deficient mice promote a large-vessel vasculitis.[4]
  - An association with parvovirus B19 has also been proposed.[5]

Pathophysiology

- **Cell-mediated processes** appear to drive GCA pathology.
  - T cells in particular may play an important role, as the majority of vessel-infiltrating lymphocytes are CD4 T cells.[6]
  - In addition to T cells, alterations of dendritic cell function have been identified.[7]
  - Macrophages play multiple roles, such as secretion of interleukin (IL)-1, IL-6, and transforming growth factor (TGF)-β; promoting oxidative damage; producing nitric oxide; and generating giant cells.[6]
  - Components of the humoral immune response appear to be less important. B cells are not found in GCA lesions, and hypergammaglobulinemia and autoantibodies are not found in patient sera.[6]
- Cytokines, particularly **IL-6**, may play an underappreciated role in disease activity.
  - IL-6 levels strongly correlate with disease activity.[8]
  - mRNA levels of interferon-γ (IFN-γ) and IL-1β within involved arteries correlate with ischemic symptoms (vision compromise or jaw claudication), while serum IL-2 levels associate with PMR.[9]
- The pathology within vasculitic lesions of GCA explains the mechanism of vascular compromise.
  - The vasculitic lesion contains a mononuclear cell infiltrate comprised of T cells and macrophages that is present initially in the adventitia, and subsequently in all layers of the arterial wall. As the inflammatory response progresses, the media of the arterial wall thins while the intima becomes hyperplastic. This is a mechanism of vascular compromise, in addition to platelet aggregation.
  - The infiltrates may be granulomatous (particularly in the media), being characterized by the presence of histiocytes and multinucleated giant cells.
    - **While the presence of giant cells led to the naming of this disease, they are typically absent.**

- When present, they are found close to the fragmented internal elastic lamina. This correlates with elevated platelet-derived growth factor (PDGF) levels and increased risk of ischemic complications.[10]
  - The presence of fibrinoid necrosis should suggest another type of vasculitic process.

Risk Factors

- Age is the greatest risk factor for both GCA.
- Female gender is associated with GCA.
- Ethnicity is another risk factor for GCA development. Patients of Northern European descent are 2.5- to 4-fold more likely than Southern Europeans, and 7.5- to 25-fold more likely than Hispanics and African-Americans to develop GCA.[11]

Prevention

No known preventive measures have been identified for GCA.

DIAGNOSIS

- It is rare to have GCA in individuals <50 years of age.
- **Headache is the most common presenting symptom for GCA, while jaw claudication mostly highly predicts a positive temporal artery biopsy.**
- Anyone suspected to have GCA should be started on high-dose oral or intravenous glucocorticoid therapy, even if the temporal artery biopsy has not yet been performed.
- If the temporal artery biopsy is negative, but suspicion for GCA remains high, treat as if the patient has GCA and consider biopsy of the other temporal artery.
- GCA should also be considered in patients >50 years of age with fever of unknown origin.

Clinical Presentation

History

- In **GCA,** the onset of symptoms tends to be **gradual** rather than abrupt.
- **Cranial arteritis:** 80% to 90% of all GCA cases present with cranial arteritis.
  - **Headache:** over half of the patients will have a chief complaint of headache.
    - Characterized as throbbing, sharp, or dull.
    - Located classically over the temporal regions, but can be seen over the occipital or frontal lobes, or be generalized.
  - **Temporal tenderness:** Individuals may also complain about temporal tenderness when wearing eyeglasses or lying on a pillow.
  - **Jaw claudication:** 50% of patients will complain of fatigue or pain while eating, or trismus-like symptoms.
    - Patients may not recognize the significance of this, so they must be asked directly.
    - Symptoms are due to reduced blood flow through the extracranial branches of the carotid artery supplying the masseter or temporalis muscles.
    - A striking feature of GCA-associated jaw claudication is how quickly fatigue begins upon chewing, and how disabling the pain can be.

- Jaw claudication may be the most specific symptom for cranial arteritis. Fifty-four percent of those with jaw claudication had a positive temporal artery biopsy, while only three percent of those with a negative biopsy had jaw claudication.[12]
○ **Systemic complaints:**
  - 50% will have low-grade fever (>37.7 °C), while 15% have fevers >39 °C.[13]
  - 15% of elderly patients with fever of unknown origin are diagnosed with GCA.[13]
  - 10% of patients will have constitutional symptoms or laboratory evidence of inflammation as the only symptoms/signs of GCA.[14]
○ **Visual complaints:** a wide variety of manifestations occur in GCA.
  - **Vision loss is sudden, painless and usually permanent.**
  - **Amaurosis fugax** is a temporary monocular loss of vision caused by focal ophthalmic artery lesions. This leads to transient ischemia of the retina, choroid, or optic nerve, or a combination of the above. Patients will report **visual blurring** (associated with heat, exercise, or posture) and **diplopia.** If left untreated, the other eye will likely be affected in 1 to 2 weeks.
  - **Anterior ischemic optic neuropathy** (AION) may follow an episode of amaurosis fugax. It is due to compromise of blood flow through the posterior ciliary artery leading to acute ischemia of the optic nerve head. Typically presenting unilaterally, the other eye can be affected within days or weeks if left untreated. **While AION is the most common ocular presentation of GCA, only 5% of AION patients have GCA.**
  - **Posterior ischemic optic neuropathy is a rare** (approximately 5%) etiology for the cause of blindness in GCA. This is due to compromised blood flow to the retrobulbar portion of the optic nerve.
  - Despite effective therapy, vision loss occurs in one or both eyes in 15% to 20% of GCA patients. This is due in part to the fact that blindness may be the presenting symptom.
  - **Diplopia** can occur not only from amaurosis fugax, but also from ischemic injury to the oculomotor system or extraocular muscles, paresis of ocular motor nerves, and brainstem disease.
  - **Bitemporal hemianopia** occurs when arteries supplying the optic chiasm are damaged.
  - **Homonymous hemianopia** (vision defect involving either the two right or left halves of the visual field) results from damage to vessels feeding the retrochiasmal visual sensory pathways. In GCA, this most commonly occurs from lesions in the vertebrobasilar circulation, leading to occipital lobe infarction.
  - **Visual hallucinations** can be induced by glucocorticoid-associated psychosis or from Charles Bonnet syndrome (the presence of visual hallucinations in psychologically normal patients due to vision loss from peripheral or central vision pathway lesions).
○ **Musculoskeletal complaints:**
  - **PMR** (see later for symptoms) is observed in 40% to 50% of GCA patients, but only 15% of PMR patients have GCA. Five percent of patients considered to have isolated PMR will have a positive temporal artery biopsy.
  - **Peripheral synovitis and peripheral edema** of the distal extremities are also seen in a minority of GCA patients. These symptoms can mimic

seronegative rheumatoid arthritis (RA) or remitting seronegative symmetrical synovitis with pitting edema (RS3PE) (see Differential Diagnosis).

- ○ **Neurologic complaints:** Neurologic manifestations occur in 20% to 30%.
  - ■ **Transient ischemic attacks (TIAs) and strokes** are typically due to extradural internal carotid (less common) or vertebral artery (more common) vasculitic lesions. Aortic dissection can also compromise blood flow through these vessels leading to symptoms.
  - ■ **Vertigo and hearing loss** can also occur with vertebral or carotid artery involvement.
  - ■ **Intracranial vasculitis** is extremely rare (<1%).
- • **Large-vessel GCA:** Represents 10% to 15% of all GCA cases, and typically lacks cranial involvement. These patients are marginally younger (mean age = 66 years), have fewer complaints of headache, and more likely to present with arm claudication. Fifty percent of these patients will have had a negative temporal artery biopsy.
  - ○ **Aortic arch syndrome:** Observed with involvement of the subclavian and axillary arteries.
    - ■ **Arm claudication** is the most common symptom, seen in 51% of large-vessel GCA patients.
    - ■ **Absent or asymmetric pulses and paresthesias** may also be seen.
  - ○ **Aortitis**
    - ■ Active aortitis was observed in 50% of GCA patients postmortem as well as at surgery, most commonly affects the **ascending aorta**, which can lead to dilatation of the aortic valve.
    - ■ **Aneurysms** (particularly thoracic, can present similarly to Takayasu's arteritis [see Chapter 21, Takayasu's Arteritis]) and **dissections** (due to chronic aortitis) are the most significant complications.
  - ○ There is a 17-fold increased incidence of thoracic aortic aneurysm development, which occurs in approximately 10% of GCA patients.[15]
  - ○ Similarities between GCA and Takayasu's arteritis highlight the possibility that they are part of a spectrum of the same disease.

Physical Examination
- • **GCA** patients are typically **chronically ill** appearing, often with **fever.**
- • **Temporal artery abnormalities:**
  - ○ **Decreased or absent pulses:** If pulse was absent, likelihood ratio (LR) of a positive temporal artery biopsy was 2.7 over a patient without this finding.[16]
  - ○ **Tender or thickened artery:** If the patient had a prominent or enlarged temporal artery, the LR = 4.3; if tender, LR = 2.6.[16]
  - ○ Even in the absence of physical examination findings relative to the temporal artery, 33% will still have a positive temporal artery biopsy.[17]
- • **Ophthalmologic findings:**
  - ○ May be normal in those with amaurosis fugax.
  - ○ Cotton wool spots can be seen at areas of vascular lesions.
  - ○ **Swollen pale optic disc with blurred margins** in those with acute vision loss from AION.
  - ○ Optic atrophy and pale, flat disc in those with permanent blindness from AION. These patients will also have a relative afferent pupillary defect (Marcus Gunn pupil manifested by positive swinging flashlight sign).

- **Cardiovascular findings:**
  - ○ **Bruits** may be heard on auscultation of supraclavicular, carotid, axillary, brachial, and femoral areas.
  - ○ **Aortic regurgitation murmur** may indicate an ascending aortic aneurysm.
  - ○ **Diminished pulses** in the extremities may be associated with asymmetric blood pressures in affected extremities.
- **Musculoskeletal** (see Polymyalgia Rheumatica later).

Diagnostic Criteria

- No true diagnostic criteria exist for GCA. The ACR criteria, though, can influence the decision to proceed with subsequent temporal artery biopsy.
- The following clinical findings were effective in distinguishing GCA from other forms of vasculitis[18,19]:
  - ○ Age ≥50 years at time of disease onset.
  - ○ Localized headache of new onset.
  - ○ Tenderness or decreased pulse of temporal artery.
  - ○ Erythrocyte sedimentation rate (ESR) >50 mm/hour.
  - ○ Biopsy revealing necrotizing arteritis with a predominance of mononuclear cells or a granulomatous process with multinucleated giant cells.
- If a patient has an existing diagnosis of vasculitis, the presence of three of these five criteria is associated with 94% sensitivity and 91% specificity for the diagnosis of GCA.[18]
- There is a 95% probability for a negative temporal artery biopsy with the following findings[20]:
  - ○ ESR <40 mm/hour.
  - ○ No jaw claudication.
  - ○ No temporal artery tenderness.
  - ○ Presence of synovitis.

Differential Diagnosis

- The differential diagnosis for GCA includes:
  - ○ Other large-vessel vasculitides (such as Takayasu's arteritis, which does not involve the temporal artery).
  - ○ Polyarteritis nodosa, Wegener's granulomatosis or CNS vasculitis (if involving the temporal artery).
  - ○ Amyloidosis (presenting as jaw or arm claudication if vascular involvement of the temporal or subclavian artery occurs).
  - ○ Nonarteritic anterior ischemic optic neuropathy (NAAION) has low inflammatory markers and is associated with hypertension, diabetes mellitus, and sildenafil use.

Diagnostic Testing

Laboratories

- No single laboratory test is pathognomonic for diagnosing GCA, but they can strongly suggest the presence of disease. Laboratory abnormalities resolve with glucocorticoid treatment.
- Complete blood count (CBC)
  - ○ **Normocytic anemia** is usually present at diagnosis of GCA. Interestingly, the white blood cell (WBC) count is generally normal despite systemic signs of inflammation.

- Comprehensive metabolic panel (CMP)
  - **Transaminitis and an elevation in alkaline phosphatase** are seen in 25% to 35% of GCA patients; serum albumin levels are usually normal.[21]
- ESR and C-reactive protein (CRP)
  - **Significant elevations of ESR and CRP** values are characteristically seen in GCA.
  - In GCA, a normal ESR reduces the probability of a positive temporal artery biopsy by 5-fold.[16] An ESR <40 mm/hour correlates to fewer systemic systems, but does not reduce the likelihood of visual loss in those with GCA.
  - In GCA, the CRP usually correlates with ESR values.
- IL-6
  - **IL-6 concentrations closely correlate with clinical disease** in GCA and more strongly predict relapse than ESR. IL-6 testing is not yet widespread, and its clinical usefulness is unclear.[8]

Imaging
- **For GCA-associated cranial arteritis, imaging is typically not necessary.** Magnetic resonance angiography (MRA) has been utilized to identify areas of temporal artery inflammation, helping to guide temporal artery biopsy.
- **If large-vessel GCA is suspected, the study of choice is MRA.** Aortic, carotid, subclavian, and other large vessels can be visualized for the presence of vessel wall edema.
  - While MRA has been investigated in tracking disease activity and in the evaluation of response to treatment, vessel wall edema has not been always associated with disease activity or helpful in identifying new lesions. Therefore, its use should always be in conjunction with clinical findings in the setting of GCA.
  - While currently investigational, the future use of positron emission tomography (PET) may be beneficial in the identification of large-vessel GCA.
- The role of conventional angiography has been limited with the use of MRA. It does play a role in those with large-vessel GCA in all the four extremities where peripheral blood pressure measurements are unreliable. Aortography with central aortic pressure measurements may be useful in this setting.
- Ultrasound has shown mixed success in GCA, and is unreliable at this time.

Diagnostic Procedures
- **Temporal artery biopsy** is the gold standard in establishing the diagnosis of GCA, and should be done in all patients suspected to have GCA.
- Sensitivity of temporal artery biopsy is 94%.[18]
- The predictive value of a positive biopsy was significantly increased in patients with jaw claudication, and higher yet with the addition of headache, scalp tenderness or vision changes.[22]
- A 2-cm length of the temporal artery should be obtained unless the artery is visibly abnormal, where a smaller segment can yield the diagnosis. Complications are rare with this procedure.
- Full tissue processing should be performed, as there may be "skip" lesions.
- Controversy exists whether to obtain unilateral or bilateral temporal artery biopsy samples.
  - Unilateral biopsy is usually sufficient to diagnose GCA, missing only 13% of cases compared to bilateral biopsies.[23,24]

- We suggest the following algorithm to decide on unilateral versus bilateral temporal artery biopsies (as proposed by the European League Against Rheumatism)[25]:
  - If an obvious temporal artery abnormality is present on examination, or headache is unilateral, biopsy of that vessel should be performed.
  - If there are no localizing hints, obtain a unilateral temporal artery biopsy.
  - If the unilateral biopsy result is negative, and clinical suspicion remains high, biopsy of the contralateral temporal artery should be considered.
  - Patient preference may play a role in the decision to obtain a simultaneous bilateral biopsy.
  - Regardless, **treatment for GCA should be initiated before the biopsy is scheduled.** The inflammatory infiltrate resolves slowly after starting prednisone, usually not resolving for weeks to months.
- Recognize that **negative biopsies do not exclude the possibility of large-vessel GCA** (look for arm claudication in those patients).
- Biopsy of other vessels: Temporal arteries are typically biopsied since they are easily accessible. If other vessels are abnormal (such as the facial or occipital arteries), then those can also be biopsied.

TREATMENT

The goal of treatment for GCA is to avoid AION. Unfortunately, once vision has been lost, the likelihood of significant visual improvement is small (<10%). **Thus, prevention of vision loss is of paramount importance.**

Medications

Glucocorticoids

- The standard of care is **glucocorticoids,** despite the lack of placebo-controlled studies. Its efficacy in GCA has been established through many years of use and the known consequences of untreated disease.
- **Glucocorticoids must be started immediately once a patient has been suspected to have GCA,** even before the diagnosis has been confirmed. This is especially true if the patient has recent or potential vascular complications. **Nevertheless, temporal artery biopsies should be obtained as quickly as possible.**
- The optimal initial dose is unclear, but virtually all cases should be started on a minimum of **prednisone 40 to 60 mg PO daily.**
- Daily dosing is more efficacious than alternate day dosing. Splitting a single daily dose into multiple doses during the day is no more effective than single daily dosing.
- The use of **intravenous glucocorticoids** (15 mg/kg/day of methylprednisolone for three doses) has been investigated in a small randomized, double-blind, placebo-controlled study, concluding that those receiving methylprednisolone had[26]:
  - Higher rates of sustained remission following the discontinuation of glucocorticoid therapy.
  - Higher likelihood of achieving and maintaining low doses of prednisone (≤5 mg/day) at 9, 12, and 15 months following initial loading dose.
  - Lower median total glucocorticoid dose (excluding the initial loading dose).

○ Those with vision loss at diagnosis did not improve significantly with parenteral glucocorticoids.

○ In summary, while the use of parenteral glucocorticoids for those with visual dysfunction has not been rigorously tested, we believe that it is appropriate to use pulse-dose glucocorticoids for these patients.

- **Patients should be maintained on the starting dose of glucocorticoids for at least 2 to 4 weeks or whenever disease activity resolves, whichever comes later.** A slow taper should follow this over the next 9 to 18 months.

  ○ Typically, patients will report **resolution of symptoms 24 to 48 hours after treatment initiation** (with the exception of vision loss from AION). Laboratory measures of inflammation will also begin to normalize during this time.

  ○ The tapering of prednisone should be done with the goal of avoiding flares.

  ○ **A reasonable initial goal for prednisone tapering is to reach 20 mg/day at 2 months of therapy.**

  ○ The tapering schedule will slow down after this. Usually, once 10 mg/day is reached, decrease the dose by 1 mg every month, so that the full course of treatment is 9 to 12 months in total.

  ○ **If a patient flares during the tapering process, redosing with the initial starting dose should be done with a slower tapering schedule afterwards.**

  ○ Patients rarely flare at doses >15 mg/day, but unfortunately commonly do below this dose.

Aspirin

The use of **daily low-dose aspirin** to reduce the risk of vision loss, TIA, and stroke has been recommended.[27] This benefit appears to be due to its antiplatelet effect.

Other Medications

- Methotrexate (MTX)
  ○ Data from three randomized trials tested whether MTX can be used as a steroid-sparing agent with conflicting results.[28–30]
  ○ The use of MTX for GCA is not recommended at this time.
- Infliximab
  ○ One randomized trial showed a lack of efficacy for tumor necrosis factor (TNF) inhibition in GCA.[31]
- Tocilizumab, a monoclonal anti–IL-6 antibody, has shown efficacy in a few case reports.[32]

COMPLICATIONS

- Other than visual loss, no long-term complications typically occur directly from GCA as the disease is self-limited over months or years.
- Most complications occur as a result of prolonged glucocorticoid use, and should be addressed as necessary. One should **anticipate side effects from prolonged use of prednisone therapy** (see Chapter 9, Drugs Used for the Treatment of Rheumatic Diseases).
  ○ Hyperglycemia, weight gain, infection, hypertension, and other side effects must be monitored.
  ○ Loss of bone integrity or frank **osteoporosis** can also occur. Screen with bone density scans and prophylactic treatment with calcium, vitamin D, and an appropriate osteoporotic medication (see Chapter 48, Osteoporosis).

REFERRAL

- Those suspected with GCA should be immediately referred to a rheumatologist. If there is strong suspicion of disease or if there are vision symptoms, inpatient management with rheumatology consultation is warranted.
- Anyone requiring prolonged glucocorticoid use should be referred to a rheumatologist for medication toxicity monitoring.

PATIENT EDUCATION

- Patients must be informed of the side effects associated with prednisone and appropriately managed to avoid long-term complications.
- Recognition of symptoms of GCA must be emphasized to patients to aid in flare identification.

MONITORING/FOLLOW-UP

- **Monitoring for disease activity is challenging in GCA.** It can be difficult to assess the presence of flares in the setting of a prednisone taper.
- Following **ESR and CRP** is very useful, but they are imperfect markers of disease activity, as not everyone mirrors clinical activity with these labs.
  - **When the ESR or CRP is elevated, question the patient regarding any symptoms related to GCA. Close follow-up is warranted in this setting.**
  - IL-6 may prove to be a more reliable measure of disease activity than ESR, although the clinical usefulness of this assay has not been thoroughly assessed.[8]
- Yearly chest radiography to evaluate for aortic aneurysms should be done for at least 10 years following the initial diagnosis. If dilatation is present, chest CT every 6 to 12 months should be performed.

OUTCOME/PROGNOSIS

- Prognosis is typically very good in those with timely and appropriate treatment.
- Some may need life-long low-dose glucocorticoid therapy for suppressing GCA disease activity.
- In those without visual compromise, new presentation of vision loss is uncommon once treatment has begun (<1%).
- In those with preexisting visual defects from GCA, the incidence of contralateral vision loss is estimated to be 13% over the next 5 years, even with appropriate treatment.[33] Age >80 is the most significant risk factor for this outcome.
- Overall survival appears not to be affected in those with GCA.

POLYMYALGIA RHEUMATICA

GENERAL PRINCIPLES

- PMR is a musculoskeletal syndrome seen in individuals **>50 years of age** manifested by **symmetric pain and stiffness in the muscles of the neck, torso, shoulders, and hip girdle for at least 4 weeks.**

○ It is associated with signs of systemic inflammation, elevated ESR and CRP, and anemia.

○ **PMR is closely related to GCA,** and is often considered a form of GCA that lacks fully developed vasculitis.

○ PMR responds very well to low-dose oral glucocorticoid therapy.

Definition

PMR is a syndrome characterized by symmetric aching and morning stiffness on the shoulder and hip girdles, neck and torso in individuals >50 years old with an ESR >50 mm/hour.

Epidemiology

- PMR is seen almost exclusively in older individuals. **Mean age at diagnosis is >70 years.**
- Like, GCA, it is rare to have PMR in individuals <50 years old.
- Women are affected —two to three times more often than men.
- 15% of PMR patients develop GCA.

Etiology

- The pathogenesis of PMR is unknown.
- Genetic factors have been correlated with PMR.
  ○ A polymorphism in the second hypervariable region of HLA-DRB1 (the region of HLA that binds to antigen) has been associated with PMR.[2]
  ○ Other genetic polymorphisms in intracellular adhesion molecule (ICAM)-1, TNF-α, vascular endothelial growth factor (VEGF), or carriage of certain alleles, such as the PI^{A2} allele of the platelet glycoprotein IIIa gene, may also be associated with PMR.[34–37]

Pathophysiology

The pathophysiology driving PMR is unknown.

Risk Factors

- Age is the greatest risk factor for PMR.
- Female gender is associated with PMR.

Prevention

No known preventive measures have been identified for PMR.

DIAGNOSIS

Clinical Presentation

History

- **PMR** is characterized by the subacute or chronic onset of symmetric morning stiffness and achiness of the shoulder and hip girdles, neck, and torso.
- **Morning stiffness** and tenderness last >30 minutes, leading to difficulties dressing or turning over in bed. It is thought to be due to bursitis and/or synovitis.
- Pain occurs in **shoulders** more than in hips or neck. It is worse with movement and can interfere with sleep. It may be associated with subjective weakness.

- Sleep is often disrupted.
- **Systemic symptoms** occur in up to 40% of patients, and include malaise, depression, anorexia and weight loss, and fever (almost always low grade unless GCA is present).

Physical Examination

- **Pain** with active range of motion of shoulders, neck, and hips.
- **Tenderness to palpation of shoulders.**
- **Synovitis occurs** in knees, wrists, and metacarpophalangeal (MCP) joint, and is typically mild, asymmetric, and nonerosive. It is also seen in 15% to 20% of GCA patients.
- **Tenosynovitis** and **peripheral edema** occur most commonly in hands, wrists, ankles, and the dorsum of feet, and are thought to represent regional tenosynovitis. Carpal tunnel syndrome is seen in 10% to 15% of patients.

Diagnostic Criteria

- No diagnostic criteria exist for PMR, but the following have been suggested to strongly support the diagnosis[19]:
  - Age >50.
  - ESR >40, or elevated CRP in the setting of normal ESR.
  - One month duration of morning stiffness >30 minutes and bilateral aching of the two of the following three areas: neck/torso, shoulders/proximal arms, and hip/proximal thighs.
  - Prompt responsiveness (within 3 days) to low-dose glucocorticoid therapy (10–20 mg/day prednisone) has been suggested by some as another criterion.

Differential Diagnosis

- **Early seronegative RA** is the most common alternative diagnosis in patients presenting with symptoms consistent with PMR.
  - RA patients will have more swollen joints of the hands, wrists and feet and usually only a partial response to low-dose prednisone compared to PMR patients. PMR patients will have complete resolution of any swollen joints and a more rapid decrease in acute phase reactants with low-dose prednisone.
  - Nevertheless, there is considerable symptom overlap between seronegative RA and PMR, making the diagnosis difficult at times.
- Other diagnoses mimicking PMR include:
  - Remitting seronegative symmetric synovitis with pitting edema (RS3PE)
  - Bursitis/tendonitis
  - Spondyloarthropathy
  - Calcium pyrophosphate deposition disease (CPPD)
  - Hypothyroidism
  - Fibromyalgia and depression
  - Malignancy (such as multiple myeloma)
  - Infective endocarditis
  - Inflammatory myopathy (pain is usually not a feature; creatine kinase is normal in PMR)
  - Parkinson disease
  - Hyperparathyroidism

Diagnostic Testing

Laboratories

- Similar to GCA, no single laboratory test independently diagnoses PMR, but can strongly suggest the presence of disease. Laboratory abnormalities resolve with glucocorticoid treatment.
- **Normocytic anemia** is usually present at diagnosis of PMR. The WBC count is generally normal despite systemic signs of inflammation.
- **ESR and CRP are typically significantly elevated.**

Imaging

- For PMR, imaging is typically not required. Nevertheless, **MRI** and **ultrasound** have been shown to demonstrate inflammation of extraarticular synovial structures such as tenosynovitis or shoulder bursitis with effusion.
- Plain films of affected joints do not usually reveal abnormalities.

Diagnostic Procedures

No invasive diagnostic procedures aid in the diagnosis of PMR.

T R E A T M E N T

Medications

- The goal of treatment is resolution of symptoms.
- **A prompt response (within 24–48 hours) to glucocorticoid therapy is highly characteristic of PMR.**

Prednisone

- Initial dosing of **prednisone 15 mg PO daily** is sufficient for most patients, but this may range from 10 to 20 mg/day.[38]
  - ○ Symptom reduction should be evident within 3 days of treatment, often overnight.
  - ○ **Maintain the initial dose of prednisone for 2 to 4 weeks.**
  - ○ If symptoms are not well controlled, increase prednisone by 5 mg/day up to 30 mg/day.
  - ○ **An alternative diagnosis should be entertained if little or no symptom relief is obtained with prednisone dose of 20 mg/day or higher.**
- Generally, maintenance dosing and prednisone tapering protocols lack consensus. We recommend:
  - ○ For those receiving ≥15 mg/day, reduce prednisone by 5 mg/day every 2 to 4 weeks to 15 mg/day.
  - ○ For those receiving 10 to 15 mg/day, reduce by 2.5 mg/day every month.
  - ○ For those receiving ≤10 mg/day, reduce by 1 mg/day every month.
  - ○ **Flares typically occur if tapering is too rapid.** Restart prednisone at approximately the last dose that achieved complete symptom control, and restart tapering at a slower rate (every 2–3 months).
  - ○ If a flare occurs off prednisone, the patient may need to completely restart the initial dosing and tapering protocol.
  - ○ Continue low-dose prednisone for at least 1 year to minimize the risk of relapse after discontinuation.

Other Therapies
- MTX
  - Inconsistent results have been observed in those receiving MTX with prednisone compared to prednisone alone. Its use in PMR is typically not recommended.
- Etanercept
  - In two very small observational studies and one small randomized trial, etanercept has demonstrated modest efficacy.[39–41]
- Infliximab
  - In contrast to etanercept, infliximab in combination with prednisone did not demonstrate superiority compared to prednisone alone. *Ann Intern Med.* 2007;146:631–639.[42]
- Nonsteroidal antiinflammatory drugs (NSAIDs)
  - NSAIDs may be effective in some as glucocorticoid-sparing therapy, but drug-related side effects limit their use in this elderly patient population.
  - NSAIDs may be used as adjunct therapy with low-dose prednisone for osteoarthritis or tendonitis pain, but great care must be used to avoid gastrointestinal side effects. Concurrent proton-pump inhibitor (PPI) administration should be strongly encouraged.

COMPLICATIONS

- No long-term complications typically occur directly from GCA or PMR as the disease is self-limited over months or years.
- Most complications occur as a result of prolonged glucocorticoid use, and should be addressed as necessary. **One should anticipate side effects from prolonged use of prednisone therapy** (see Chapter 9, Drugs Used for the Treatment of Rheumatic Diseases).
  - Hyperglycemia, weight gain, infection, hypertension, and other side effects must be monitored.
  - Loss of bone integrity or frank **osteoporosis** can also occur. Screen with bone density scans and prophylactic treatment with calcium, vitamin D, and an appropriate osteoporotic medication (see Chapter 48, Osteoporosis).

REFERRAL

Anyone requiring prolonged glucocorticoid use should be referred to a rheumatologist for medication toxicity monitoring.

Patient Education
- Patients must be informed of the side effects associated with prednisone and appropriately managed to avoid long-term complications.
- Recognition of symptoms of GCA must be emphasized to PMR patients.

MONITORING/FOLLOW-UP

- Monitoring for symptoms in PMR is the best method for picking up flares. Interpretation of ESR and CRP values must be done in the context of the patient's clinical presentation.
- **Those with PMR should be continuously monitored for symptoms of GCA.** 4.4% of those with "isolated" PMR had positive temporal artery biopsies.

OUTCOME/PROGNOSIS

- Overall survival appears not to be affected in those with PMR.
- Glucocorticoid therapy for PMR typically lasts for 2 to 3 years, but some may need long-term low-dose (<10 mg/day) treatment. Spontaneous relapse occurs in up to 25% of patients regardless of glucocorticoid dosing, particularly in the first two years.

REFERENCES

1. Jennette JC, Falk RJ, Andrassy K, et al. Nomenclature of systemic vasculitides. Proposal of an international consensus conference. *Arthritis Rheum.* 1994;37:187–192.
2. Weyand CM, Hunder NN, Hicok KC, et al. HLA-DRB1 alleles in polymyalgia rheumatica, giant cell arteritis, and rheumatoid arthritis. *Arthritis Rheum.* 1994;37:514–520.
3. Petursdottir V, Johansson H, Nordbord E, et al. The epidemiology of biopsy-positive giant cell arteritis: special reference to cyclic fluctuations. *Rheumatology (Oxford).* 1999;38:1208–1212.
4. Weck KE, Dal Canto AJ, Gould JD, et al. Murine gamma-herpesvirus 68 causes severe large-vessel arteritis in mice lacking interferon-gamma responsiveness: a new model for virus-induced vascular disease. *Nat Med.* 1997;3:1346–1353.
5. Gabriel SE, Espy M, Erdman DD, et al. The role of parvovirus B19 in the pathogenesis of giant cell arteritis: a preliminary evaluation. *Arthritis Rheum.* 1999;42:1255–1258.
6. Weyand CM, Goronzy JJ. Medium- and large-vessel vasculitis. *N Eng J Med.* 2003;349:160–169.
7. Ma-Krupa W, Jeon MS, Spoerl S, et al. Activation of arterial wall dendritic cells and breakdown of self-tolerance in giant cell arteritis. *J Exp Med.* 2004;199:173–183.
8. Roche NE, Fulbright JW, Wagner AD, et al. Correlation of interleukin-6 production and disease activity in polymyalgia rheumatica and giant cell arteritis. *Arthritis Rheum.* 1993;36:1286–1294.
9. Weyand CM, Tetzlaff N, Björnsson J, et al. Disease patterns and tissue cytokine profiles in giant cell arteritis. *Arthritis Rheum.* 1997;40:19–26.
10. Kaiser M, Weyand CM, Björnsson J, et al. Platelet-derived growth factor, intimal hyperplasia, and ischemic complications in giant cell arteritis. *Arthritis Rheum.* 1998;41:623–633.
11. Hunder GG. Giant cell arteritis and polymyalgia rheumatica. *Med Clin North Am.* 1997;81:195–219.
12. Hall S, Persellin S, Lie JT, et al. The therapeutic impact of temporal artery biopsy. *Lancet.* 1983;2:1217–1220.
13. Calamia KT, Hunder GG. Giant cell arteritis (temporal arteritis) presenting as fever of undetermined origin. *Arthritis Rheum.* 1981;24:1414–1418.
14. Gonzalez-Fay MA, Barros S, Lopez-Diaz ME, et al. Giant cell arteritis: disease patterns of clinical presentation in a series of 240 patients. *Medicine (Baltimore).* 2005;84:269–276.

15. Evans JM, O'Fallon WM, Hender GG. Increased incidence of aortic aneurysm and dissection in giant cell (temporal) arteritis. A population-based study. *Ann Intern Med.* 1995; 122:202–207.

16. Smetana GW, Shmerling RH. Does this patient have temporal arteritis. *JAMA.* 2002; 287:92–101.

17. Manna R, Cristiano G, Todaro L, et al. Microscopic haematuria: a diagnostic aid in giant-cell arteritis? *Lancet.* 1997;350:1226.

18. Hunder GG, Bloch DA, Michel BA, et al. The American College of Rheumatology 1990 criteria for the classification of giant cell arteritis. *Arthritis Rheum.* 1990;33:1122–1128.

19. Salvarani C, Cantini F, Hunder GG. Polymyalgia rheumatica and giant-cell arteritis. *Lancet.* 2008;372:234–245.

20. Gabriel SE, O'Fallon WM, Achkar AA, et al. The use of clinical characteristics to predict the results of temporal artery biopsy among patients with suspected giant cell arteritis. *J Rheumatol.* 1995;22:93–96.

21. Hazleman B. Laboratory investigations useful in the evaluation of polymyalgia rheumatica (PMR) and giant cell arteritis (GCA). *Clin Exp Rheumatol.* 2000;18:S29–S31.

22. Younge BR, Cook BE Jr, Bartley GB, et al. Initiation of glucocorticoid therapy: before or after temporal artery biopsy? *Mayo Clin Proc.* 2004;79:483–491.

23. Pless M, Rizzo JF 3rd, Lamkin JC, et al. Concordance of bilateral temporal artery biopsy in giant cell arteritis. *J Neuroophthalmol.* 2000;20:216–218.

24. Breuer GS, Nesher G, Nesher R. Rate of discordant findings in bilateral temporal artery biopsy to diagnose giant cell arteritis. *J Rheumatol.* 2009;36:794–796.

25. Mukhtyar C, Guillevin L, Cid MC, et al. EULAR recommendations for the management of large vessel vasculitis. *Ann Rheum Dis.* 2009;68:318–323.

26. Mazlumzadeh M, Hunder GG, Easley KA, et al. Treatment of giant cell arteritis using induction therapy with high-dose glucocorticoids: a double-blind, placebo-controlled, randomized prospective clinical trial. *Arthritis Rheum.* 2006;54:3310–3318.

27. Lee MS, Smith SD, Galor A, et al. Antiplatelet and anticoagulant therapy in patients with giant cell arteritis. *Arthritis Rheum.* 2006;54:3306–3309.

28. Jover JA, Hernández-Garcia C, Morado IC, et al. Combined treatment of giant-cell arteritis with methotrexate and prednisone. a randomized, double-blind, placebo-controlled trial. *Ann Intern Med.* 2001;134:106–114.

29. Spiera RF, Mitnick HJ, Kupersmith M, et al. A prospective, double-blind, randomized, placebo controlled trial of methotrexate in the treatment of giant cell arteritis (GCA). *Clin Exp Rheumatol.* 2001;19:495–501.

30. Hoffman GS, Cid MD, Hellmann DB, et al. A multicenter, randomized, double-blind, placebo-controlled trial of adjuvant methotrexate treatment for giant cell arteritis. *Arthritis Rheum.* 2002;46:1309–1318.

31. Martínez-Taboada VM, Rodríguez-Valverde V, Carreño L, et al. A double-blind placebo controlled trial of etanercept in patients with giant cell arteritis and corticosteroid side effects. *Ann Rheum Dis.* 2008;67:625–630.

32. Seitz M, Reichenbach S, Bonel HM. Rapid induction of remission in large vessel vasculitis by IL-6 blockade. A case series. *Swiss Med Wkly.* 2011;141:w13156.

33. Aiello PD, Trautmann JC, McPhee TJ, et al. Visual prognosis in giant cell arteritis. *Ophthalmology.* 1993;100:550–555.

34. Salvarani C, Casali B, Boiardi L, et al. Intercellular adhesion molecule 1 gene polymorphisms in polymyalgia rheumatica/giant cell arteritis: association with disease risk and severity. *J Rheumatol.* 2000;27:1215–1221.

35. Mattey DL, Hajeer AH, Dababneh A, et al. Association of giant cell arteritis and polymyalgia rheumatica with different tumor necrosis factor microsatellite polymorphisms. *Arthritis Rheum.* 2000;43:1749–1755.

36. Meliconi R, Pulsatelli L, Dolzani P, et al. Vascular endothelial growth factor production in polymyalgia rheumatica. *Arthritis Rheum.* 2000;43:2472–2480.

37. Salvarani D, Casali B, Farnetti E, et al. PlA1/A2 polymorphism of the platelet glycoprotein receptor IIIA and risk of cranial ischemic complications in giant cell arteritis. *Arthritis Rheum.* 2007;56:3502–3508.

38. Dasgupta B, Borg FA, Hassan N, et al. BSR and BHPR guidelines for the management of polymyalgia rheumatica. *Rheumatology (Oxford)*. 2010;49:186–190.
39. Catanoso MG, Macchioni P, Boiardi L, et al. Treatment of refractory polymyalgia rheumatica with etanercept: an open pilot study. *Arthritis Rheum*. 2007;57:1514–1519.
40. Corrao S, Pistone G, Scaglione R, et al. Fast recovery with etanercept in patients affected by polymyalgia rheumatica and decompensated diabetes: a case-series study. *Clin Rheumatol*. 2009;28:89–92.
41. Kreiner F, Galbo H. Effect of etanercept in polymyalgia rheumatica: a randomized controlled trial. *Arthritis Res Ther*. 2010;12:R176.
42. Salvarani C, Macchioni P, Manzini C, et al. Infliximab plus prednisone or placebo plus prednisone for the initial treatment of polymyalgia rheumatica: a randomized trial. *Ann Intern Med*. 2007;146:631–639.

Polyarteritis Nodosa

23

Maria C. Gonzalez-Mayda and
John P. Atkinson

GENERAL PRINCIPLES

- Formal diagnosis of polyarteritis nodosa (PAN) requires the presence of three out of the ten criteria listed in Table 23-1. Of these, a biopsy or angiogram demonstrating vasculitis of small- to medium-sized vessels particularly helps solidify the diagnosis.
- Mesenteric and renal angiography is sensitive and specific for PAN with gastro-intestinal (GI) and kidney involvement.
- Classic PAN spares the lungs and glomeruli.

Definition

Defined by the Chapel Hill Consensus Conference as a necrotizing inflammation of medium- or small-sized arteries, without glomerulonephritis or vasculitis of the arterioles, capillaries, or venules.[1]

Epidemiology

- Affects men more frequently than women, between ages 40 to 60, with peak around 50 years of age.
- Classic PAN is rare with an estimated annual incidence rate of 2.0 to 9.0 per million.

Etiology

- Most cases of PAN are **idiopathic.**
- A substantial minority of cases are caused by the **Hepatitis B virus** (HBV).
  - The prevalence rates of PAN are higher in populations with endemic HBV infection. Consequently, the widespread use of HBV vaccines has decreased the rate of HBV-related PAN.
- PAN has also been linked to other viral infections, especially **HIV and Hepatitis C virus** (HCV).
  - In a cohort of 161 patients with HCV-related vasculitis, 31 of them (19.3%) were classified as having PAN.[3]
  - HCV-PAN was associated with a more acute and severe clinical presentation as well as a higher rate of clinical remission when compared to HCV-related mixed cryoglobulinemia (HCV-MC).
  - When compared to HBV-PAN, HCV-PAN was seen more frequently in an older female population, with a higher prevalence of skin involvement and relapse rate, and a worse prognosis.
- Myelodysplastic syndrome (MDS), chronic myelomonocytic leukemia, and hairy cell leukemia have been linked to PAN.

TABLE 23-1	AMERICAN COLLEGE OF RHEUMATOLOGY 1990 CRITERIA FOR POLYARTERITIS NODOSA

The presence of at least three of the following ten are required:

- Unintentional weight loss >4 kg since the start of illness
- Livedo reticularis
- Testicular pain or tenderness not due to infection, trauma, or other causes
- Diffuse myalgias, weakness, or leg tenderness
- Mononeuropathy or polyneuropathy
- Diastolic blood pressure >90 mm Hg
- Blood urea nitrogen >40 mg/dL or creatinine >1.5 mg/dL, not due to dehydration, medications, or obstruction
- Hepatitis B virus infection
- Abnormal angiogram showing aneurysms or occlusions of visceral arteries, not due to atherosclerosis, fibromuscular dysplasia, or non-inflammatory disease
- Biopsy of small- or medium-sized vessels demonstrating an artery containing polymorphonuclear leukocytes and mononuclear leukocytes in the vessel wall.

Adapted from: Lightfoot RW Jr, Michel BA, Bloch DA. The American College of Rheumatology 1990 criteria for the classification of polyarteritis nodosa. *Arthritis Rheum.* 1990;33:1088–1093.

Pathophysiology

- The mechanism of PAN is not well understood but typically involves circulating foreign antigens, antibodies, Fc receptors, and complement.
- It appears to involve immune complex–mediated damage to vessel walls.
- In those patients with HBV-related PAN, hepatitis B surface antigen/antibody interaction triggers activation of the complement cascade and Fcγ receptors.
- The clinical symptoms of PAN result from systemic manifestations secondary to the release of cytokines as well as from local inflammation and vessel damage.
- The pathologic lesion is a **focal segmental necrotizing vasculitis of medium- and small-sized arteries.** This inflammation commonly leads to disruption of the elastic lamina of the vessel wall with subsequent weakening and formation of **microaneurysms,** endothelial dysfunction, thrombosis, and stenosis.

DIAGNOSIS

Clinical Presentation

- The presentation of PAN may be nonspecific.
- Most of the patients develop **systemic symptoms of inflammation** (e.g., malaise, arthralgias, myalgias, fever, and/or weight loss) along with localized signs and symptoms of vasculitis (e.g., peripheral neuropathy and GI, testicular and/or cutaneous manifestations).

- Most of the patients present with acute illness and severe manifestations.
- HBV-related PAN:
  - Patients tend to be <40 years old and have a more acute and fulminant form of PAN than those with PAN without HBV.
  - Malignant hypertension (HTN), renal infarction, and orchitis are more common in HBV-related PAN.
  - PAN tends to precede hepatitis which is usually clinically silent at the time of the vasculitis.
  - Seroconversion often leads to remission of PAN.
- Limited forms of PAN:
  - **Cutaneous PAN** (CPAN) refers to a chronic cutaneous vasculitis of medium vessels with histologic features similar to PAN but without systemic vascular involvement.
    - These patients also usually present with extra-cutaneous manifestations, which include myalgias, arthralgias, malaise, fever, and neuropathy.
    - Clinical manifestations of CPAN include **livedo reticularis, tender subcutaneous nodules, ulcers, and necrosis.**
    - A workup to exclude systemic involvement is required before the diagnosis of CPAN can be made.
    - Treatment ranges from nonsteroidal antiinflammatory drugs (NSAIDs) and colchicine to steroids and other immunosuppressive agents, depending on the severity of symptoms.
    - Its course tends to be chronic with remissions and relapses. Overall, it has a favorable prognosis, and **rarely converts into systemic PAN.**
  - Rarely, microaneurysms and stenoses **limited to single organs without systemic involvement** occur.[4]

History

- Given the systemic involvement in PAN, a thorough history and a detailed review of systems are indicated.
- **Skin:** Inquire about the appearance of tender, erythematous nodules, bullous or vesicular lesions, ulcerations, and/or digital ischemia/gangrene.
- **Musculoskeletal:** Inquire about myalgias, muscle weakness, and claudication.
- **Cardiovascular:** Inquire about hypertension, chest pain, and dyspnea on exertion as microaneurysm and thrombi formation as well as myocardial ischemia and coronary dissection may occur secondary to PAN.
- **GI:** Inquire about abdominal pain, especially after a meal, nausea, vomiting, diarrhea, and melena.
  - Pain may be intermittent or continuous. This may be indicative of mesenteric vasculitis with subsequent bowel wall ischemia, ulceration, and/or perforation.
  - The most commonly involved portion is the small bowel.
- **Kidney:** Renal ischemia secondary to vasculitis of the medium-sized muscular arteries leads to **hypertension** through the activation of the renin–angiotensin system.
  - Hematuria has been reported; however, red blood cell (RBC) casts and other signs of glomerulonephritis are not common in PAN.
  - Their presence along with pulmonary symptoms such as hemoptysis merits consideration of a vasculitis affecting primarily the smaller vessels such as microscopic polyangiitis (MPA) or Wegener's granulomatosis.

- **Neurologic:** The most common symptom is **mononeuritis multiplex,** present in >70% of patients, which may be the presenting symptom.
  - ○ Characterized by an asymmetric sensory and motor peripheral neuropathy caused by ischemia and inflammation to the vasa nervorum supplying the affected nerve.
  - ○ The lower limbs, especially the sciatic nerve and its peroneal and tibial branches, are most commonly affected.
  - ○ Hypoesthesia or hyperesthesia and pain are present in the areas of motor deficits.
  - ○ The motor deficits may be abrupt and may precede the sensory symptoms.
  - ○ Cranial nerve and central nervous system (CNS) involvement are rare but may include cranial nerve palsies and hemorrhagic or ischemic strokes.
- **Acute inflammatory orchitis:** PAN should be considered in the differential diagnosis.

Physical Examination
- A thorough physical examination is necessary in order to determine which organs are involved and the extent of vascular lesions.
- It is also important to seek the presence of additional disease processes that may be mimicking PAN.
- **Skin:** Cutaneous manifestations of classic PAN are uncommon and variable. They include palpable purpura, which is usually papular/petechial and sometimes bullous or vesicular, livedo reticularis, tender subcutaneous nodules, and distal gangrene.
- **GI:** The stool should be checked for occult blood.
- **Renal:** New onset hypertension may be indicative of renal involvement.
- **Neurologic:** Test especially for motor weakness and sensory deficits.

Diagnostic Criteria

- The diagnosis of PAN is based on the presence of systemic features as well as either an abnormal angiogram demonstrating the presence of aneurysms or thrombosis and/or a biopsy showing vasculitic involvement of the small- or medium-sized vessels.
- The American College of Rheumatology criteria are presented in Table 23-1.

Differential Diagnosis

- **Multiple conditions can mimic PAN,** which is why a broad differential must be considered and evaluated during your workup. These include the following:
  - ○ **Viral infections** such as hepatitis B and C, HIV, cytomegalovirus (CMV), parvovirus B19, and human T-cell lymphotropic virus 1 (HTLV-1).
  - ○ **Connective tissue diseases** (e.g., systemic lupus erythematosus, rheumatoid arthritis, Sjögren's syndrome, mixed connective tissue disease, and systemic sclerosis) may present like PAN.
  - ○ **Bacterial endocarditis, cholesterol embolization, sepsis, and malignancy** should also be excluded.
  - ○ **Antineutrophil cytoplasmic antibody (ANCA)-associated vasculitides** such as MPA may have signs and symptoms similar to PAN, but are distinguished by small-vessel vasculitis in the pulmonary and renal vasculature, normal visceral angiography, presence of ANCA and the greater tendency to relapse (see Chapter 26, Microscopic Polyangiitis).

○ PAN has been associated with MDS, chronic myelomonocytic leukemia, and hairy cell leukemia. The course of MDS tends to be more severe if associated with PAN.

Diagnostic Testing

Laboratories
- Erythrocyte sedimentation rate (ESR) >50 mm/hour and an elevated C-reactive protein (CRP) >10 mg/L.
- Leukocytosis.
- Hypereosinophilia (seen in 10%–30% of patients).
- Normocytic normochromic anemia of chronic inflammation.
- Mild renal insufficiency, hypertension, non-nephrotic range proteinuria, and mild hematuria.
  ○ **Active urinary sediment is not a feature of PAN.**
- Check hepatitis serologies and investigate other causes of PAN as appropriate.
- Positive tests for ANCA are uncommon with PAN (<30%).

Imaging
- **Visceral angiography** may be useful to demonstrate **microaneurysms and stenoses in small- to medium-sized vessels,** usually in the renal, mesenteric, and/or hepatic arterial systems.
- Angiography may also be helpful, before hepatic or renal biopsies, to identify microaneurysms and minimize the risk of visceral bleeding.
- **Coronary angiography** can also reveal microaneurysms in the coronary arteries.
- In patients with coronary arteritis, a spiral CT scan as well as cardiac MRI scans may better visualize aneurysms and myocardial ischemia.[5]

Diagnostic Procedures
- Seek biopsies of the affected organ, if possible.
- Although skin is not routinely involved in PAN, a biopsy is indicated if lesions are present.
- Full thickness skin biopsy is recommended because it requires tissue as deep as the subcutaneous fat to capture the small- and medium-sized muscular-walled arteries involved in PAN.
- Another potential site to biopsy is the sural nerve, especially if a lower extremity neuropathy is present.
- A muscle biopsy of the gastrocnemius muscle should be done concurrently, as it increases the yield of finding vessel involvement with PAN if the sural nerve biopsy is negative.

TREATMENT

- Depends on the presence of HBV as well as the assessment of disease activity.
- The French Cooperative Study Group (FCSG) for PAN devised a **five-factor score for determining prognosis.**[6]
- **The five parameters predicting higher mortality are:**
  ○ Proteinuria >1 g/day.
  ○ Serum creatinine >1.58 mg/dL (140 μmol/L).
  ○ Cardiomyopathy.
  ○ GI involvement.
  ○ CNS involvement.

Medications

First Line

- First line treatment includes **oral or intravenous corticosteroids.**
- PAN without HBV and with none of the five factors above at the time of diagnosis can be treated with **oral prednisone** (1 mg/kg/day is a commonly used starting dose).
- **Pulse IV methylprednisolone** (1 gm daily for 3–5 days) is usually employed if there are severe, life-threatening manifestations of vasculitis.
- The addition of immunosuppressants such as cyclophosphamide and azathioprine has prolonged the survival rates of patients with PAN.
  - **Pulse cyclophosphamide,** in addition to corticosteroids, induces remission with fewer side effects in patients with no poor prognostic factors than oral cyclophosphamide.
  - Treat patients with a factor score ≥1 with pulse IV methylprednisolone (1000 mg/ day for 3–5 days) followed by oral prednisone, (1 mg/kg/day), and pulse IV cyclophosphamide 0.5 to 2.5 g every week to every month depending on the patient's condition, renal function, response to previous therapy and hematologic data.
  - Reserve oral cyclophosphamide for patients failing IV cyclophosphamide or for those with fulminant manifestations.
  - Taper prednisone slowly after the patient's clinical status improves and the ESR returns to normal, usually in approximately 1 month. The dose may be dropped by about 25% every 2 to 4 weeks.
  - IV cyclophosphamide therapy should in most cases not exceed 1 year when combined with corticosteroids.
  - Patients receiving cyclophosphamide should receive prophylaxis for *Pneumocystis jiroveci* pneumonia with oral trimethoprim 160 mg/sulfamethoxazole 800 mg, three times per week.
  - Once remission has been achieved with steroids and IV cyclophosphamide, use azathioprine or methotrexate for 12 to 18 months for maintenance therapy.[7]

Second Line

- Consider **plasma exchange** in refractory cases.
- Management of HBV-related PAN involves treatment of both vasculitis and HBV infection.
  - **Use steroids in the first few weeks to control the vasculitis,** then stop them abruptly to enhance viral clearance and increase the rate of seroconversion of HBV e antigen to HBV e antibody. Continued use of steroids and other immunosuppressants jeopardizes viral clearance and promotes chronic infection.[8,9]
  - Standard anti-HBV agents (e.g., interferon-α 2b, lamivudine) are used in conjunction.
  - If seroconversion occurs, remission can be obtained and relapses are rare.

Other Non-Pharmacologic Therapies

In patients with PAN associated with HBV infection, plasma exchange has been used after corticosteroids are withdrawn to control the symptoms.[9]

COMPLICATIONS

Complications of PAN vary and depend on which organ systems are involved as well as how much damage has occurred before treatment.

REFERRAL

Patients with suspected PAN should be immediately referred to a rheumatologist for further management and treatment.

MONITORING/FOLLOW-UP

- Follow-up involves clinical and laboratory assessment of disease status and monitoring of medication side effects and toxicities.
- In patients with HBV-related PAN, consultation with a hepatologist is strongly advised.

OUTCOME/PROGNOSIS

- PAN tends to be monophasic.
- Prognosis depends on the number of five-factor score risk factors present.[6]
  - Patients with no risk factors have 88% 5-year survival rate.
  - Patients with one risk factor have 74% 5-year survival rate.
  - Patients with ≥2 risk factors have 54% 5-year survival rate.

REFERENCES

1. Jennette JC, Falk RJ, Andrassy K, et al. Nomenclature of systemic vasculitides: Proposal of an international consensus conference. *Arthritis Rheum.* 1994;37:187–192.
2. Lightfoot RW Jr, Michel BA, Bloch DA. The American College of Rheumatology 1990 criteria for the classification of polyarteritis nodosa. *Arthritis Rheum.* 1990;33:1088–1093.
3. Saadoun D, Terrier B, Semoun O, et al. Hepatitis C virus-associated polyarteritis nodosa. *Arthritis Care Res (Hoboken).* 2011;63:427–435.
4. Maillard-Lefebvre H, Launay D, Mouquet F, et al. Polyarteritis nodosa-related coronary aneurysms. *J Rheumatol.* 2008;35:933–934.
5. Kobayashi H, Yokoe I, Hattan N, et al. Cardiac magnetic resonance imaging in polyarteritis nodosa. *J Rheumatol.* 2010;37:2427–2429.
6. Guillevin L, Lhote F, Gayroud M, et al. Prognostic factors in polyarteritis nodosa and Churg–Strauss syndrome: A prospective study in 342 patients. *Medicine (Baltimore).* 1996;75:17–28.
7. Guillevin L, Pagnoux C. Therapeutic strategies for systemic necrotizing vasculitides. *Allergol Int.* 2007;56:105–111.
8. Guillevin L, Lhote F. Treatment of polyarteritis nodosa and microscopic polyangiitis. *Arthritis Rheum.* 1998;41:2100–2105.
9. Guillevin L, Mahr A, Cohen P, et al. Short-term corticosteroids then lamivudine and plasma exchanges to treat hepatitis B virus-related polyarteritis nodosa. *Arthritis Rheum.* 2004; 51:482–487.

Wegener's Granulomatosis

24

Jeffrey Sparks and John P. Atkinson

GENERAL PRINCIPLES

- Wegener's granulomatosis (WG) is a systemic vasculitis usually associated with **antineutrophil cytoplasmic antibodies (ANCA).**
- WG most often affects the **respiratory tract and then the kidney.**
- Treatment involves immunosuppressants and is individually tailored primarily on the basis of severity of end-organ involvement.

Definition

WG, also known as ANCA-associated granulomatous vasculitis, is defined by the Chapel Hill Consensus Conference as a granulomatous inflammation involving the respiratory tract and vasculitis affecting small- to medium-sized vessels, commonly with a necrotizing glomerulonephritis.[1]

Classification

- The European League Against Rheumatism (EULAR) recommends classification based upon disease severity.[2]
- **Localized:** upper and/or lower respiratory tract disease, without any other systemic involvement or constitutional symptoms.
- **Early systemic:** without organ-threatening or life-threatening disease.
- **Generalized:** renal or other organ-threatening disease, serum creatinine <5.6 mg/dL.
- **Severe:** renal or other vital organ failure, serum creatinine ≥5.6 mg/dL.
- **Refractory:** progressive disease unresponsive to glucocorticoids alone (common) and cyclophosphamide (uncommon).

Epidemiology

- WG affects men and women equally. WG affects mostly Caucasians. The peak age of onset is in the 65 to 74 range, though there is wide variation.
- The prevalence has been estimated to be about 10 to 20 cases per million, although this may underestimate the true prevalence. Milder and more limited forms are being recognized with the availability of ANCA testing.
- The incidence has been estimated to be about 3 to 14 cases per million.

Pathophysiology

- **ANCA is positive in WG about 80% to 90% of the time.** The c-ANCA in WG has been identified as an **antibody to proteinase-3** (anti-PR3), a cytoplasmic glycoprotein present in active form in monocytes and endothelial cells and in the azurophil granules of neutrophils. PR3 is involved in neutrophil migration and cytokine modulation.

- The role of c-ANCA in the pathogenesis of WG is controversial. Although animal studies show that serum anti-PR3 antibodies result in lesions similar to those found in WG, antibodies to PR-3 are not present in all cases.
- **WG is a pauci-immune syndrome** in which immune complex deposition and complement activation are not prominent features.

DIAGNOSIS

Clinical Presentation

Initial Phase

- The initial phase is characterized by chronic inflammation, usually in the upper airways. Sinusitis develops as the initial symptom in >50% of patients and develops in >85% of patients at some time during the course of illness. Other nasal symptoms include sinus obstruction, mucosal swelling, hearing loss, ulcers, septal perforations, epistaxis, serosanguinous discharge and saddle nose deformity. The sinusitis is commonly progressive and refractory to the usual therapies and severe. Sinus biopsies rarely show granulomatous inflammation.
- Granulomatous inflammation may occur in the oral cavity, retrobulbar space and trachea, especially if mass-type lesions are present.
- Laryngotracheal disease can be asymptomatic or present as hoarseness, stridor or acute airway obstruction. Subglottic stenosis occurs in approximately 15% of adults and 50% of children.
- Myalgias and arthralgias are common presenting symptoms.

Generalized Phase

- The generalized phase is characterized by **systemic signs and symptoms of small-vessel vasculitis. Fever and weight loss are common.**
- **Pulmonary disease** is a cardinal feature. Cough, hemoptysis, and pleuritis are common. Pulmonary hemorrhage, infiltrates, cavities, nodules, pleural effusions, and mediastinal lymphadenopathy may be present.
- **Renal disease develops in approximately 80% of patients, usually after other manifestations.** The disease progression can be rapid once glomerulonephritis develops.
- WG may affect any segment of the urinary tract. Hematuria without RBC casts usually indicates nonrenal urinary tract involvement.
- Although most patients experience **arthralgias,** some patients exhibit **migratory polyarthritis.**
  - The pattern of joint involvement is variable and includes monoarticular, oligoarticular, and polyarticular.
  - Presentation with symmetric polyarthritis can be mistaken for rheumatoid arthritis (RA), especially if a positive value for rheumatoid factor (RF) is obtained.
  - Low titers of RF are seen in 20% to 40% of patients with WG.
- **Neurologic disease** develops in approximately 50% of patients but is rarely a presenting feature.
  - **Mononeuritis multiplex and symmetric polyneuropathy** are the most common patterns.
  - **Cranial neuropathies** also occur, with II (optic neuritis), VI, and VII being the most common.
- **Common gastrointestinal (GI) manifestations** are abdominal pain, diarrhea, and bleeding from ulcerations in both the small and large intestines.

TABLE 24-1	AMERICAN COLLEGE OF RHEUMATOLOGY 1990 CRITERIA FOR WEGENER'S GRANULOMATOSIS

The presence of at least two of the following ten are required:
- Nasal or oral inflammation (painful or painless ulcers, purulent or bloody nasal discharge)
- Abnormal chest radiograph (nodules, fixed infiltrates, or cavities)
- Hematuria or red blood cell casts in urine sediment
- Pathologic evidence of granulomas, leukocytoclastic vasculitis, and necrosis

Adapted from: Leavitt RY, Fauci AS, Bloch DA, et al. The American College of Rheumatology 1990 criteria for the classification of Wegener's granulomatosis. *Arthritis Rheum.* 1990;33: 1101–1107.

- **Cutaneous manifestations** are typical of the small-vessel vasculitis and include palpable purpura, ulcers, subcutaneous nodules, papules, and vesicles. They tend to parallel disease activity.
- WG can also have **ocular manifestations,** including keratoconjunctivitis, scleritis, episcleritis, pseudotumor of the orbit, conjunctivitis, and uveitis.

Diagnostic Criteria

The American College of Rheumatology 1990 classification criteria for WG are presented in Table 24-1.

Differential Diagnosis

- **Cocaine,** especially when inhaled with the adulterant **levamisole,** can induce pseudovasculitis with nasal, upper airway, and lesions that are similar to WG. ANCA reacting with human neutrophil elastase (HNE) have been reported to distinguish the cocaine-related syndrome from a true autoimmune vasculitis.[3]
- The differential diagnosis of WG should be considered carefully. Inappropriate diagnosis of WG and subsequent **treatment with potent immunosuppressants may prove fatal if the underlying disease is infectious.** Conditions to be considered include the following:
  - ○ Granulomatous diseases (tuberculosis, histoplasmosis, blastomycosis, coccidioidomycosis, sarcoidosis).
  - ○ Neoplastic diseases (lymphomas, head and neck malignancies, metastatic adenocarcinoma).
  - ○ Connective tissue diseases (systemic lupus erythematosus, relapsing polychondritis, antiphospholipid antibody syndrome, scleroderma, mixed connective tissue disease, Still's disease).
  - ○ Small-vessel vasculitides.
  - ○ Goodpasture's disease.

Diagnostic Testing

Laboratories
- The presence of **c-ANCA and, more specifically, anti-PR3 antibodies,** supports the diagnosis, although c-ANCA may be negative in earlier and less fulminant forms of WG.
- **Elevated serum creatinine and blood urea nitrate (BUN)** indicate renal impairment.

- Urinalysis may show hematuria and microscopy may reveal red blood cell (RBC) casts, indicating glomerulonephritis.
- Markers of inflammation, including elevated **erythrocyte sedimentation rate (ESR), C-reactive protein (CRP)**, leukocytosis, and thrombocytosis, are commonly present in WG.
- **Anemia of chronic disease** is common in WG.
- Leukopenia and thrombocytopenia are rarely present in untreated WG and should prompt a search for other disorders.
- Complement levels are typically normal or slightly elevated.

Imaging
- **Chest imaging:**
  - Perform chest radiography on all patients suspected of having WG; asymptomatic patients may have significant radiologic abnormalities.
  - Use chest CT scans in patients with hemoptysis with clear plain films, as early pulmonary hemorrhage, small areas of cavitation, nodules and interstitial disease may not be visible on plain films. Chest CT should be considered in patients with abnormal plain films to further define the extent of disease.[4]
- **Sinus imaging:**
  - Sinus CT scans are superior to plain sinus films to define the extent of disease.

Diagnostic Procedures
- **Pulmonary function tests** with flow volume loops may be useful to define irreversible extrathoracic or intrathoracic obstruction caused by airway inflammation leading to tracheal stenosis or collapse.
- **Bronchoscopy** is useful when pulmonary hemorrhage is present or suspected. Transbronchial biopsy, bronchoalveolar lavage, and endoscopic inspection of lesions detected on imaging may be useful in helping to establish the diagnosis of WG, and also in ruling out infectious mimics.
- The yield of **tissue diagnosis** for WG depends on the biopsy site, specimen size and the manner in which the tissue is collected.
  - **Open lung biopsies** with adequate tissue are most often diagnostic, showing the hallmark features of **vasculitis, necrosis, and granulomatous inflammation.** The yield of open lung biopsy is highest when larger samples are obtained and is frequently diagnostic, especially if lesions are radiographically evident.
  - **Transbronchial biopsies are rarely diagnostic;** however, when used in combination with bronchoalveolar lavage and cultures, they are useful for ruling out infections that mimic or complicate WG.
  - **Renal biopsy** shows **pauci-immune, focal and segmental glomerulonephritis (FSGN)** with occasional medium-vessel vasculitis, and rarely granulomatous changes. Immunofluorescence studies are negative or weakly positive for antibody and complement deposition.
  - **Head and neck biopsies,** especially sinus biopsies, tend to show chronic, nonspecific inflammation and are rarely diagnostic. Most specimens are compatible with, but not diagnostic of, WG, as they show acute and chronic inflammation.

TREATMENT

- Base the treatment plan on the objective presence of activity, its site, and severity.
- Lungs, kidney, neuropathic, and vision-threatening ocular disease usually merit high-dose corticosteroids and immunosuppressants.
- **Corticosteroids alone are inadequate in systemic disease, especially in patients with renal involvement.**

Medications
- **Induction therapy:**
  - **Oral prednisone,** 1 mg/kg daily dose.
  - **Oral cyclophosphamide,** approximately 2 mg/kg.
  - IV methylprednisolone (1000 mg) and higher doses of oral cyclophosphamide (3–5 mg/kg) may be used for the first three days in cases of immediately life-threatening fulminant disease (e.g., pulmonary hemorrhage or rapidly progressive glomerulonephritis).
  - Monthly IV cyclophosphamide has less toxic complications compared to daily oral cyclophosphamide but may have a higher rate of relapse.
  - MESNA may be given with oral cyclophosphamide to reduce bladder toxicity.
  - **Rituximab,** weekly for four weeks, with corticosteroids has been shown to be noninferior to cyclophosphamide and may be superior in preventing relapse.[5]
- **Maintenance therapy:**
  - Once a remission has been achieved, switch to **oral methotrexate** (20–25 mg/week) and then taper steroids.
  - Prednisone and methotrexate (20–25 mg/week) may be used for patients with significant cyclophosphamide-related side effects or who do not have immediately life-threatening disease.
  - **Azathioprine,** 2 mg/kg, is an alternative to methotrexate for maintenance therapy.
  - **Trimethoprim/sulfamethoxazole** (TMP/SMX), 160 mg/800 mg three times a week, for *Pneumocystis jiroveci* pneumonia (PCP) prophylaxis while on immunosuppressants.
- **Limited upper airway involvement:**
  - Local therapy with nasal irrigation and nasal steroids may be given.
  - TMP/SMX may also be effective.
  - Subglottic stenosis is treated with mechanical dilatation and intratracheal injection of a long-acting steroid.
- IV immune globulin and plasmapheresis are generally not thought to be effective, though plasma exchange is sometimes used for severe pulmonary hemorrhage, renal vasculitis or concomitant anti-glomerular basement membrane (GBM) disease.

MONITORING/FOLLOW-UP

- Follow-up should include laboratory and radiographic studies of upper airway and lung and renal function.

- ANCA and anti-PR3 antibody levels correlate roughly with disease activity in large groups of patients, but direct studies of organ function should be the primary guide to therapy.[6]
- TMP/SMX, 160 mg/800 mg bid, for 24 months during remission has been shown to prevent relapses.
- Monitor for toxicity of treatment modalities and opportunistic infections.
- Patients with WG have a high rate of deep vein thrombosis.

OUTCOME/PROGNOSIS

- There is considerable variability, mostly depending on the presentation. WG limited to the upper airway has a better prognosis and higher response rate to treatment than generalized and severe WG.
- **Alveolar hemorrhage and severe renal failure portend the worst prognosis.**
- **Relapse occurs in as many as 50% of patients.**
- Untreated patients have a survival rate of only 20% at 2 years. However, the 2-year survival rate for treated patients is about 90%.
- Morbidity of treated WG is related to irreversible organ damage, treatment toxicity, and opportunistic infections.

REFERENCES

1. Jennette JC, Falk RJ, Andrassy K, et al. Nomenclature of systemic vasculitides. Proposal of an international consensus conference. *Arthritis Rheum.* 1994;37:187–192.
2. Mukhtyar C, Guillevin L, Cid MC, et al. EULAR recommendations for the management of primary small and medium vessel vasculitis. *Ann Rheum Dis.* 2009;68:310–317.
3. Walsh NM, Green PJ, Burlingame RW, et al. Cocaine-related retiform purpura: Evidence to incriminate the adulterant, levamisole. *J Cutan Pathol.* 2010;37:1212–1219.
4. Leavitt RY, Fauci AS, Bloch DA, et al. The American College of Rheumatology 1990 criteria for the classification of Wegener's granulomatosis. *Arthritis Rheum.* 1990;33:1101–1107.
5. Stone JH, Merkel PA, Spiera R, et al. Rituximab versus cyclophosphamide for ANCA-associated vasculitis. *N Engl J Med.* 2010;363:221–232.
6. Finkielman JD, Merkel PA, Schroeder D, et al. Antiproteinase 3 antineutrophil cytoplasmic antibodies and disease activity in Wegener granulomatosis. *Ann Intern Med.* 2007;147:611–619.

25

Churg–Strauss Syndrome

Lesley Davila and John P. Atkinson

GENERAL PRINCIPLES

Definition

The Chapel Hill Consensus Conference defines **Churg–Strauss Syndrome (CSS)**, also known as **allergic granulomatosis and angiitis,** as an eosinophil-rich, granulomatous inflammation involving the respiratory tract and necrotizing vasculitis affecting small- to medium-sized vessels associated with **asthma and peripheral eosinophilia.**

Epidemiology

- CSS is a rare disease with an annual incidence of approximately 2.4 cases per million.
- CSS affects the sexes equally.
- The asthma associated with CSS usually begins in the fourth or fifth decade but can occur at any age.

Pathophysiology

- The two diagnostic lesions are **arterial and venous vasculitis** and **extravascular necrotizing granulomas,** usually with eosinophilic infiltration of tissue. These findings coexist temporally only in few patients.
- The signs and symptoms of CSS are caused by the effects these lesions have on the involved organ system at a given time and by the systemic effects of inflammation.
- The most commonly affected organ systems (in decreasing order) are pulmonary, neurologic, cutaneous, otorhinolaryngeal, musculoskeletal, GI, cardiac, and renal.
- **Antineutrophil cytoplasmic antibody (ANCA),** in particular, the perinuclear **antimyeloperoxidase (anti-MPO) variant,** has been associated with CSS in 40% to 60% of patients, but its role in pathogenesis is not well understood.

Risk Factors

- An association with leukotriene modifiers (zafirlukast and montelukast) has been recognized in patients with steroid-dependent asthma who were tapered from corticosteroids after initiation of the leukotriene modifier.
- Most of these patients had milder airway obstruction and a greater incidence of acute dilated cardiomyopathy than other patients with CSS.
- It is unclear whether the leukotriene modifiers induced the disease or the steroid tapering led to expression of patients with preexisting CSS. The latter seems more likely.[1]

DIAGNOSIS

Clinical Presentation

- **Three phases** of CSS are described:
  - ○ The first is a **prodrome** beginning in childhood and lasting up to 30 years characterized by **allergic rhinitis, sinusitis, and nasal polyposis. Asthma** develops later in life at an average age of 35 years. The asthma is usually severe and requires systemic corticosteroids.
  - ○ The second phase is characterized by **peripheral blood and tissue eosinophilia.** Löffler's syndrome (transient, pulmonary, and acute eosinophilic infiltrates), chronic eosinophilic pneumonia, and eosinophilic gastroenteritis are common. The pulmonary infiltrates tend to be peripheral, patchy, parenchymal, migratory, and transient and may be associated with eosinophilic pulmonary effusions. However, these are neither sensitive nor specific pulmonary patterns.
  - ○ The third phase is characterized by **small-vessel vasculitis,** with a mean time of onset of 3 years after the development of asthma. The symptoms are usually nonspecific, representing constitutional manifestations of systemic inflammation (e.g., myalgias, arthralgias, fatigue, and weight loss). Asthma usually worsens during this phase.
- **Organ system involvement:**
  - ○ **Pulmonary manifestations** include **asthma, which is present in over 95% of patients with CSS.** Asthma is usually difficult to treat and requires corticosteroids. It usually develops years before other organ involvement. Later on, eosinophilic pulmonary infiltrates, effusions, and rarely pulmonary hemorrhage may develop.[2]
  - ○ **Cutaneous signs** are similar to those of other vasculitides and include palpable purpura of the lower extremities, subcutaneous nodules of the scalp and lower extremities, livedo reticularis, and infarction.
  - ○ **Neurologic manifestations** are similar to those of polyarteritis nodosa (PAN), with **mononeuritis multiplex** in about two-thirds of cases. Distal, usually symmetric, **peripheral neuropathies** are also common. Cranial nerve palsies are less common, with ischemic optic neuritis being the most common. Cerebral infarctions are rare.
  - ○ **Cardiac disease is the most common cause of death. Eosinophilic myocarditis and coronary vasculitis** are the most frequent cardiac lesions and can lead to severe heart failure or myocardial infarction (MI). Pericardial effusions are also common, but only occasionally lead to hemodynamic compromise. Endomyocardial fibrosis is rare.
  - ○ **Gastrointestinal (GI) tract manifestations** account for a substantial number of deaths and include tissue eosinophilic infiltration and/or mesenteric vasculitis with resultant ischemia, infarction, and perforation.
  - ○ **Renal involvement tends to be mild.** The most common manifestations are hematuria, albuminuria, and focal segmental necrotizing glomerulonephritis, although severe necrotizing glomerulonephritis has been described.

Diagnostic Criteria

The American College of Rheumatology 1990 criteria for CSS are presented in Table 25-1.[3]

TABLE 25-1	THE AMERICAN COLLEGE OF RHEUMATOLOGY 1990 CRITERIA FOR CHURG–STRAUSS SYNDROME

The presence of at least four of the following six are required:

- Asthma
- Eosinophilia >10%
- Mononeuropathy or polyneuropathy attributable to a systemic vasculitis
- Migratory or transient infiltrates on chest radiography
- Paranasal sinus abnormality (acute or chronic paranasal pain or radiographic opacification of paranasal sinuses)
- Extravascular eosinophils on biopsy

Adapted from: Masi AT, Hunder GC, Lie JT. The American College of Rheumatology 1990 criteria for the classification of Churg-Strauss syndrome (allergic granulomatosis and angiitis). *Arthritis Rheum.* 1990;33:1094–1100.

Differential Diagnosis

- The differential diagnosis includes PAN, microscopic polyangiitis (MPA), Wegener's granulomatosis (WG), chronic eosinophilic pneumonia, and idiopathic hypereosinophilic syndrome (IHS).
  - ○ **PAN** usually spares the glomeruli and lungs, demonstrates arterial microaneurysms and stenoses, and tends to be ANCA negative.
  - ○ **MPA** causes necrotizing vasculitis of arterioles, venules, and capillaries without granulomas. It often involves the glomeruli and lungs.
  - ○ The key clinical, laboratory, and histologic findings usually make the distinction between WG and CSS straightforward.
  - ○ **Chronic eosinophilic pneumonia** commonly has no extrapulmonary findings, affects women, and no granulomatous or vasculitic component.
  - ○ **IHS** typically has endomyocardial fibrosis and no vasculitic, granulomatous, asthmatic, or allergic component. IHS responds poorly to systemic steroids.

Diagnostic Testing

A patient with late-onset and worsening asthma, peripheral eosinophilia and transient migratory lung infiltrates should raise suspicion for CSS.

Laboratories

- Laboratory data supporting CSS include **peripheral eosinophilia** (usually 5000–9000 eosinophils/μL), elevated erythrocyte sedimentation rate (ESR), thrombocytosis, and **elevated IgE** levels.
- A positive **p-ANCA**, specifically **anti-MPO** antibody, supports the diagnosis, but its absence does not rule out CSS.
- Urine protein and plasma creatinine and assessment of cardiac function provide prognostic information.

Diagnostic Procedures

- Biopsies of skin, nerve, or lung lesions may be highly suggestive.
- They may also be nonspecific or helpful in sorting through the differential diagnosis.

TREATMENT

Medications

- Initial therapy to induce remission of CSS includes the following options:
  - The response to **oral prednisone**, 1 mg/kg daily, is dramatic. Within 1 month, most patients are clinically improved and have a decreasing if not normal eosinophil count and ESR. Steroids should be tapered once the ESR has normalized.
  - **Pulse IV methylprednisolone**, 1000 mg daily for 3 days, is used for life-threatening disease.
  - Studies suggest that combination therapy with **cyclophosphamide** (usually 0.6 g/m^2 monthly IV doses with adjustments based on laboratory response or 2 mg/kg qd PO doses) has increased efficacy in those patients who have signs and symptoms of severe or life-threatening disease. IV cyclophosphamide is preferred for initial therapy, with oral administration reserved for severe disease or relapses.
  - For milder disease, **methotrexate or azathioprine** may be used in combination with corticosteroids to induce disease remission.
- **Long-term therapy** to maintain remission and allow reduction of corticosteroid dose is often used in patients with CSS.
  - Usually **azathioprine or methotrexate** is employed after induction of remission (6–12 months) or if patients are in remission, but require >10 to 20 mg of prednisone.
  - Methotrexate is used more cautiously as it can cause hypersensitivity pneumonitis that is difficult to distinguish from a reoccurrence of CSS.[4]
- Mycophenolate mofetil, rituximab, hydroxyurea, and mepolizumab have also been used for the treatment of steroid-resistant CSS.[5–8]

COMPLICATIONS

- Complications of treatment are usually from opportunistic infections or related to long-term use of corticosteroids.
- Patients receiving cyclophosphamide should receive prophylaxis for *Pneumocystis jiroveci* pneumonia with oral trimethoprim 160 mg/sulfamethoxazole 800 mg, three times per week.
- When cyclophosphamide is administered intravenously, mercaptoethane sulfonate (MESNA) should be given to reduce the risk of drug-induced cystitis (dosing of MESNA is the same as that of cyclophosphamide). Half of the dose is administered prior to the cyclophosphamide infusion, and the other half is infused 2 hours following the cyclophosphamide infusion.
- Corticosteroids should be weaned as quickly as appropriate and patients should be evaluated for osteoporosis, diabetes, and hypertension and warned about weight gain.

MONITORING/FOLLOW-UP

- Follow-up involves clinical and laboratory assessment of disease status and monitoring of medication side effects and toxicities.

- Perform frequent eosinophil counts, as increases in counts tend to precede flares of CSS.

OUTCOME/PROGNOSIS

- With the use of steroids and immunosuppressants, remission rates have been >75%.
- Factors associated with lower 5-year survival rates include proteinuria >1 g/day, creatinine >1.6 mg/dL, cardiomyopathy, and GI tract or CNS involvement.

REFERENCES

1. Weller PF, Plaut M, Taggart V, et al. The relationship of asthma therapy and Churg-Strauss syndrome: NIH workshop summary report. *J Allergy Clin Immunol.* 2001;108:175–183.
2. Lhote FC, Guillevin L. Polyarteritis nodosa, microscopic polyangiitis, and Churg-Strauss syndrome. Clinical aspects and treatment. *Rheum Dis Clin North Am.* 1995;21:911–947.
3. Masi AT, Hunder GC, Lie JT. The American College of Rheumatology 1990 criteria for the classification of Churg-Strauss syndrome (allergic granulomatosis and angiitis). *Arthritis Rheum.* 1990;33:1094–1100.
4. De Groot K, Rasmussen N, Bacon PA, et al. Randomized trial of cyclophosphamide versus methotrexate for induction of remission in early systemic antineutrophil cytoplasmic antibody-associated vasculitis. *Arthritis Rheum.* 2005;52:2461–2469.
5. Assaf C, Mewis G, Orfanos CE, et al. Churg-Strauss syndrome: Successful treatment with mycophenolate mofetil. *Br J Dermatol.* 2004;150:598–600.
6. Jones RB, Ferraro AJ, Chaudhry AN, et al. A multicenter survey of rituximab therapy for refractory antineutrophil cytoplasmic antibody–associated vasculitis. *Arthritis Rheum.* 2009;60:2156–2168.
7. Lee RU, Stevenson DD. Hydroxyurea in the treatment of Churg-Strauss syndrome. *J Allergy Clin Immunol.* 2009;124:1110–1111.
8. Kim S, Marigowda G, Oren E, et al. Mepolizumab as a steroid-sparing treatment option in patients with Churg-Strauss syndrome. *J Allergy Clin Immunol.* 2010;125:1336–1343.

Microscopic Polyangiitis

26

Kristine A. Kuhn and John P. Atkinson

GENERAL PRINCIPLES

Microscopic polyangiitis (MPA) is a **small vessel vasculitis** initially termed a microscopic form of polyarteritis nodosa (PAN) because of its clinical similarity to PAN, with the additional involvement of arterioles, capillaries, and venules giving rise to glomerulonephritis.[1,2] However, unlike PAN, MPA is not associated with hepatitis B.

Definition

- MPA is defined by the Chapel Hill Consensus Conference as a necrotizing vasculitis with few or no immune deposits (**pauci-immune**) affecting **small vessels such as capillaries, arterioles, and venules.** Medium vessels may also be involved. These may result in **necrotizing glomerulonephritis and pulmonary capillaritis.**[1]
- Involvement of small vessels distinguishes MPA from PAN.

Classification

MPA is classified as a small vessel vasculitis. See Chapter 20 for further review of the classification of vasculitides.

Epidemiology

- The incidence of MPA in Europe is 2 to 11 cases per million. MPA is 2 to 3 times more frequent than Wegener's granulomatosis (WG) in Southern Europe, while in Northern Europe WG is more prevalent.
- In Asia, there is a much greater incidence of MPA compared to WG. Kuwait has the greatest incidence at 24 cases per million. The prevalence in other non-Caucasian populations is less well defined.
- The mean age is 50 to 70 years.

Etiology

- The etiology of MPA is not well established. Several environmental triggers have been implicated, but these do not explain the majority of cases.
- **Infections:**
  - Some individuals with glomerulonephritis secondary to MPA have antibodies directed to human lysosomal membrane protein-2 (LAMP-2). The epitope recognized by anti-LAMP-2 antibodies is homologous to type 1 fimbrial adhesin (FimH), an adhesion protein produced by Gram negative bacteria. Rats immunized with FimH produce anti-LAMP antibodies and develop crescentic glomerulonephritis.[3]
  - Parvovirus B19 infection may induce antineutrophil cytoplasmic antibodies (ANCA), but these antibodies typically are transient.[4]

- **Drugs:**
  - Medications including hydralazine, minocycline, tumor necrosis factor (TNF) antagonists, penicillamine, sulfasalazine, and propylthiouracil (PTU) have resulted in anti-myeloperoxidase (MPO)–ANCA seropositivity and clinical vasculitis.
  - **PTU-induced MPA is the most recognized form of drug-induced vasculitis.** One-fifth of patients taking PTU will develop ANCA seropositivity, and of these, about one-forth will develop overt vasculitis. Both the ANCA seropositivity and clinical vasculitis will resolve with cessation of PTU.
- **Silica:**
  - About 20% to 40% of patients with ANCA-associated vasculitis have been exposed to silica, and about 20% of perinuclear (p)-ANCA positive individuals have been exposed to silica.
  - The odds ratio for silica exposure for vasculitis ranges from 2 to 14.[5]

Pathophysiology

- ANCA may participate in the pathogenesis of MPA in a two-step process:
  - Low levels of inflammatory cytokines such as interleukin (IL)-1 and TNF-α prime neutrophils to express MPO on their surface.
  - Antibodies to MPO–ANCA bind neutrophils via the surface MPO antigen and/or Fc receptors. Neutrophils become activated causing release of reactive oxygen species and lytic enzymes.
- This process only occurs if neutrophils are attached to a surface such as a vessel wall.
- The model fails to address patients with MPA who are ANCA negative.

Risk Factors

- No specific environmental risk factors have been identified for idiopathic MPA, although infections and other environmental triggers have been suggested.
- Drugs such as hydralazine, minocycline, TNF antagonists, penicillamine, sulfasalazine, and PTU can induce MPA, but the risk is low.
- Genetic risk factors have not been identified.

DIAGNOSIS

Diagnosis is based on clinical, serologic and pathologic findings.[2]

Clinical Presentation

- The most common manifestations of MPA are constitutional, renal, pulmonary, gastrointestinal (GI), cutaneous, musculoskeletal, and neurologic. Onset may be acute or indolent.
- **Constitutional symptoms** (e.g., weakness, weight loss, fevers, malaise, and arthralgias) are present in >70% of patients.
- **Renal involvement** occurs in >80% and can range from asymptomatic active urinary sediment to end-stage renal failure requiring hemodialysis.
- **Pulmonary manifestations** occur in 25% to 55% and include cough, dyspnea, hemoptysis, and pleuritic chest pain. **Pulmonary hemorrhage** occurs in approximately 25% of patients and may be due to either capillaritis or bronchial arteritis. Patients may also present with findings suggesting interstitial fibrosis.

- **Cutaneous manifestations** exist in 30% to 60%. **Palpable purpura** is the most common finding but livedo reticularis, nodules, urticarial, and ulcers from skin necrosis may also be found.
- **Abdominal pain** (30%–60%) and GI bleeding (20%–30%) may be present; however, severe hemorrhage, ulcerations, ischemia, and perforation are less likely to occur in MPA than PAN.
- One- to two-thirds of patients will have **neurologic manifestations** such as **peripheral neuropathy and mononeuritis multiplex,** and, less commonly, central nervous system (CNS) manifestations of pachymeningitis and cerebral infarctions (hemorrhagic or ischemic).

Differential Diagnosis

- Both small and medium-vessel vasculitides are included in the differential diagnosis of MPA.[1]
  - **Pauci-immune immunofluorescence on histology** differentiates MPA from the immune-complex mediated small vessel vasculitides, cryoglobulinemic vasculitis, and Henoch–Schönlein purpura.
  - Lack of granulomas on histopathology distinguishes MPA from WG.
  - The presence of asthma and eosinophilia suggests Churg–Strauss syndrome.
- Distinguishing between MPA and PAN can be difficult. Table 26-1 compares these two diseases.[6]

TABLE 26-1	DISTINGUISHING FEATURES OF PAN AND MPA	
Manifestation	PAN	MPA
Vasculitis	Necrotizing, medium- and small-sized arteries, may sometimes involve arterioles, rarely granulomatous	Necrotizing small vessels, may sometimes involve small- and medium-sized arteries, no granulomas
Renal	Renal vasculitis with renovascular hypertension, infarcts, and microaneurysms; no RPGN	RPGN very common
Pulmonary	No hemorrhage	Hemorrhage common
Peripheral neuropathy	Present in 50%–80%	Present in 10%–50%
Relapses	Rare	Frequent
Lab data	ANCA positive in <20%, HBV may be present but uncommon, angiography commonly illustrates microaneurysms and stenoses	ANCA positive in 50–80%, HBV not present, normal angiography

ANCA, antineutrophil cytoplasmic antibody; HBV, hepatitis B virus; RPGN, rapidly progressive glomerulonephritis.

Adapted from: Guillevin L, Lhote F. Distinguishing polyarteritis nodosa from microscopic polyangiitis and implications for treatment. *Curr Opin Rheumatol* 1995;7:20–24.

○ Involvement of capillaries, arterioles, and venules distinguishes MPA from PAN.

○ **ANCA associates with MPA, but not with PAN. PAN is associated with hepatitis B, while MPA is not.**

• Other conditions to consider include Goodpasture's syndrome and vasculitis associated with other connective tissue diseases (e.g., systemic lupus erythematosus and rheumatoid arthritis).

Diagnostic Testing

The diagnostic workup of MPA includes assessment of renal, pulmonary, and nerve function (e.g., serum creatinine, urinalysis, spirometry, chest radiography, and nerve conduction studies).

Laboratories

• Common laboratory findings include elevated erythrocyte sedimentation rate (ESR) and C-reactive protein (CRP), leukocytosis, thrombocytosis, and normochromic normocytic anemia of chronic inflammation.

• Evaluation of renal function may reveal an elevated blood urea nitrogen (BUN) and creatinine and an **active urinary sediment** (proteinuria, hematuria, red blood cell [RBC] casts and leukocyturia).

• C3 and C4 levels are normal or elevated.

• ANCA testing, either by indirect immunofluorescence or enzyme-linked immunosorbent assay (ELISA) for specific antigens (i.e., proteinase 3 [PR3] and MPO) is not uniformly standardized; therefore, diagnostic performance will vary by laboratory.

○ ANCA is present in about 75% of patients, usually p-ANCA/anti-MPO.[7]

○ ANCA positivity should be confirmed with ELISA testing form anti-MPO and anti-PR3 antibodies.[8]

○ In the appropriate clinical setting, p-ANCA has 98% specificity for MPA.[9]

○ The sensitivity of anti-MPO antibodies ranges broadly depending on the kit used and the cut off value selected.[9]

• Low titer rheumatoid factor (RF) and antinuclear antibodies (ANAs) may also be present.

Imaging

• **Chest radiography** should be performed to evaluate for pulmonary manifestations. Patchy diffuse opacities are found in the setting of alveolar hemorrhage.

• **CT of the chest** demonstrates ground-glass opacifications in the setting of alveolar hemorrhage, and septal thickening and honeycombing may be present with interstitial fibrosis.

• **Mesenteric angiography** may be performed if necessary to differentiate PAN from MPA.

• Other organ-specific imaging may be required for evaluation of complications.

Diagnostic Procedures

• Almost all patients need **renal biopsies.**

○ **Focal segmental glomerulonephritis** is found in nearly 100% of patients with renal disease.

○ Glomerular crescents, frank vasculitis, fibrinoid necrosis, interstitial nephritis, and tubular atrophy may also be observed.

- ○ **The immunofluorescence pattern is pauci-immune,** with minimal immunoglobulin and complement in glomeruli.
- **Bronchoscopy with transbronchial biopsy and bronchoalveolar lavage** (BAL) is useful in demonstrating capillaritis and ruling out infectious causes of pulmonary hemorrhage.
  - ○ BAL fluid is usually grossly hemorrhagic and histology demonstrates hemosiderin-laden macrophages.
  - ○ Biopsy of tissue in hemorrhagic areas can demonstrate necrotizing alveolar capillaritis with pauci-immune immunofluorescence. Other histologic patterns may demonstrate intra-alveolar and interstitial red blood cells, fibrinoid necrosis, and intra-alveolar hemosiderosis.
- **Cutaneous biopsies** demonstrate **leukocytoclastic vasculitis.** Again, immunofluorescence demonstrates a pauci-immune pattern.
- **Nerve conduction velocity** (NCV) studies can identify peripheral neuropathies manifested as acute axonopathy, and **sural nerve biopsy** demonstrates necrotizing vasculitis in nearly 80% of patients with abnormal NCV studies.

TREATMENT

- Treatment is divided into two phases: induction and then maintenance of remission.
  - ○ **Glucocorticoids** are given at **induction** and a prolonged taper is prescribed.
  - ○ **Induction** of remission is established with **cyclophosphamide or rituximab,** while **maintenance** therapy is provided with **azathioprine or methotrexate.**
- Supportive measures with hemodialysis and mechanical ventilation may be required.
- Plasmapheresis may be considered in refractory cases.

Medications
Glucocorticoids
- Initially, methylprednisolone 1000 mg IV daily for 3 days is followed by prednisone orally at 1 mg/kg daily and then tapered slowly over 12 to 18 months.
- Relapses of MPA are common and usually occur during tapering of prednisone doses. Relapses are usually milder than the initial presentation and can often be treated with increased doses of prednisone.
- **Glucocorticoid monotherapy is not recommended,** as remission rates are lower than when given cyclophosphamide.

Cyclophosphamide
- Cyclophosphamide is given as a daily oral regimen or monthly IV infusions.
  - ○ Daily oral cyclophosphamide is given as 2 mg/kg (up to a maximum 200 mg) PO daily for 3 to 6 months followed by maintenance therapy with either azathioprine or methotrexate.
  - ○ Alternatively, it may be given 0.5 to 1.0 g/m^2 IV once monthly for up to 12 months (usually until remission is induced). Again, this is followed by maintenance therapy with azathioprine or methotrexate.
- There is no difference in efficacy between the two regimens. However, the cumulative dose of cyclophosphamide is higher when given orally, which may lead to increased toxicity. This drug should only be given by a physician familiar with its use.

Azathioprine
- Once remission has been induced, substitution of cyclophosphamide with azathioprine has been shown to be effective at the maintenance of remission while reducing the exposure to cyclophosphamide.
- Azathioprine is given 2 mg/kg PO daily to complete a total of 18 months of therapy (from induction).

Methotrexate
Methotrexate given 25 mg PO once weekly for 12 months is similar in efficacy and safety to azathioprine for the maintenance of remission in MPA.[10]

Rituximab
- Compared to cyclophosphamide, rituximab is equally efficacious in the induction of remission for the treatment of MPA and without differences in adverse events.[11] However, long-term data are not well established.
- Rituximab is usually given as an IV infusion of 375 mg/m^2 once weekly for 4 weeks.

Mycophenolate Mofetil
Studies have failed to demonstrate that mycophenolate mofetil 2000 mg PO daily is equally efficacious to azathioprine as maintenance therapy for ANCA-associated vasculitides.[12] Therefore, it is considered a second line agent.

Other Non-pharmacologic Therapies
- **Plasmapheresis** may be indicated in refractory cases of ANCA-associated glomerulonephritis.
- In addition to pulse steroids and cyclophosphamide, plasma exchange reduced the number of patients requiring hemodialysis.
- Plasmapheresis did not affect overall mortality, though.[13]

COMPLICATIONS

- MPA can lead to end-organ failure. Complications depend upon the organ(s) affected. Most commonly renal and pulmonary failure occurs.
- Therapy-specific complications may occur.

REFERRAL

- Patients should be referred to a rheumatologist for diagnosis, treatment, and management of MPA.
- Referral to other specialists should be considered based on specific organ involvement (e.g., nephrologist for renal disease).

PATIENT EDUCATION

Patients should be educated on the disease manifestations, complications, and treatment options for their disease.

MONITORING/FOLLOW-UP

- Follow-up involves the clinical and laboratory assessment of disease activity (complete blood count, renal function, urinary sediment and acute phase reactants) as well as monitoring of medication toxicities.
- Patients in remission should be monitored at least every 3 to 6 months for relapse.
- There is controversy as to whether ANCA levels are useful in monitoring disease activity. It is not recommended. More important are the assessments for end organ damage.

OUTCOME/PROGNOSIS

- About 20% of patients progress to end-stage renal failure. A normal serum creatinine at diagnosis carries a more favorable prognosis.[2]
- Alveolar hemorrhage and pulmonary fibrosis carry a poor prognosis; patients are nine times more likely to die. Also, higher relapse rates occur in those with pulmonary disease.

REFERENCES

1. Jennette JC, Falk RJ, Andrassy K, et al. Nomenclature of systemic vasculitides. Proposal of an international consensus conference. *Arthritis Rheum.* 1994;37:187–192.
2. Chung SA, Seo P. Microscopic polyangiitis. *Rheum Dis Clin North Am.* 2010;36:545–558.
3. Kain R, Exner M, Randes R, et al. Molecular mimicry in pauci-immune focal necrotizing glomerulonephritis. *Nat Med.* 2008;14:1088–1096.
4. Hermann J, Demel U, Stunzner D, et al. Clinical interpretation of antineutrophil cytoplasmic antibodies: Parvovirus B19 infection as a pitfall. *Ann Rheum Dis.* 2005;64:641–643.
5. Hogan SL, Satterly KK, Dooley MA, et al. Silica exposure in anti-neutrophil cytoplasmic autoantibody-associated glomerulonephritis and lupus nephritis. *J Am Soc Nephrol.* 2001; 12:134–142.
6. Guillevin L, Lhote F. Distinguishing polyarteritis nodosa from microscopic polyangiitis and implications for treatment. *Curr Opin Rheumatol.* 1995;7:20–24.
7. Guillevin L, Durand-Gasselin B, Cevallos R, et al. Microscopic polyangiitis: clinical and laboratory findings in eight-five patients. *Arthritis Rheum.* 1999;42:421–430.
8. Savige J, Gillis D, Benson E, et al. International Consensus Statement on Testing and Reporting of Antineutrophil Cytoplasmic Antibodies (ANCA). *Am J Clin Pathol.* 1999; 111:507–513.
9. Holle JU, Hellmich B, Backes M, et al. Variation in performance characteristics of commercial enzyme immunoassay kits for detection of antineutrophil cytoplasmic antibodies: what is the optimal cut off? *Ann Rheum Dis.* 2005;64:1773–1779.
10. Pagnoux C, Mahr A, Hamidou MA, et al. Azathioprine or methotrexate maintenance for ANCA-associated vasculitis. *N Engl J Med.* 2008;359:2790–2803.
11. Stone JH, Merkel PA, Spiera R, et al. Rituximab versus cyclophosphamide for ANCA-associated vasculitis. *N Engl J Med.* 2010;363:221–232.
12. Hiemstra TF, Walsh M, Mahr A, et al. Mycophenolate mofetil vs azathioprine for remission maintenance in antineutrophil cytoplasmic antibody-associated vasculitis: a randomized controlled trial. *JAMA.* 2010;304:2381–2388.
13. Jayne DR, Gaskin G, Rasmussen N, et al. Randomized trial of plasma exchange or high-dosage methylprednisolone as adjunctive therapy for severe renal vasculitis. *J Am Soc Nephrol.* 2007;18:2180–2188.

Henoch–Schönlein Purpura

27

Amy Archer and John P. Atkinson

GENERAL PRINCIPLES

Definition

Henoch–Schönlein purpura (HSP) is defined as a **vasculitis with IgA-dominant immune deposits affecting small vessels**, including capillaries, venules, and arterioles (Chapel Hill Consensus Conference).[1]

Epidemiology

- The annual incidence is 14 cases per 100,000 people.
- Although HSP can be seen at any age, the majority of patients are children less than 10 years old. The mean age at presentation is 6.
- HSP is slightly more common in males.
- HSP presents most commonly in the fall and winter months, often after a respiratory infection.

Etiology

- Although many cases of HSP follow respiratory infections, it may also be associated with the administration of drugs and vaccines. No single dominant etiologic agent has been identified.
- There may be genetic susceptibility with particular HLA alleles.[2]

Pathophysiology

- HSP is characterized by the deposition of IgA-dominant immune complexes in the walls of arterioles, capillaries, and post-capillary venules with resultant complement activation and **leukocytoclastic vasculitis.**
  - Skin and gastrointestinal (GI) manifestations are a direct result of **immune-complex driven inflammation** leading to tissue damage and extravasation of blood cells.
  - Renal biopsies demonstrate glomerulonephritis with prominent mesangial immune complex deposition.
- Aberrant glycosylation in the hinge region of the IgA1 subtype may play a role in pathogenesis.[3]

Associated Conditions

HSP clinical picture develops in about 3% to 7% of patients with familial Mediterranean fever.[4,5]

DIAGNOSIS

Clinical Presentation

- HSP primarily affects the **skin, kidneys, and GI tract.**
- Is often associated with **arthralgias and arthritis.**
- Occasionally, it affects the pulmonary vasculature, resulting in pulmonary capillaritis and **alveolar hemorrhage.**
- Coronary vessel vasculitis and neurologic sequelae are rare.
- There are two main distinctions between children and adults that present with HSP.[6]
  - **Intussusception** is rare in adults.
  - Adults have a greater risk of developing **severe renal disease.**

History

- The typical presentation of HSP is a child with **colicky abdominal pain** associated with **nausea** and **vomiting** as well as **lower extremity arthritis.** The skin lesions may also be early manifestations.
- The initial presentation is often then followed by **bloody diarrhea and palpable purpura,** affecting predominantly the lower extremities and buttocks.
- Boys may present with **orchitis.**
- Rare presentations occur with headache or seizures.
- Symptoms of HSP are usually preceded by an **upper respiratory tract infection** (e.g., fever, rhinorrhea, and cough).

Physical Examination

- **Palpable purpura**
  - In children, purpura may be preceded by a transient urticaria, angioedema, and maculopapular rash.
  - The purpura tends to occur in crops in regions on the **legs and buttocks.** However, purpura can present in other areas of the body and often presents before other manifestations of HSP.
  - Individual lesions are 2 to 10 mm in diameter, typically last several days and resolve more quickly with bed rest.
- **Arthritis**
  - Arthritis is the second most common manifestation of HSP and presents in 75% of patients.
  - The **knees, ankles, and feet** are typically involved.
  - While joints are usually warm and painful, joint effusions are not consistently present.
- **Gastrointestinal**
  - Abdominal pain, nausea, and vomiting
  - **Guaiac-positive stool** is seen in about half of the patients, but hemorrhage is rare.
- **Genitourinary**
  - Pain, tenderness, and swelling of the **testicle and/or scrotum** are less common manifestations of HSP.
- **Neurologic**
  - Rare reports of focal neurologic deficits, ataxia, central and peripheral neuropathy.

TABLE 27-1	AMERICAN COLLEGE OF RHEUMATOLOGY 1990 CRITERIA FOR THE CLASSIFICATION OF HENOCH–SCHÖNLEIN PURPURA

The presence of at least two of the following four are required:

- Palpable purpura, not related to thrombocytopenia
- Age ≤20 years
- Bowel angina, defined as either diffuse abdominal pain that is worsened by meals or the diagnosis of bowel ischemia, usually with bloody diarrhea.
- Histologic changes showing granulocytes in the walls of arterioles or venules

—

Adapted from: Mills JA, Michel BA, Bloch DA, et al. The American College of Rheumatology 1990 criteria for the classification of Henoch–Schönlein purpura. *Arthritis Rheum.* 1990; 33:1114–1121.

Diagnostic Criteria

- American College of Rheumatology 1990 criteria for the classification of HSP are presented in Table 27-1.[7]
- In 2006 the European League against Rheumatism and Pediatric Rheumatology European Society published new criteria for pediatric HSP and these are presented in Table 27-2.[8]
- For typical presentations of HSP in children, it is necessary to **exclude sepsis, thrombocytopenia, and clotting disorders.**
- In adults, further studies are needed to rule out other causes of small vessel vasculitis.

Differential Diagnosis

The differential diagnosis includes other causes of small-vessel vasculitis (Wegener's granulomatosis, microscopic polyangiitis, cryoglobulinemic vasculitis, and leukocytoclastic angiitis), polyarteritis nodosa (in cases of unusually chronic or severe HSP), systemic lupus erythematosus, thrombotic thrombocytopenic purpura/hemolytic-uremic syndrome, exanthematous drug eruption, purpura fulminans, and septic vasculitis.

TABLE 27-2	2006 THE EUROPEAN LEAGUE AGAINST RHEUMATISM AND PEDIATRIC RHEUMATOLOGY EUROPEAN SOCIETY CLASSIFICATION CRITERIA FOR HENOCH–SCHÖNLEIN PURPURA

Palpable purpura with at least one of the following:

- Diffuse abdominal pain
- Biopsy with predominant IgA
- Acute arthritis/arthralgias
- Hematuria or proteinuria

—

Adapted from: Ozen S, Ruperto N, Dillon MJ, et al. EULAR/PReS endorsed consensus criteria for the classification of childhood vasculitides. *Ann Rheum Dis.* 2006;65:936–941.

Diagnostic Testing

Laboratories
- Urinalysis: The most common renal manifestation is microscopic hematuria but up to one-third of patients with nephritis have gross hematuria.
- Serum **creatinine** should be checked.
- Erythrocyte sedimentation rate (ESR) may be elevated.
- Complete blood count should be checked for possible leukocytosis and to ensure a normal platelet count.
- Coagulation studies to **rule out coagulopathies.**
- **Antinuclear antibodies** (ANA) and **antineutrophil cytoplasmic antibody** (ANCA).
- Immunoglobulins: **IgA may be elevated** in up to 72% of children with HSP.[9]

Imaging
- **Abdominal plain films**
  - May have dilated loops of bowel.
  - Can be used in combination with chest radiography to evaluate for perforation.
- **Abdominal ultrasound**
  - More effective means of identifying ileoileal intussusception.
- Doppler flow and/or radionuclide studies
  - Utilized in patients presenting with scrotal pain.
- Head CT/MRI
  - Utilized in rare cases of neurologic presentation to evaluate intracerebral hemorrhage.

Diagnostic Procedures
- Renal biopsy:
  - In children renal biopsy is recommended when there is impaired renal function or marked proteinuria, as histologic lesions are prognostic indicators.
  - **In adults a biopsy may be needed to rule out other causes of small-vessel vasculitis.**
  - Mild disease often demonstrates **focal mesangial proliferation with IgA-dominant immune complex deposition and C3 deposits in the mesangial matrix.**
  - In patients with more severe renal disease, such as nephrotic range proteinuria, there is likely to be marked **cellular proliferation and crescentic glomerulonephritis.**
- Skin biopsy:
  - In adults a skin biopsy may be needed to confirm the diagnosis of HSP.
  - Biopsies will demonstrate small-vessel **leukocytoclastic vasculitis,** most prominent in the post-capillary venules.
  - Immunofluorescence studies show **IgA-dominant immune complex deposition in combination with C3 deposits.**

TREATMENT

Most patients completely recover without specific therapy.

Medications

- **Angiotensin converting enzyme (ACE) inhibitors** should be considered in cases of proteinuria or as a first line agent in patients with hypertension.
- Nonsteroidal antiinflammatory drugs (NSAIDs) are generally sufficient to relieve arthralgias and arthritis, but often are avoided due to side effects.
- **Corticosteroids**
  - May be used for severe joint pain.
  - May be used in severe abdominal pain, especially when intussusception is suspected.
  - **Do not have a role in the treatment of purpura** as there is no decrease in the duration of the skin lesion or frequency of recurrences.
  - **Do not appear to have a role in preventing nephritis.**[10]
- Several treatment regimens for renal disease have been suggested including corticosteroids, azathioprine, cyclophosphamide, cyclosporine, mycophenolate mofetil, plasmapheresis, IV immunoglobulin, and rituximab.

Surgical Management

Those patients that progress to end-stage renal disease are candidates for a renal transplant, although the disease can reoccur following transplant.

COMPLICATIONS

GI involvement has the potential for serious complications including **intussusception** (typically ileoileal), **infarction, massive hemorrhage, and perforation.**

MONITORING/FOLLOW-UP

- In patients with mild renal disease, measurement of blood pressure, serum creatinine, and urinalysis should be obtained at least weekly while the disease is clinically active and once a month for 3 months when the disease remits.
- Females who were diagnosed with HSP in childhood are at increased risk of proteinuria and hypertension during pregnancy and need to be carefully monitored during this time.

OUTCOME/PROGNOSIS

- HSP resolves within 2 to 4 weeks in over 80% of childhood cases.
- Children generally have milder disease and are less likely to have nephritis.
- **HSP is more severe and prolonged in adults,** with renal failure and nephritis occurring more frequently.
- **Recurrence of symptoms occurs in one-third** of patients; resolution in these patients often occurs within 4 months.
- Approximately 30% to 50% of patients with nephritis have persistent urinary abnormalities after long-term follow-up.
- Long-term prognosis of HSP depends on the severity of renal impairment. Only 1% of patients develop end-stage renal disease.
  - Patients with gross hematuria, nephrotic syndrome, or hypertension are more likely to progress to end-stage renal disease (ESRD).
  - If a renal biopsy has crescents involving >50% of the glomeruli, there is increased rate of chronic renal failure and ESRD.

REFERENCES

1. Jennette JC, Falk RJ, Andrassy K, et al. Nomenclature of systemic vasculitides. Proposal of an international consensus conference. *Arthritis Rheum.* 1994;37:187–192.
2. Soylemezoglu O, Peru H, Gonen S, et al. HLA-DRB1 alleles and Henoch–Schönlein purpura: Susceptibility and severity of disease. *J Rheumatol.* 2008;35:1165–1168.
3. Novak J, Moldoveanu Z, Yanagihara T, et al. IgA nephropathy and Henoch–Schoenlein purpura nephritis: Aberrant glycosylation of IgA1, formation of IgA1-containing immune complexes, and activation of mesangial cells. *Contrib Nephrol.* 2007;157:134–138.
4. Ozodogan H, Arisoy N, Kasapçapur O, et al. Vasculitis in familial Mediterranean fever. *J Rheumatol.* 1997;24:323–327.
5. Aksu K, Keser G. Coexistence of vasculitides with familial Mediterranean fever. *Rheumatol Int.* 2011;31:1263–1274.
6. Pillebout E, Thervet E, Hill G, et al. Henoch–Schönlein purpura in adults: Outcome and prognostic factors. *J Am Soc Nephrol.* 2002;13:1271–1278.
7. Mills JA, Michel BA, Bloch DA, et al. The American College of Rheumatology 1990 criteria for the classification of Henoch–Schönlein purpura. *Arthritis Rheum.* 1990;33:1114–1121.
8. Ozen S, Ruperto N, Dillon MJ, et al. EULAR/PReS endorsed consensus criteria for the classification of childhood vasculitides. *Ann Rheum Dis.* 2006;65:936–941.
9. Fretzayas A, Sionti I, Moustaki M, et al. Clinical impact of altered immunoglobulin levels in Henoch–Schönlein purpura. *Pediatr Int.* 2009;51:381–384.
10. Chartapisak W, Opastiraku S, Willis NS, et al. Prevention and treatment of renal disease in Henoch–Schönlein purpura: A systematic review. *Arch Dis Child.* 2009;94:132–137.

Cryoglobulinemia and Cryoglobulinemic Vasculitis

28

Reeti Joshi and John P. Atkinson

GENERAL PRINCIPLES

- Cryoglobulins are serum proteins that undergo precipitation upon refrigeration of serum and redissolve on warming to 37°C.
- They are typically composed of **immunoglobulins** and **complement** fragments.
- This phenomenon was first described by Wintrobe and Bruell in 1933 and later named "cryoprecipitation."
- About 20 years later, Metzler described the classic clinical triad of purpura, arthralgias, and asthenia.
- Cryoglobulinemia refers to presence of circulating cryoglobulins.[1,2]
- Cryoglobulinemic vasculitis (CV) is defined as a vasculitis secondary to deposition of cryoglobulins in small vessels such as arterioles, venules, and capillaries (Chapel Hill Consensus Conference).[1-3]
- An important caveat is that **cryoglobulinemia does not necessarily lead to CV.**

Classification

- Cryoglobulins are commonly classified as per Brouet et al.[1,2,4,5]
  - ○ **Type I: Isolated monoclonal immunoglobulins** IgG or IgM.
    - Frequently associated with myeloma and Waldenström's macroglobulinemia, chronic lymphocytic leukemia (CLL) and B-cell non-Hodgkin lymphomas.
    - Serum levels are often high (5–30 mg/mL) and they usually readily precipitate in cold.
  - ○ **Type II: Immune complexes of polyclonal or monoclonal IgM rheumatoid factor directed against polyclonal IgG**
    - Most are IgM–IgG, although IgG–IgG and IgG–IgA can occur.
    - Serum levels are usually high, 40% with levels >5 mg/mL.
    - Primarily associated with hepatitis C virus (HCV).
  - ○ **Type III: Polyclonal IgM rheumatoid factor directed against polyclonal IgG**
    - These are consistently heterogeneous (always polyclonal).
    - More difficult to detect because they precipitate slowly and tend to be present in much smaller quantities (50–1000 μg/dL).
    - Associated with HCV to a lesser extent compared to Type II cryoglobulins.
- **Type II and III are considered "mixed cryoglobulins" (MC)** as they contain a mixture of IgM and IgG.
- Type II and III are associated with HCV, other viral and bacterial infections (HIV, hepatitis B virus [HBV]), endocarditis, autoimmune disease (e.g., rheumatoid arthritis [RA], systemic lupus erythematosus [SLE], and systemic sclerosis), and lymphoproliferative disorders.
- Essential mixed cryoglobulinemia refers to cases with no identifiable cause; however, after the identification of HBV and HCV, a large majority of these cases were shown to be related to these infections.

Epidemiology

- The laboratory assessment of MC is not standardized and requires expertise beyond the abilities of most labs. Furthermore, improper handling of samples leads to false negatives. Consequently, the actual prevalence may be underestimated.
- Prevalence of "essential" MC is reported to be approximately 1:100,000; however, **very few cases are truly "essential"** (no identifiable cause).
- Estimates of MC prevalence in HCV infection vary widely, ranging from 10% to 70%.
- Female-to-male ratio is 3:1.
- Several groups have focused on HLA alleles. Studies from France, Italy, and China have associated DRB1*11 alleles and DR3, DR5, and DR6 serological clusters with MC. A group in Japan found no significant association between HLA and HCV MC.[2]

Cryoglobulinemic Vasculitis in Chronic Hepatitis C Infection

- The natural history and prognosis of MC vasculitis are variable and highly dependent on renal involvement and overall extent of vasculitic lesions.
- CV is usually associated with advanced age, longer duration of HCV infection, type II MC, a higher MC serum level, and clonal B-cell expansions in both the blood and liver.[4]
- The worse prognostic factors are being older than 60 years at diagnosis and renal involvement.
- The overall 5-year survival after the diagnosis of vasculitis ranges from 50% to 90% in cases with renal involvement. Even in the absence of significant renal failure, increased mortality from liver involvement, cardiovascular disease, infection, and lymphoma has been reported.

Pathophysiology

- Clinical and histological features indicate vascular deposits of cryoglobulins leading to cold induced symptoms of vascular insufficiency secondary to occlusion of various small vessels. This is commonly seen in patients with Type I or II cryoglobulins.
- Circulating immune complexes are present in occluded blood vessel walls as well as in serum.
- The monoclonal rheumatoid factors (mRF) that bear the WA cross-idiotype are responsible for most cases of CV in patients with HCV infection.
- HCV exerts a chronic stimulus on the immune system and provides a chronic intravascular antigenic source.
- A pathogenic factor in MC is thought to be the production of IgM by B-cell clones.
- **Cutaneous vasculitis and glomerulonephritis are typically seen in Type II and III cryoglobulins.**
- Vasculitic lesions in different organs with HCV may vary. For example, while complexes of HCV RNA, monoclonal IgM-RF, IgG, and complement components are detected in skin, demonstration of HCV proteins in kidneys remains difficult.
- Low C4 is found in patients with CV.
- Cryoglobulinemic neuropathy may be caused by vasculitis of vasa nervorum as well as immunologically mediated demyelination, hyperviscosity, and microvascular occlusion.

• Vasculitis of intramuscular or cerebral arteries may cause paresis or plegia, strokes, or a diffuse encephalopathy.

Associated Conditions

Infections
• Viral: hepatitis A virus (HAV), HBV, HIV, HCV, Epstein–Barr virus (EBV), cytomegalovirus (CMV).
• Bacterial: syphilis, leprosy, Q-fever, streptococcal infections, infectious endocarditis.
• Fungal: coccidiomycosis.
• Parasitic: leishmaniasis, toxoplasmosis, echinococcosis, malaria, schistosomiasis, and trypanosomiasis.

Hematologic/Oncologic
• Hodgkin's and non-Hodgkin's lymphoma.
• Chronic myelogenous leukemia and CLL.
• Multiple myeloma.
• Waldenström's macroglobulinemia.
• Myelodysplastic syndrome.
• Myeloproliferative diseases.
• Castleman's disease.
• Thrombotic thrombocytopenic purpura.

Autoimmune Diseases
• Sjögren's syndrome.
• RA.
• SLE.
• Systemic sclerosis.
• Giant cell arteritis.
• Inflammatory bowel disease.
• Sarcoidosis.
• Dermatomyositis/polymyositis.
• Autoimmune thyroiditis.

DIAGNOSIS

Diagnosis of cryoglobulinemia is by clinical and lab parameters. CV has different presentations based on organ systems affected.

Clinical Features

• **Type I cryoglobulinemia:**
  ○ Type I is rarely implicated in clinical symptoms related to vasculitis and tends to cause **signs of peripheral vascular occlusion and hyperviscosity.** Raynaud's phenomenon, purpura, acrocyanosis, dystrophic manifestation, ulcers, and gangrene may be seen.
  ○ Hematologic abnormalities may be present due to the underlying disease.
  ○ High cryocrit and cryoglobulins may only be a casual finding.
• **Mixed Cryoglobulinemia (MC):**
  ○ MC syndrome is characterized by the triad of **purpura, weakness, and arthralgias.**

○ **Multisystem organ involvement** including chronic hepatitis, membranoprolif-
erative glomerulonephritis (MPGN), and peripheral neuropathy due to leukocytoclastic vasculitis of small- and medium-sized vessels is frequently observed.

History and Physical Examination
- The history should be aimed primarily at identifying an underlying disease.
- General symptoms included Raynaud's phenomenon, acrocyanosis, rashes pre-
cipitated by cold, and sicca symptoms.

Cutaneous Manifestations
- **Purpura** is the main manifestation of CV.
- Palpable purpura is usually found on lower extremities.
- About 70% patients have this cutaneous finding, which may be transient or
may progress to **ulcers and gangrene.**

Arthralgias/Arthritis
- Affects small **distal joints, oligoarticular, and nonerosive** pattern usually seen
in MC.
- Often sensitive to low doses of steroids, with or without hydroxychloroquine.
- In HCV associated MC, rarely an erosive symmetrical polyarthritis may develop.
- An overlap syndrome of RA and MC must be considered.
- Anti-cyclic citrullinated protein (CCP) antibodies may represent an important
diagnostic tool as they are not increased in MC while RF positivity is seen in
30% to 70% of patients with HCV, even in the absence of RA.

Symmetric Peripheral Neuropathy
- Symmetric peripheral neuropathy is the most common neurologic manifestation.
- It is more frequent in Type III cryoglobulinemia.
- It may have an acute or subacute presentation, usually accompanied by cutane-
ous disease.
- It is typically, a **sensory axonal neuropathy in glove and stocking pattern.**
- Symmetric or asymmetric motor and/or sensory polyneuropathy is common.
- Mononeuritis multiplex may also be seen.
- Causes of neuropathy:
  ○ Vasculitis of vasa nervosum.
  ○ Hyperviscosity with occlusion of microcirculation.
  ○ Immune-mediated demyelination.

Renal Disease
- Most common in type II cryoglobulinemia, being observed in 30% to 60% of
MC and portending a poor prognosis.
- HCV RNA detected in kidney of affected patients.
- **Non-nephrotic range proteinuria, hematuria, and hypertension.** This rarely
presents as an acute nephritis/nephritic syndrome.
- **Type I MPGN** accounts for 80% of type II cryoglobulinemic nephropathy.
There is thickening of glomerular basement membrane and cellular prolifera-
tion on biopsy.
- Distinguishing histological features in cryoglobulinemic MPGN:
  ○ Marked influx of circulating macrophages
  ○ Intraluminal thrombi of precipitated cryoglobulins
  ○ Fingerprint subendothelial deposits by electron microscopy
  ○ IgM deposition in capillary loops by immunofluorescence.

- Less common presentations:
  - ○ Mild mesangial membranous nephropathy
  - ○ Acute vasculitis of small- and medium-sized renal vessels
  - ○ Thrombotic microangiopathy
  - ○ Occasionally oliguria and rapidly progressive acute renal failure is seen.

Liver Disease
- Diffuse lymphoid infiltration of liver (lupoid hepatitis).
- Usually related to HCV.
- Levels of cryoglobulins typically decrease as cirrhosis progresses.
- Autoimmune hepatitis may share a number of extrahepatic features including leukocytoclastic vasculitis, hypocomplementemia, glomerulonephritis, and anti-smooth muscle antibodies, further confounding the diagnosis.

Rare Findings
- Lymphadenopathy.
- Mesenteric vasculitis.
- Subclinical pulmonary fibrosis.
- Coronary vasculitis.
- Pulmonary vasculitis, pleurisy, dyspnea, cough, and hemoptysis are often overlooked.

Diagnostic Criteria

- The American College of Rheumatology does not have a set of criteria for CV.
- The Gruppo Italiano di Studio delle Crioglobulinemie published a system for defining and characterizing the cryoglobulinemic syndrome; this is presented in Table 28-1.[6]

Diagnostic Testing

Laboratories
- Cryoglobulins are heterogeneous in composition, thermal properties, and efficiency of complement activation.

TABLE 28-1	PROPOSED SYSTEM FOR DEFINING AND CHARACTERIZING THE CRYOGLOBULINEMIC SYNDROME

- Cryocrit >1% for at least 6 months.
- At least two of the following: purpura, arthralgia, weakness
- C4 <8 mg/dL.
- Positive rheumatoid factor (monoclonal or polyclonal).
- Secondary, if associated with connective tissue diseases, chronic liver diseases, lymphoproliferative diseases, infections.
- Essential, if without an identifiable underlying cause.
- Assess the extent of the vasculitis: hepatic/renal involvement, neuropathies.
- Identification of microlymphoma-like nodules in the bone marrow.

Adapted from: Invernizzi F, Pietrogrande M, Sagramoso B. Classification of the cryoglobulinemic syndrome. *Clin Exp Rheumatol.* 1995;13:S123–S128.

- Serum concentrations do not necessarily correlate with severity.
- Sample collection is a critical step.
- A negative test should not exclude the disease; if clinical suspicion remains high, the test should be repeated.
- If a cryoprecipitate is present, it should be resolubilized and subject to both quantitative analysis (cryocrit estimation, immunoglobulin and C4 levels, rheumatoid factor) and qualitative analysis (serum protein electrophoresis and immunofixation).[7]
- Tests for both HCV antibody and HCV RNA should be done, even if hepatic enzymes are normal.
- Negative HCV test may rarely be due to HCV RNA concentrated in circulating cryoglobulin immune complexes.
- Other lab findings include elevated erythrocyte sedimentation rate (ESR), low C4 with normal or slightly low C3, normocytic normochromic anemia, and RF. Total hemolytic complement may be zero due to cold activation. (complement activation may occur after the sample is obtained).[7]

TREATMENT

- Asymptomatic patients with detectable cryoglobulins can simply be monitored.
- Patients with mild to moderate disease, such as arthralgias, asthenia, and purpura, may be treated with low to medium dose prednisone (10–30 mg/day).
- Moderate to severe disease, including glomerulonephritis and cutaneous vasculitis are treated with low to medium dose prednisone and, if HCV positive, pegylated IFN and ribavirin.
- Patients with life-threatening manifestations including rapidly progressing glomerulonephritis, sensorimotor neuropathy, and extensive or visceral vasculitis, should receive plasma exchange and high dose steroids plus cyclophosphamide or rituximab or, if they have hepatitis C, should receive sequential therapy with rituximab followed by pegylated IFN and ribavirin.[1]
- Due to the complexity of etiopathogenesis, the **treatment of HCV-associated MC is particularly challenging.**
  ○ Three important factors should be considered: HCV infection, the presence of an autoimmune disorder, and possible neoplastic associations.
  ○ The most effective treatment for HCV MC is **eradication of underlying HCV infection** (i.e., removal of the antigen driving the process).
  ○ In patients with sustained virologic response to anti-HCV therapy, the symptoms of MC and evidence of B-cell lymphoproliferative disorders almost always disappear.
  ○ HCV relapse is associated with recurrence of symptoms.
  ○ The eradication of HCV with pegylated IFN/ribavirin leads to resolution of MC associated splenic villous lymphomas and immunocytomas.[8,9]
  ○ Current standard of care for HCV is pegylated IFN in combination with ribavirin. However, the care is complicated in that there are several different genotypes of HCV, each with a variable response to treatment.
  ○ Sustained virologic response of 45% to 50% is noted in genotypes 1 and 4, 70% to 80% in genotypes 2 and 3.

- Other therapies for cryoglobulinemia (type II) have relied on cytotoxic agents or apheresis, although no controlled trials have been undertaken for either agent.
- There is a concern with immunosuppression leading to worsening of underlying infectious disease.
- Due to risk of lymphoproliferative disease development, cytotoxic agents are not preferred but have been used (e.g., chlorambucil in CLL-induced cryoglobulinemia).[10]

Medications

Cyclophosphamide

- Cyclophosphamide is typically used in severe cases and remains the first line cytotoxic agent.
- For severe life-threatening disease, use daily oral cyclophosphamide with pulse steroids and plasmapheresis (doses similar to those used for Wegener's granulomatosis).
- Severe but non–life-threatening disease may be treated with monthly pulse IV cyclophosphamide along with oral prednisone.
- Once remission of severe disease is achieved, employ daily oral prednisone with weekly oral methotrexate or azathioprine.
- Treatment of underlying causes such as RA or lymphoma is essential in preventing relapse.

Rituximab

- Systemic B-cell depletion with rituximab, a chimeric monoclonal antibody against CD20 antigen, has been utilized successfully in patients with several autoimmune diseases.
- Several case reports and small uncontrolled case series have reported variable success with rituximab in cryoglobulinemia and CV.[11,12]
- Recent treatment guidelines for mixed cryoglobulinemia syndrome in HCV infected patients suggests that HCV viral load and liver function be carefully monitored in patients receiving rituximab, and antiviral prophylaxis should be given to HBV carriers.
- Type 1 cryoglobulinemia appears to have a lower response rate than MC.
- In one meta-analysis, 128 patients with CV were reviewed.[11]
  - In most studies, rituximab was administered intravenously at doses of 375 mg/m^2 weekly for 4 weeks, sometimes followed by two extra infusions at 1 and 2 months. This higher dose was associated with more side effects. A lower dose of 250 mg/m^2 at days 1 and 8 showed a response rate of 80% in six patients with HCV induced MC.
  - Neuropathy and renal involvement were more resistant to treatment whereas skin and joint disease responded quickly.
  - Side effects were reported in 27 out of 128 patients, including infection, serum sickness, thrombosis of retinal arteries, and development of cold agglutinin disease.

Colchicine

- The rationale underlying the use of colchicine (1mg/day) to treat MC is based on the drug's activity in reducing immunoglobulin secretion.
- In a small open study, it had favorable effects on purpura, weakness, and leg ulcers. Minor gastrointestinal side effects are common at this dose.[13]

Other Non-Pharmacologic Therapies
Plasmapheresis
- This should be reserved for life-threatening forms of disease including vasculitis, glomerulonephritis, severe central nervous system disease, malignant hypertension, vascular insufficiency with distal necrosis, and hyperviscosity syndrome.
- Concomitant immunosuppressive therapy must be instituted to prevent rebound antibody formation and relapse of disease after withdrawal of plasmapheresis.
  - A protocol typically includes methylprednisolone 1 g daily for 3 days followed by oral prednisone and cyclophosphamide (doses similar to those used for treatment of Wegener's granulomatosis).
- Plasmapheresis, exchanging one plasma volume three times weekly for 2 to 3 weeks is generally used. Replacement fluid can be 5% albumin, which must be warmed to prevent precipitation of cryoglobulins.
- Optimal methods for assessment of efficacy are not clear as cryocrit may not correlate with disease intensity. Clinical examination is used to guide further therapy. Skin, arthritic, and renal manifestations can improve rapidly whereas cryoglobulinemic neuropathy does not remit in short-term therapy.[14]

REFERENCES

1. Ferri C. Mixed Cryoglobulinemia. *Orphanet J Rare Dis.* 2008;3:25.
2. Charles ED, Dustin LB. Hepatitis C virus-induced Cryoglobulinemia. *Kidney Int.* 2009; 76:818–824.
3. Jennette JC, Falk RJ, Andrassy K, et al. Nomenclature of systemic vasculitides. Proposal of an international consensus conference. *Arthritis Rheum.* 1994;37:187–192.
4. Saadoun D, Landau D, Calabrese L, et al. Hepatitis C-associate mixed cryoglobulinemia: A crossroad between autoimmunity and lymphoproliferation. *Rheumatol (Oxford).* 2007;46: 1234–1242.
5. Brouet JC, Clauvel JP, Danon F, et al. Biologic and clinical significance of cryoglobulins. A report of 86 cases. *Am J Med.* 1974;57:775–788.
6. Invernizzi F, Pietrogrande M, Sagramoso B. Classification of the cryoglobulinemic syndrome. *Clin Exp Rheumatol.* 1995;13:S123–S128.
7. Sargur R, White P, Egner W. Cryoglobulin evaluation: best practice? *Ann Biochem.* 2010;47:8–16.
8. Pietrogrande M, DeVita S, Zignego A, et al. Recommendations for the management of mixed cryoglobulinemia syndrome in Hepatitis C virus-infected patients. *Autoimmun Rev.* 2011;10:444–454.
9. Iannuzella F, Vaglio A, Garini G. Management of Hepatitis C Virus related Mixed Cryoglobulinemia. *Am J Med.* 2010;123:400–408.
10. Pietrogrande M, Meroni M, Fusi A, et al. Therapeutical approach to the mild cryoglobulinemic syndrome : Results from a retrospective cohort study. *Ann Rheum Dis.* 2006;70:65–72.
11. Wink F, Houtmann P, Jansen T. Rituximab in cryoglobulinaemic vasculitis, evidence for its effectivity: A case report and review of literature. *Clin Rheumatol.* 2011;30:293–300.
12. Terrier B, Launay D, Kaplanski G, et al. Safety and efficacy of rituximab in nonviral cryoglobulinemia vasculitis: Data from the French Autoimmunity and Rituximab registry. *Arthritis Care Res (Hoboken).* 2010;62:1787–1795.
13. Monti G, Saccardo F, Rinaldi G, et al. Cochicine in the treatment of mixed cryoglobulinemia. *Clin Exp Rheumatol.* 1995;13:S197–S199.
14. Foessel L, Besancenot J, Bertrand M, et al. Clinical spectrum, treatment and outcome of patients with type II mixed cryoglobulinemia without evidence of hepatitis C infection. *J Rheumatol.* 2011;38:1–8.

Cutaneous Vasculitis

29

Michael L. Sams and John P. Atkinson

GENERAL PRINCIPLES

Definitions

- Cutaneous vasculitis (CV) is a **small-vessel vasculitis affecting the skin.** However, small-vessel vasculitis is often not specific to just the small-vessels and there **may be overlap involvement of the medium-sized vessels.**
- There are multiple different names for CV which leads to confusion. **Leukocytoclastic vasculitis** (LCV) is often used to refer to CV. However, it is a pathologic term and refers to the nuclear "dust" due to degranulation of neutrophils seen under light microscopy. **Leukocytoclasia is nonspecific** and LCV may be seen with multiple types of CV.
- **Necrotizing vasculitis is synonymous with LCV.**
- **Cutaneous leukocytoclastic angiitis (CLA)** refers to isolated CV without systemic vasculitis or glomerulonephritis. It has also been referred to as **primary cutaneous small vessel vasculitis (PCSVV).**[1]
- **Hypersensitivity vasculitis** is a CV of the small vessels (arterioles and venules) secondary to an immune response to an exogenous substance. However, there is often no clear evidence of an ongoing immune response or an inciting agent. CLA may be the preferred term over hypersensitivity vasculitis.
- **Lymphocytic vasculitis** is also a CV but is different histologically from LCV as it features a lymphocytic infiltrate. It is more commonly observed with vasculitis due to the connective tissue disorders and Behçet's disease (BD).

Etiology

- There are multiple causes of CV. (Table 29-1).
- **One-third of cases of CV are idiopathic.**
- The most common cause of CV is **drug-induced.** Typically it does not involve other organs and presents as CLA.
- **Urticarial vasculitis** results in an urticarial-like rash that lasts longer than 24 to 48 hours. The lesions may progress to a purpuric stage and after resolution, there is postinflammatory hyperpigmentation. There are two types of urticarial vasculitis: the **normocomplementemic form** and the **hypocomplementemic form.** The latter is often associated with systemic lupus erythematosus (SLE).[2]
- **Viral infections** including both hepatitis B and C as well as HIV have also been linked to vasculitis. In the case of hepatitis C virus (HCV), **mixed cryoglobulins** (Types II and III) deposit in the small and medium vessels leading to inflammation.

TABLE 29-1 CAUSES OF CUTANEOUS VASCULITIS SYNDROMES

Cutaneous leukocytoclastic angiitis:
Usually idiopathic or drug-induced

Drugs (most common cause):
Penicillins, sulfonamides, allopurinol, thiazides, quinolones, propylthiouracil, hydantoins, nonsteroidal anti-inflammatory drugs (NSAIDs), and many others

Infections:
Bacterial: *Streptococcus, Neisseria, Chlamydia, Staphylococcus,* endocarditis
Viral: Hepatitis C (through type II and III cryoglobulins), HIV

Erythema elevatum diutinum:
Many potential associations including infections (e.g., *Streptococcus,* HIV), rheumatologic conditions (e.g., rheumatoid arthritis, relapsing polychondritis), and inflammatory bowel disease

Connective tissue diseases:
Rheumatoid arthritis, systemic lupus erythematosus, Sjögren's syndrome

Systemic vasculitides:
Henoch–Schönlein purpura, polyarteritis nodosa (classic and cutaneous), urticarial vasculitis, Behçet's disease, cryoglobulinemia (type II and III), Wegener's granulomatosis, Churg–Strauss syndrome, microscopic polyangiitis

Malignancy:
Lymphoma, leukemia, solid tumors (e.g., lung, colon, breast, renal, prostate)

Inflammatory bowel disease

Idiopathic

- **Connective tissue diseases** may present with CV. The disorders prone to this include SLE, Sjögren's syndrome, and rheumatoid arthritis (RA) (rheumatoid vasculitis). The resulting vasculitis can also be lymphocytic.
- There are multiple **systemic vasculitides** that present with cutaneous involvement. These include all three of the antineutrophil cytoplasmic antibody (ANCA)-associated vasculitides, BD, Henoch–Schönlein purpura (HSP), polyarteritis nodosa (PAN), and cutaneous PAN (vasculitic changes as with PAN but limited to the skin). As mentioned, hypocomplementemic urticarial vasculitis is often associated with SLE.
- **Erythema elevatum diutinum** is a specific form of chronic CV typified by papules and nodules on the extensor surfaces of the extremities. The cause, while unknown, is presumed to be immune complex related. Early lesions show LCV. Many potential associations have been made including infections and various rheumatologic disorders.[3]
- **Lymphoma, leukemia,** and even **solid tumors** have been associated with CV. However, malignancy accounts for less than 5% of cases.
- **Hypercoagulable states,** while not an inflammatory process, may appear on physical examination of the skin like a vasculitis due to the ischemia and damage to the vessel.

Pathophysiology

- The pathophysiology of CV depends on the etiology.
- Certain infections cause direct invasion of blood vessels (e.g., *Neisseria, Rickettsia*) or may induce immune complex deposition (e.g., hepatitis B virus infection).
- Other vasculitides may also be immune-complex mediated (drug-induced or rheumatoid vasculitis) or due to immunoglobulin deposition (e.g., IgA in HSP). ANCA-associated vasculitis may involve the skin in addition to other organs but the role of these antibodies in these cases is unclear.
- The size of the vessel involved dictates the clinical findings. With small-vessel vasculitis **palpable purpura** is common but **non-palpable purpura, urticaria, pustules, vesicles, superficial ulcerations, and splinter hemorrhages** all occur.
- When medium-sized vessels are involved skin changes include **nodules, livedo reticularis, digital infarctions, ulcers, and papulonecrotic lesions.** These differences reflect the greater area of ischemia due to obstruction of a larger blood vessel.
- The majority of CV is classified as small-vessel vasculitides.
- Common types of medium-sized vasculitis include PAN, cutaneous PAN, rheumatoid vasculitis, and Buerger's disease.

DIAGNOSIS

- The approach to vasculitis of the skin is to answer the following questions:
  - ○ Are the skin findings due to vasculitis?
  - ○ What is the etiology?
  - ○ Are other organ systems involved?

Clinical Presentation

History

- CV usually appears suddenly and the lesions are often painless. In contrast, urticarial vasculitic lesions are often painful and burning rather than pruritic-like allergic urticaria. Myalgias or arthralgias may accompany the skin lesions.
- A history of a connective tissue disease (e.g., RA, SLE, Sjögren's syndrome) is important, as are symptoms of an underlying systemic disease (e.g., fever, weight loss, hematuria, abdominal pain, joint pain, focal or generalized weakness).
- Often CV is the first sign of a serious illness.
- Examine the medication list for possible etiologic agents, as **drugs are the most common cause.** Drug-induced vasculitis usually develops 7 to 21 days after starting a drug. Almost any drug can cause a vasculitic reaction and the most common ones are listed in Table 29-1. Drug reactions typically resolve spontaneously upon discontinuing the medication.

Physical Examination

- **Palpable purpura is the classic lesion of CV.** Nonpalpable purpura, nodules, urticaria, vesicles, and shallow or deep ulcerations are also seen, sometimes in combination.
- Lesions usually occur in the lower extremities or in dependent locations. However, urticarial vasculitis is more common on the trunk and proximal extremities.

TABLE 29-2	AMERICAN COLLEGE OF RHEUMATOLOGY 1990 CRITERIA FOR HYPERSENSITIVITY VASCULITIS

The presence of at least three of the following five are required:

- Age >16 years
- Use of a possibly causative drug related temporally to symptoms
- Palpable purpura
- Maculopapular rash
- Biopsy demonstrating granulocytes around the arteriole or venule

—

Adapted from: Calabrese LH, Michel BA, Bloch DA, et al. The American College of Rheumatology 1990 criteria for the classification of hypersensitivity vasculitis. *Arthritis Rheum.* 1990;33: 1108–1113.

- The physical examination aims to identify other organ system involvement and should include a musculoskeletal examination looking for arthritis.
  - A neurologic examination is important to identify focal or diffuse weakness that may occur due to mononeuritis multiplex.
  - Palpate for enlarged lymph nodes that may suggest infection or underlying malignancy.
  - Auscultate the heart for murmurs and inspect the nails if endocarditis is suspected.

Diagnostic Criteria

The American College of Rheumatology criteria for hypersensitivity vasculitis are presented in Table 29-2.[4]

Differential Diagnosis

Multiple processes in the skin can result in non-blanching purpura, ulcerations, and urticaria. See Table 29-3 for common nonvasculitic causes of these findings.

Diagnostic Testing

Laboratories

- Investigate renal involvement with **chemistries** and **urinalysis.**
- A **hepatic function panel** can be helpful.
- **Blood cultures** (and cultures from other sites) are mandatory in cases with fever, as infections, including endocarditis, can cause vasculitis.
- The **erythrocyte sedimentation rate** (**ESR**) is often elevated but is nonspecific. Testing for systemic markers of disease is not recommended unless there is clinical suspicion.
- Specific labs to help diagnose systemic causes include but are not limited to antinuclear antibodies (ANA), anti-double stranded DNA (dsDNA), rheumatoid factor (RF), ANCA, hepatitis serologies, cryoglobulin determination, C3, C4, CH50, SSA, SSB, and urine protein electrophoresis (UPEP).

Imaging

Chest radiographs or CT scans may be needed to evaluate the lungs and the upper respiratory tract and rule out systemic disease.

TABLE 29-3 MIMICS OF CUTANEOUS VASCULITIS

Hypercoagulable states:
Antiphospholipid syndrome

Monoclonal cryoglobulins (Type I): Associated with multiple myeloma and
   Waldenström's macroglobulinemia; may cause hyperviscosity
Warfarin-induced skin necrosis
Protein C and S deficiency
Thrombocytosis

Emboli:
Cholesterol
Endocarditis
Scurvy
Pyoderma gangrenosum
Sweet's syndrome
Calciphylaxis

Other causes of purpura:
Thrombotic thrombocytopenia purpura
Idiopathic thrombocytopenia purpura
Other causes of thrombocytopenia
Other coagulation disorders

Diagnostic Procedures

Skin Biopsy

- A skin biopsy is essential to confirm the diagnosis.
- Indications for biopsy include symptoms of systemic disease or continual formation of new lesions for more than 3 weeks.
- If possible, perform biopsies within 24 to 48 hours after the appearance of a lesion. Biopsies performed before or after this time typically show a nonspecific lymphocytic infiltrate.[5]
- Ulcerated sites should be avoided. When it is necessary to biopsy an ulcerated site, the edge should be sampled.
- A punch biopsy provides the appropriate depth for examination, especially for deeper medium-sized vessels.
- Examine specimens under light microscopy and direct immunofluorescence.
- Under light microscopy, the affected blood vessels are characterized by **fibrinoid necrosis** of the vessel wall with an **inflammatory infiltrate within and around the vessel wall.**
  ○ When the infiltrate is only perivascular, the diagnosis of vasculitis cannot be made reliably.
  ○ Hemorrhage and fragments of leukocytes (**leukocytoclasia**) are also seen.
  ○ Cutaneous vasculitic lesions associated with connective tissue diseases often have lymphocytic infiltration.
  ○ Prominence of eosinophils is suggestive of Churg–Strauss syndrome.
  ○ Urticarial lesions have an LCV histopathology.

- **Direct immunofluorescence** may reveal **immunoglobulin and complement deposition** on the vessel wall.
  - In particular, IgA deposition is characteristic of HSP. C3 fragments may also be aggregated with IgA.
  - **ANCA-associated vasculitides are considered pauci-immune** as few immune reactants are present on immunofluorescence.
  - Rheumatoid vasculitis reveals a granular IgM and C3 deposition suggesting immune-complex mediated disease.

TREATMENT

- In the absence of other organ involvement and underlying diseases, treatment of CV is symptomatic.
  - **Antihistamines and nonsteroidal antiinflammatory drugs (NSAIDs)** may be helpful.
  - Some severe cases may require **corticosteroids.**
  - If drug-induced vasculitis is suspected, **stop the offending drug.** Most cases of drug-induced CV resolve within 2–3 weeks to a few months upon stopping the offending medication.
- For chronic disease, steroid sparing agents may be used.
- **The treatment of CV, as a manifestation of an underlying disorder, varies according to the type of disorder and other organ involvement.**

MONITORING/FOLLOW-UP

Follow-up is important as CV can be the first manifestation of a systemic disease or malignancy.

REFERENCES

1. Russell JP, Gibson LE. Primary cutaneous small vessel vasculitis: Approach to diagnosis and treatment. *Int J Dermatol.* 2006;45:3–13.
2. Davis MD, Brewer JD. Urticarial vasculitis and hypocomplementemic urticarial vasculitis syndrome. *Immunol Allergy Clin North Am.* 2004;24:183–213.
3. Gibson LE, el-Azhary RA. Erythema elevatum diutinum. *Clin Dermatol.* 2000;18:295–299.
4. Calabrese LH, Michel BA, Bloch DA, et al. The American College of Rheumatology 1990 criteria for the classification of hypersensitivity vasculitis. *Arthritis Rheum.* 1990;33:1108–1113.
5. Stone JH, Nousari HC. "Essential" cutaneous vasculitis: What every rheumatologist should know about vasculitis of the skin. *Curr Opin Rheumatol.* 2001;13:23–34.

Thromboangiitis Obliterans

30

Rebecca Brinker and John P. Atkinson

GENERAL PRINCIPLES

- **Thromboangiitis obliterans** (TAO), or **Buerger's disease,** is a chronic, recurring inflammatory occlusive disease of medium- and small-sized vessels in the upper and lower extremities.
- It is characterized by segmental, nonatherosclerotic, thrombotic vessel stenosis, and occlusion with subsequent limb ischemia and necrosis or thrombophlebitis.

Epidemiology

- TAO tends to affect **male smokers <40 years of age.**
- In 1986 the United States prevalence rate of TAO was approximately 12.6 cases per 100,000.
- It is seen with at higher frequency among countries of the "old Silk Route," such as India, Israel, Japan, and Manipur.
- The highest prevalence is in **Jewish men of Ashkenazi descent.**

Pathophysiology

- The exact etiology of TAO is unknown but is clearly related to tobacco use.
- There is cellular, inflammatory thrombus occluding the lumen, with sparing of the blood vessel wall.
- Increased cellular immunity to Type I and III collagens has been demonstrated.[1]
- There may be a role for prothrombotic factors in the pathophysiology of TAO.
  - Prothrombin gene mutation 20210 and anticardiolipin antibodies are associated with an increased risk of the disorder.[2]
- TAO may be pathologically divided into three phases:[3]
  - Acute: Occlusive highly cellular inflammatory thrombi in distal limb arteries or veins composed of polymorphonuclear leukocytes, micro-abscesses, and multinucleated giant cells.
  - Intermediate: Organization of thrombus.
  - Chronic: Organized thrombus and vascular fibrosis are now prominent, without inflammatory infiltrate. At this stage the biopsy is nonspecific and these findings are common in other types of vascular occlusive disease.

Risk Factors

- **Smoking,** especially heavy smokers (>1.5 packs per day) and those who use raw tobacco.
- There have been case reports of TAO in patients who use smokeless tobacco, snuff, or cigars.
- Possibly chronic anaerobic periodontal infections.[4]
- Chronic arsenic poisoning.

Prevention
- Abstinence of tobacco use is the only known preventative measure.
- No clear evidence that second-hand smoke increases prevalence.

DIAGNOSIS

- **Definitive diagnosis is by biopsy** of the affected limb revealing pathology consistent with an acute phase lesion in the vessels of the affected limb in the appropriate clinical setting.
- Other causes of distal extremity ischemia must be ruled out.

Clinical Presentation
- Typically seen in **male smokers**, <40 years of age.
- Ischemia usually starts at distal fingertips or toes and progresses proximally.
- **Ischemic findings and symptoms** may occur (e.g., claudication or ulcerations).
  - Ulcerations are a more common initial symptom because TAO has the tendency to affect smaller arteries first.
- **Pain at rest and sensory deficits** are very common and are usually secondary to ischemic neuritis.
- **Migratory superficial thrombophlebitis** and **Raynaud's phenomenon** are present in about 40% of patients.[3,5]
- Signs of peripheral vascular disease (e.g., extremity poikilothermia, pallor, pulselessness, and paresthesia) are present in the affected as well as unaffected limbs.
- TAO rarely affects the cerebral, coronary, mesenteric, pulmonary, iliac or renal arteries, or the aorta. However, if these arteries are affected, ischemic symptoms in the affected organ may be seen.

History
- Digital pain, ulceration, or color changes from blood vessel obstruction and eventual tissue necrosis.
- Claudication of upper or lower extremities with use.
- Superficial thrombophlebitis may occur before digital ischemia.
- Symptoms and color changes consistent with Raynaud's phenomenon.
- Nonspecific, episodic, joint pains in the extremities may be observed months to years before the occlusive phase of the disease.
  - Most commonly affected joints are wrists and knees.

Physical Examination
- Digital ulcerations and necrosis that is usually bilateral.
- Claudication with exercise of the extremity in question.
- Raynaud's phenomenon.
- Superficial thrombophlebitis.
- Altered Allen's test (used to evaluate radial and ulnar perfusion of the hand).[5]

Diagnostic Criteria
- The American College of Rheumatology does not have diagnostic or classification criteria for TAO. However, several authors have suggested such criteria and most propose a combination of clinical, angiographic, and histopathologic, as well as exclusionary findings.
- Commonly used criteria of Olin and colleagues are presented in Table 30-1.[5]

TABLE 30-1	CRITERIA FOR THROMBOANGIITIS OBLITERANS

- Age of onset <45 years
- Current or recent tobacco use
- Distal extremity ischemia manifested as claudication, rest pain, ulceration, or gangrene plus consistent noninvasive vascular testing
- Consistent angiographic findings
- Exclusion of proximal sources of emboli (by echocardiography and arteriography)
- Exclusion of autoimmune diseases, hypercoagulable states, diabetes mellitus

Adapted from: Olin JW. Thromboangiitis obliterans (Buerger's disease) *N Engl J Med.* 2000; 343:864–869.

Differential Diagnosis

- Thrombotic or embolic disease.
- Peripheral vascular disease.
- Cholesterol embolic disease.
- Trauma.
- Hypercoagulable states.
- Infection.
- Raynaud's disease.
- Small vessel vasculitis.

Diagnostic Testing

There is no definitive laboratory or radiographic test to diagnose TAO. However, disease mimics must be ruled out.

Laboratory
- Test for systemic vasculitis or other autoimmune disorders associated with vasculitis. Consider checking antinuclear antibodies (ANA), antineutrophil cytoplasmic antibodies (ANCA), rheumatoid factor (RF), anti-cyclic citrullinated protein antibodies (CCP), complement levels, Scl-70 antibodies, and antiphospholipid antibodies.
  - Autoimmune serologies should be negative. However, few patients with TAO may have a low titer positive antiphospholipid screen.
- Evaluate for possible hypercoagulable states.
- Unlike some other vasculitides, TAO does not have laboratory signs of systemic inflammation (e.g., elevated erythrocyte sedimentation rate [ESR] and C-reactive protein [CRP], thrombocytosis, normochromic normocytic anemia).
- Screen for diabetes mellitus.

Imaging
Transthoracic echocardiography (TTE) with follow-up transesophageal echocardiography (TEE) if there is suspicion of intra-cardiac thrombus.

Diagnostic Procedures
Arteriography
- Perform angiography of **all the four limbs,** even those without clinical evidence of occlusive disease.
- Arteriogram should reveal normal proximal arteries with **distal segmental occlusive disease of small- and medium-sized vessels** (e.g., palmar, plantar,

tibial, peroneal, radial, ulnar, or digital arteries) with severe distal disease and collateralization around the occlusion ("corkscrew" collaterals).

- These findings are not pathognomonic as they may be seen in hypercoagulable states, autoimmune diseases, and vasculitis.
- Disease-modifying interventions may also be taken during this diagnostic study.

TREATMENT

- Crucial to the treatment of TAO is **complete smoking cessation.**
- It is inconclusive, but unlikely, that second-hand smoke causes disease exacerbation or progression.
- With complete tobacco cessation, patients can largely avoid amputation.[6] Patients may still have claudication or Raynaud's phenomenon.
- Nicotine replacement therapy may also perpetuate disease activity.[3,5]
- Many medications are under investigation for treatment, but none have been proven to be as beneficial as smoking cessation.

Medications

- Smoking cessation aids:
  - Do not use nicotine replacement therapy as this may duplicate disease activity.
  - Consider some FDA approved non-nicotine containing medications such as **bupropion or varenicline.**
- The following medications are investigational. Most have been tried in the acute and chronic phases of the disease.
  - There is no study showing overwhelming support for the use of aspirin or anticoagulation during acute or chronic phases of TAO.
  - Iloprost, a prostaglandin analog, may increase ulcer healing, decrease pain, and reduce the need for amputation.[7] These results have only been seen with IV but not oral administration. Continuation or re-initiation of smoking may completely blunt these potentially beneficial effects.
  - Thrombolytic therapy may be beneficial in a limited number of patients, but remains investigational.
  - Calcium-channel blockers, β-blockers, and sildenafil may be of benefit. However, clear cut evidence for efficacy is not available. These medications have not been studied in prospective clinical trials.
  - Medications and procedures to promote therapeutic angiogenesis are undergoing evaluation. Some of these small studies have showed promise in increasing ulcer healing and decreasing ischemic pain.

Other Non-Pharmacologic Therapies

- Epidural spinal cord stimulators are under investigation.
- Few studies evaluating the effect of autologous bone marrow mononuclear cell implantation for critical limb ischemia show short-term promising results. However the long-term efficacy, safety, and complications are not well defined.[8,9]

Surgical Management

- Ischemic digits may require amputation.
- Arterial bypass is usually not an option or recommended secondary to the mostly distal and intermittent occlusive nature of the disease.

- ○ However, in other countries, there are reports of successful surgical bypass with autologous vein or omental transfers.
- Sympathectomy may be tried in patients with resistant disease, but results are mixed and controversial.

COMPLICATIONS

- Digit ischemia and loss that may become progressive, especially if the patient continues to use tobacco products.
- Infection of necrotic tissue.

REFERRAL

Consider referral to vascular surgeon.

PATIENT EDUCATION

Educate the patient about the need to stop smoking!

OUTCOME/PROGNOSIS

- Hopefully, complete resolution with discontinuation of tobacco products.
  - ○ Even if digital ischemia resolves, some patients may have persistent Raynaud's phenomenon, claudication, or rest pain.
  - ○ If the patient continues to smoke, they are much more likely to require major amputations.
- Amputation for digital necrosis.

REFERENCES

1. Adar R, Papa MZ, Halpern Z, et al. Cellular sensitivity to collagen in thromboangiitis obliterans. *N Engl J Med.* 1983;308:1113–1116.
2. Avcu F, Akar E, Demirkiliç U, et al. The role of prothrombotic mutations in patients with Buerger's disease. *Thromb Res.* 2000;100:14–17.
3. Piazza G, Creager MA. Clinical update: Thromboangiitis obliterans. *Circulation.* 2010;121: 1858–1861.
4. Iwai T, Noue Y, Umeda M, et al. Oral bacteria in the occluded arteries of patients with Buerger disease. *J Vasc Surg.* 2005;42:107–115.
5. Olin JW. Thromboangiitis obliterans (Buerger's disease). *N Engl J Med.* 2000;343:864–869.
6. Ohta T, Ishioashi H, Hosaka M, et al. Clinical and social consequences of Buerger disease. *J Vasc Surg.* 2004;39:176–180.
7. Fiessinger JN, Schafer N. Trial of iloprost versus aspirin treatment for critical limb ischaemia of thromboangiitis obliterans. The TAO Study. *Lancet.* 1990;335:555–557.
8. Motukuru V, Suresh KR, Vivekanand V, et al. Therapeutic angiogenesis in Buerger's disease (thromboangiitis obliterans) patients with critical limb ischemia by autologous transplantation of bone marrow mononuclear cells. *J Vasc Surg.* 2008;48:53S–60S.
9. Matoba S, Tatsumi T, Murohara T, et al. Long-term clinical outcome after intramuscular implantation of bone marrow mononuclear cells (Therapeutic Angiogenesis by Cell Transplantation [TACT] trial) in patients with chronic limb ischemia. *Am Heart J.* 2008; 156:1010–1018.

Behçet's Disease

Maria C. Gonzalez-Mayda and
John P. Atkinson

GENERAL PRINCIPLES

Definition

- Behçet's disease (BD) is a systemic vasculitis characterized by **recurrent aphthous oral and genital ulcers and uveitis.**
- Skin lesions, joint complaints, vascular disease, and neurologic manifestations are also associated with BD and may be the presenting problem.
- It is relatively unique among the vasculitides in its **ability to affect vessels of any size.**

Epidemiology

- Most commonly seen along the ancient Silk Route extending from **eastern Asia to the Mediterranean basin,** but due to immigration BD has extended beyond the Silk Route to other countries.
- **Turkey has the highest prevalence** of disease, estimated at 80 to 370 cases/ 100,000 population, whereas in the United States, the prevalence is roughly 8.6/100,000 inhabitants.[1]
- BD is **more common in men** than in women, but prevalence data may be inaccurate because women in some cultures may not seek medical attention for their symptoms.
- Peak age of onset is in the mid-twenties to mid-thirties.

Pathophysiology

- BD is characterized by vascular injury, hyperfunctioning neutrophils, and immune dysfunction.
- Vascular injury consists of **vasculitis of small vessels with subsequent vascular occlusion.**
- Larger vessels demonstrate **vasculitis of the vasa vasorum with aneurysmal formation** and superimposed **hypercoagulability** resulting in thrombosis.
- Active ulcerative lesions are infiltrated by **hyperfunctioning neutrophils,** which have been stimulated by local hypersecretion of cytokines.
- **Immune dysfunction** is characterized by lymphocytic infiltration of active lesions and clonal expansion of T-cells.
- The main abnormality in BD has yet to be elucidated, but the clinical manifestations appear to be due to vasculitis of **various sized vessels** in affected organs.

Risk Factors

- HLA-B51 has been associated with BD in those countries with high prevalence rates.[2]

DIAGNOSIS

Clinical Presentation

History

- In most series, the most common symptoms at presentation of BD include oral and genital aphthosis, eye manifestations, and skin lesions.
- **Oral aphthosis** is the most common manifestation and is usually seen in patients throughout the course of the disease.
- **Genital aphthosis** occurs less frequently.
- **Ocular symptoms** include changes in visual acuity, pain, photophobia, lacrimation, floaters, and periorbital erythema.
- Approximately 10% of patients have eye involvement at presentation, while approximately 50% develop manifestations during the course of the disease.
- Ocular manifestations, as the initial symptom, are more common in females, but eye involvement tends to be more severe in males.
- **Blindness** occurs in approximately 25% of patients with eye involvement.
- **Cutaneous manifestations** of BD include erythema nodosum, pseudofolliculitis, and acneiform nodules.
- **Erythema nodosum** is observed in approximately 50% of patients in the course of disease and is more common in females.

Physical Examination

- **Oral aphthosis** begins as a raised area of redness that soon ulcerates.
  - ○ Lesions are typically round or oval shaped, painful, 2 to 10 mm in size, with a sharp erythematous border, a necrotic white-centered base, and a yellow pseudomembrane.
  - ○ They may occur on the gingiva, tongue, buccal, and labial membranes. They heal within approximately 10 days but **tend to recur frequently** during the first few years.
- **Ocular findings** include the following:
  - ○ **Anterior uveitis** which tends to be recurrent and self-limited.
    - ■ **Hypopyon,** a layer of pus in the anterior ocular chamber, may be visible. This finding is classic for anterior uveitis.
    - ■ Repeated attacks can cause iris deformity and glaucoma.
  - ○ **Retinal disease** is characterized by vasculitis leading to vaso-occlusive disease.
    - ■ Attacks are recurrent and episodic and result in painless, gradual, bilateral visual loss.
    - ■ Retinal hemorrhage, exudative lesions, and cellular infiltration of the vitreous humor are visible on examination.
- **Cutaneous manifestations** include the following:
  - ○ **Erythema nodosum:** Recurrent and painful subcutaneous nodules that tend to occur on the anterior portion of the lower legs and last for several weeks. Nodules often leave an area of hyperpigmentation and, after spontaneous resolution, they occasionally ulcerate.
  - ○ **Pseudofolliculitis and acneiform nodules** are more common in men. The lesions are found on the back, face, neck, and along the hairline, and are often precipitated by shaving.
  - ○ **Genital ulcers** are rarely the presenting symptoms of BD, but over the course of the disease they appear in approximately 75% of patients.

- They are similar in appearance to oral ulcers, but tend to be more painful, larger, last longer, recur less frequently, and often leave scars.
- In young women, the ulcers may be related temporally to the menstrual cycle and may be the only manifestation of disease during the early years.
  - The **pathergy test** is performed by using two subcutaneous pricks with blunt 20-gauge sterile needles to one arm and two subcutaneous pricks with sharp 20-gauge sterile needles to the other arm.
    - A test is considered positive if a sterile erythematous papule >2 mm forms at 48 hours.
    - Blunt needles seem to produce more positive reactions.
    - The test appears to have high specificity but sensitivity is variable.
    - Pathergy is less common in European and North American patients.
- **Articular manifestations** are common.
  - The inflammatory arthritis of BD is acute, nondeforming, nonerosive, occasionally recurrent, and rarely chronic.
  - It tends to be monoarticular, commonly affecting the knee, followed by the wrist, ankle, or elbow but it can also be oligoarticular or polyarticular.
- **Venous thrombosis** is a characteristic manifestation.
  - **Superficial thrombophlebitis and deep venous thrombosis** are common after injury to vessels, including cannulation by angiocatheters.
  - Occlusions and aneurysms of major vessels can cause organ dysfunction, hemorrhage, or infarction (e.g., Budd–Chiari syndrome or pulmonary hemorrhage).
  - Embolic events are rare.
- **Central nervous system (CNS) involvement** in BD occurs in approximately 10% to 20% of patients.
  - This is more common and more severe in males, particularly if the disease begins at a young age.
  - Manifestations including **aseptic meningitis, meningoencephalitis, focal neurologic deficits, and personality changes** tend to develop more than 5 years after the time of diagnosis.
  - Focal signs include pyramidal tract disease (e.g., spastic paralysis, Babinski sign, clonus, and speech disturbances), brain stem disease (e.g., dysphagia and fits of laughter alternating with crying), cerebellar ataxia, and pseudobulbar palsy.
  - Sensory deficits are uncommon.
  - **Intracranial venous thrombosis** can lead to intracranial hypertension, seizures, and hemorrhage.[3]
  - CNS BD tends to recur and becomes irreversible. In a study of 200 Turkish patients, 41% have a relapsing–remitting course, 28% a secondary progressive course, 10% a primary progressive course, and 21% had silent neurologic involvement.[4]
  - In the terminal stage, approximately 30% of affected BD patients with CNS manifestations may have dementia.
  - Aseptic meningitis or meningoencephalitis, early in the disease course, successfully treated with steroids, carries a good prognosis.
- **Other rare manifestations** of BD include myocardial infarction, pulmonary embolus, epididymitis and ileocecal, colonic, and esophageal ulceration.

TABLE 31-1	1990 INTERNATIONAL STUDY GROUP CLASSIFICATION CRITERIA FOR BEHÇET'S DISEASE

Recurrent (≥3 episodes in a 12-month period) oral aphthous ulceration plus two of the following four:

- Genital ulceration
- Skin manifestations (erythema nodosum, pseudofolliculitis, acneiform lesions)
- Eye inflammation (anterior/posterior uveitis, retinal vasculitis)
- Pathergy phenomenon

Adapted from: Criteria for diagnosis of Behçet's disease. International Study Group for Behçet's disease. *Lancet.* 1990;335:1078–1080.

Diagnostic Criteria

- The 1990 International Study Group classification criteria for BD are presented in Table 31-1.[5]
  - A multi-ethnic study of 300 patients showed an overall sensitivity of 90% and specificity of 95% but these varied significantly by race.[6]
- The 2006 International Criteria for Behçet's Disease are presented in Table 31-2.[7]
  - A large cohort of Iranian patients demonstrated a sensitivity of 98%, specificity of 95%, and diagnostic accuracy of 97% for these new criteria.[8]

Differential Diagnosis

- The differential diagnosis depends on the presenting clinical manifestations.
- If oral and genital ulcers are present, consider **reactive arthritis** as well as **inflammatory bowel disease.**

TABLE 31-2	2006 PROPOSED INTERNATIONAL CRITERIA FOR BEHÇET'S DISEASE

Patients who present with the following manifestations whose sum of points is three or more are considered to have Behçet's disease:

Oral aphthosis	1 point
Skin manifestations	1 point
Vascular lesions (arterial and venous thrombosis, aneurysm)	1 point
Pathergy phenomenon (test)	1 point
Genital aphthosis	2 points
Ocular lesions	2 points

Adapted from: International Team for the Revision of the International Criteria for Behçet's Disease (ITR-ICBD). Revision of the International Criteria for Behçet's Disease (ICBD). *Clin Exp Rheumatol.* 2006;24(suppl 42):S14—S15.

- If ocular manifestations and acneiform nodules are present, **seronegative arthropathies** must be considered in the differential.
- Erythema nodosum, ileocecal involvement, and ulcerative mouth lesions may suggest **Crohn's disease.**
- Sarcoidosis may also produce erythema nodosum.
- CNS involvement may mimic **multiple sclerosis** and other neurologic pathologies.

Diagnostic Testing

Laboratories
- No specific test for BD is available. Laboratory findings may include an elevated erythrocyte sedimentation rate (ESR) and mild leukocytosis.
- Cerebrospinal fluid analysis may show elevated protein and IgG and pleocytosis with high numbers of both lymphocytes and neutrophils.
- Joint fluid is inflammatory with increased neutrophils.

Imaging
If neurologic BD is suspected, MRI of the brain as well as magnetic resonance venography (MRV) can show multiple high-intensity focal lesions in the brain stem, basal ganglia, and white matter.

Diagnostic Procedures
- **A positive pathergy test is often considered diagnostic.**
- The result may not be consistent throughout the course of the disease, that is, it may appear and then disappear.
- It is important to note that a positive pathergy test is much less frequently seen in Western countries such as the United States and the United Kingdom than in Eastern countries along the Silk Road.

TREATMENT

Treatment of BD depends on which manifestations are present, how severe they are, and whether or not they are resistant to first-line treatment.

Medications

First Line
- Treatment is based on systems involved and the severity of that involvement.[9]
- **Mucocutaneous aphthosis** (oral and genital):
  - First-line treatment is **colchicine** at 1 mg/day.
  - Side effects are uncommon at this dose.
  - If there is inadequate response, the dose of colchicine may be increased; however, this may be limited by the occurrence of undesirable side effects, usually diarrhea.
- **Uveitis/retinal vasculitis:**
  - **Anterior uveitis** is treated with **topical steroid drops** (e.g., betamethasone, 1–2 drops tid) and **mydriatic agents** if the symptoms are mild and isolated. Ophthalmologic referral is indicated.
  - More severe symptoms require **systemic corticosteroids** such as 0.5 mg/kg daily of prednisone as first-line therapy.

○ **Posterior uveitis** is treated with either **methotrexate** (15 mg weekly) or **aza-thioprine** (2–3 mg/kg daily) along with **prednisone** (0.5 mg/kg daily).

○ **Retinal vasculitis** should be treated first with a combination of **IV cyclo-phosphamide** (750–1000 mg/m² of body surface once monthly), **pred-nisone** (0.5 mg/kg daily) and **azathioprine** (2–3 mg daily).

- **Neurologic involvement** is treated with IV cyclophosphamide and prednisone at 1 mg/kg daily.
- **Skin lesions** are treated the same as mucocutaneous manifestations.
- **Arthralgias/arthritis** can usually be treated with nonsteroidal anti-inflammatory drugs (NSAIDs) until resolution of symptoms.
- **Thrombosis** is treated with **anticoagulation** as normally would be done for any clot; however, for clots in larger vessels, cyclophosphamide as well as corticoste-roids are often used.
- **Gastrointestinal (GI) manifestations** are treated with low-dose **corticosteroids and sulfasalazine** as first line.

Second Line

- **Mucocutaneous aphthosis** (oral and genital): Consider switching to **levamisole** (150 mg once weekly), **dapsone** (100 mg daily), or **thalidomide** (100–400 mg daily).
  ○ If no response is noted, consider switching to **methotrexate** (7.5 mg weekly) or **azathioprine** (2–3 mg/kg daily).
  ○ Dermatology consultation may be valuable in this setting.
  ○ Add low-dose prednisolone for better results and taper as soon as possible.
  ○ If these fail, **consider biologic agents.**
  ○ In resistant cases of genital aphthosis, **intra-lesional injection of triamci-nolone acetate** may help heal the lesion.
- **Uveitis/retinal vasculitis:**
  ○ **Anterior uveitis:** Since anterior uveitis is known for recurrent attacks that can eventually lead to cataracts and glaucoma, consider switching to cytotoxic agents such as **azathioprine or methotrexate** in these cases.
  ○ **Posterior uveitis:** If no response is noted with either immunosuppressant, consider switching to another cytotoxic agent such as **chlorambucil, cyclospo-rine, or IV cyclophosphamide.** If still no response, consider a biologic agent.
  ○ **Retinal vasculitis:** Consider switching to a biologic agent.
- **Arthritis/arthralgias:** If NSAIDs are ineffective, switch to either **methotrexate or azathioprine** with low-dose corticosteroids.
- **GI manifestations:** Switch to **high-dose steroids and IV cyclophosphamide** if first-line treatment does not work.
- In patients with **refractory BD,** unresponsive to the conventional treatment of steroids and immunosuppressive agents, **anti-tumor necrosis factor (anti-TNF) agents** may be effective. Although there are no large randomized control trials on use of anti-TNF agents in BD, multiple case reports and case series suggest that agents such as infliximab and etanercept should be considered in patients with relapsing uveitis, active neurologic manifestations or other symptoms related to BD that are life threatening and/or significantly affecting their quality of life.[10]

Surgical Management

- Surgery is indicated for patients with bowel perforation or recurrent bleeding.
- Since surgical procedures can result in excessive infiltration of inflammatory cells into treated tissues, intermediate doses of steroids may be used periopera-tively to prevent poor wound healing and avoid complications.

MONITORING/FOLLOW-UP

Frequency of follow-up depends on one's assessment of disease activity and requirements for monitoring drug toxicity.

REFERENCES

1. Calamia KT, Wilson FC, Icen M, et al. Epidemiology and clinical characteristics of Behçet's disease in the US: A population-based study. *Arthritis Rheum.* 2009;61:600–604.
2. de Menthon M, Lavalley MP, Maldini C, et al. HLA-B51/B5 and the risk of Behçet's disease: A systematic review and meta-analysis of case-control genetic association studies. *Arthritis Rheum.* 2009;61:1287–1296.
3. Aguiarr de Sousa D, Mestre T, Ferro JM. Cerebral venous thrombosis in Behçet's disease: A systematic review. *J Neurol.* 2001;258:719–727.
4. Akman-Demir G, Serdaroglu P, Tasçi B. Clinical patterns of neurological involvement in Behçet's disease: Evaluation of 200 patients. The Neuro-Behçet study group. *Brain.* 1999;122:2171–2182.
5. Criteria for diagnosis of Behçet's disease. International Study Group for Behçet's disease. *Lancet.* 1990;335:1078–1080.
6. O'Neill TW, Rigby AS, Silman AJ, et al. Validation of the International Study Group criteria for Behçet's disease. *Br J Rheumatol.* 1994;33:115–117.
7. International Team for the Revision of the International Criteria for Behçet's Disease (ITR-ICBD). Revision of the International Criteria for Behçet's Disease (ICBD). *Clin Exp Rheumatol.* 2006;24(suppl 42):S14–S15.
8. Davatchi F, Sadeghi Abdollahi B, Shahram F, et al. Validation of the International Criteria for Behçet's disease (ICBD) in Iran. *Int J Rheum Dis.* 2010;13:55–60.
9. Davatchi F, Shahram F, Chams-Davatchi C, et al. How to deal with Behçet's disease in daily practice. *Int J Rheum Dis.* 2010;13:105–116.
10. Arida A, Fragiadaki K, Giavri E, et al. Anti-TNF agents for Behçet's disease: Analysis of published data on 369 patients. *Semin Arthritis Rheum.* 2010;41:61–70.

Infectious Arthritis

32

Jeffrey Sparks and Prabha Ranganathan

GENERAL PRINCIPLES

- Infectious arthritis is caused by **bacteria, fungi, mycobacteria, and viruses.**
- **Prompt joint fluid analysis and culture** is essential to the diagnosis of infectious arthritis as well as tailoring specific antibiotic therapy.
- **Empiric antibiotics** are utilized while awaiting specific culture data.
- Treatment often requires a multidisciplinary approach, involving physical therapy, orthopedic surgery, and infectious diseases consultations.

Definition

Infectious arthritis, also referred to as septic arthritis, is an **acute monoarthritis or oligoarthritis** caused by an infectious agent, most often bacteria.

Classification

- Bacterial infectious arthritis is classically divided into gonococcal and non-gonococcal arthritis.
- Other etiologies for infectious arthritis include viruses, mycobacteria, and fungi.
- Please see Chapter 33 for discussion on Lyme disease.

Epidemiology

The estimated incidence of infectious arthritis in the United States is approximately 20,000 cases annually.

Etiology

- Most cases of bacterial arthritis in adults are caused by *Staphylococcus aureus,* accounting for up to 80% of confirmed cases.[1]
- The second leading pathogen is *Streptococcus pneumoniae,* followed by **gram-negative bacteria,** although any microbial pathogen is capable of causing infectious arthritis.
- The leading cause of bacterial arthritis in young, sexually active adults is *Neisseria gonorrhoeae*, with a male to female ratio of 1:4.
- Immunocompromised patients are at increased risk for developing opportunistic mycobacterial and fungal infections.
- **Viral infections** commonly associated with arthritis include hepatitis, rubella, mumps, Epstein–Barr virus, parvovirus B19, enterovirus, adenovirus, and HIV.

Pathophysiology

- **Hematogenous spread** is the most common route by which bacteria reach the joint following inoculation through the skin or mucosa.

- Bacterial colonization usually occurs within the synovial lining, followed by bacterial proliferation in the synovial fluid.
- The presence of bacteria in the joint capsule induces an inflammatory response, recruiting leukocytes that propagate the inflammatory reaction through release of cytokines.
- Bacterial products, the release of lysosomal enzymes, immune complex deposition, complement activation, metalloproteases, and chondrocyte inhibition all contribute to articular damage.
- Non-gonococcal bacterial arthritis is typically more damaging than gonococcal arthritis.

Risk Factors

- **Intravenous drug users, immunocompromised patients,** those with **prosthetic joints or heart valves,** and **chronic debilitating diseases** (such as cancer) all have an increased risk for infectious arthritis, especially with gram-negative organisms.
- **Immunocompromised patients** are at increased risk for developing opportunistic mycobacterial and fungal infections as well.
- Advanced age and comorbid conditions such as diabetes and chronic renal insufficiency are risk factors for infectious arthritis.
- Patients with **underlying inflammatory arthritis, especially rheumatoid arthritis,** are more prone to bacterial arthritis.
- Sepsis and bacteremia can lead to seeding of joints, and increase the risk of infectious arthritis.
- Direct inoculation via arthrocentesis or arthroscopy can occur but is quite uncommon, <1%.[2]
- **Gonococcal arthritis** should be considered in sexually active young patients and patients engaging in high-risk sexual behavior. Other risk factors for gonococcal arthritis include menstruation, pregnancy, and complement deficiencies.

DIAGNOSIS

Clinical Presentation

- The **acute onset of mono- or oligoarticular arthritis,** especially in the setting of a **fever and constitutional symptoms,** should raise the suspicion of infectious arthritis.
- Delay in diagnosis can lead to rapid and severe joint destruction, causing significant morbidity and increased mortality.

History

- The most common symptoms are joint pain, swelling, and fever.[3]
- Fever occurs in most patients, although up to 20% of patients may be afebrile. Chills and rigors are unusual.
- 50% of cases involve the **knee,** followed by the hip, shoulder, wrist, ankle, elbow, and small joints of the hands and feet. Up to 20% of cases may present with **polyarticular symptoms.**
- **Intravenous drug abusers** tend to develop infectious arthritis in joints of the axial skeleton including **sternoclavicular and costochondral joints.**
- History should focus on risk factors, recent trauma or procedures, high-risk sexual behavior, and the presence of prosthetic joints.

Physical Examination

- The joint examination should include checking the ability to bear weight, range of motion, and signs of soft tissue swelling, warmth, erythema, edema, and synovitis within and around suspected joints.
- As hematogenous spread to the joint often occurs from distant sites, physical examination should focus on identifying infection in such sites including the skin, respiratory, cardiac, and genitourinary system.
- The respiratory examination should focus on evaluation for **pneumonia, pharyngitis, and sinusitis.**
- The cardiac examination should include evaluation for **new murmurs or friction rubs.**
- The genitourinary examination should include evaluation for **flank pain, urethritis, and cervicitis.**
- A careful skin examination should be performed for signs of cellulitis. **Papules, pustules, bullae, or necrotic lesions** are especially suggestive of gonococcal arthritis.
- **Tenosynovitis, dermatitis, and migratory polyarthritis** are the classic triad for **disseminated gonococcal infections.** Urethritis in men is more likely to be symptomatic than cervicitis in women.

Diagnostic Criteria

The presence of a pathogen in synovial fluid culture is the most specific finding in the diagnosis of septic arthritis. However, timing of antibiotic therapy, arthrocentesis technique, and limitations in microbiologic analysis may affect culture results.

Differential Diagnosis

In addition to infectious arthritis, the differential diagnosis of acute monoarthritis includes trauma, crystalline arthritis (gout and pseudogout), early stages of inflammatory polyarthritis (e.g., rheumatoid arthritis and seronegative spondyloarthropathies), acute rheumatic fever, infectious bursitis, and Lyme disease.

Diagnostic Testing

Testing should focus on promptly establishing the diagnosis of infectious arthritis and identifying the responsible pathogen.

Laboratories

- **Blood cultures** should be obtained prior to initiation of antibiotics in an effort to isolate the responsible pathogen.
- **Inflammatory markers,** such as white blood cell (WBC) count, erythrocyte sedimentation rate (ESR), and C-reactive protein (CRP), are often elevated. The peripheral WBC count is elevated in approximately half of the affected patients.
- **Culture samples from cervix, urethra, rectum, pharynx, and skin lesions** may be helpful in isolating a pathogen, especially if gonococcal arthritis is suspected.
- Cultures for unusual organisms should be ordered in cases of suspected tuberculosis, penetrating trauma, animal bites, travel to areas endemic with particular fungal organisms, immunocompromised patients, or monoarthritis refractory to conventional antibiotic therapy.
- For Lyme disease, serologies may improve diagnostic yield.

Imaging

- **Plain radiographs** of the suspected joint can be helpful in evaluating joint destruction, bony involvement, effusions, erosions, chondrocalcinosis, and extent of disease, but are rarely helpful in the acute setting as radiographic changes of bone and joint destruction may take days to weeks to develop. Radiographic exams help exclude fractures, tumors, and osteomyelitis.
- For difficult to access joints, radiographic guidance with ultrasound, fluoroscopy, or computed tomography may be necessary for joint aspiration.
- **MRI** is useful in assessing whether there is osteomyelitis or adjacent abscess, particularly in joints such as the sternoclavicular that may be difficult to visualize on plain films.
- **Echocardiography** can be useful to evaluate for endocarditis as a source of septic emboli, especially in patients with sepsis, bacteremia, known valvulopathy, or intravenous drug abuse.

Diagnostic Procedures

Arthrocentesis

- **Prompt synovial fluid analysis is essential** for diagnosing infectious arthritis and guiding appropriate antibiotic therapy. **Arthrocentesis should be performed in any patient presenting with monoarticular joint pain with an effusion.** Entering a site with active cellulitis is to be avoided to prevent further seeding of infection.
- Aspiration of purulent drainage is highly suspicious of infectious arthritis.
- The **presence of crystals does not exclude the diagnosis of infectious arthritis.**
- **WBC counts >50,000/μL** with a **predominance of polymorphonuclear neutrophils** is consistent with infectious arthritis. The higher the WBC count, the greater the likelihood ratio (LR) for septic arthritis (>50,000/μL LR 7.7; >100,000/μL LR 28.0).[3]
- Routine **Gram stain** may show bacteria which can guide initial therapy. For non-gonococcal infections, these are positive 50% to 75% of the time.
- Chemistries such as lactate dehydrogenase (LDH), glucose, and protein have limited value, although elevated LDH and low glucose is consistent with bacterial infection.
- Special stains and culture, such as acid-fast bacillus stain and fungal cultures, are to be considered for atypical presentation or immunosuppressed patients.
- Microbiologic culture growth of an organism capable of causing infectious arthritis is most helpful in guiding antibiotic therapy. This data may take days to be finalized and may be falsely negative depending on antibiotic timing and arthrocentesis technique.
- For suspected gonococcal infection, conventional Gram stain and routine cultures are less sensitive. Cultures of synovial fluid on **chocolate agar or Thayer–Martin media** may enhance recovery.
- **Polymerase chain reaction (PCR)** of synovial fluid to detect gonococcal DNA may also increase diagnostic yield.

TREATMENT

- The mainstay of treatment of bacterial arthritis includes **intravenous antibiotics and joint drainage.**

- For non-gonococcal arthritis, initial antimicrobial therapy should be based on the results of the Gram stain and the clinical setting. **If no organisms are seen on Gram stain, broad-spectrum antibiotic coverage for both gram-positive and gram-negative organisms should be initiated.** Coverage for methicillin-resistant *Staphylococcus aureus* (MRSA) on local community rates, comorbidity, indwelling catheters, and healthcare exposure.
- The **mortality rate** associated with septic arthritis is about 10%, and as high as perhaps 50% in polyarticular disease.

Medications

Non-gonococcal Arthritis

- If MRSA coverage is not required, coverage for gram-positive organisms with anti-staphylococcal penicillin such as **oxacillin or nafcillin** is adequate.
- For MRSA coverage, empiric therapy with **vancomycin** (30 mg/kg daily IV in two divided doses) is sufficient. Dosage should be based on weight, renal function, and subsequent drug levels to ensure therapeutic dosage.
- Third-generation cephalosporins, such as **ceftriaxone** (2 g IV q24h), **ceftazidime** (1–2 g IV q8h), or **cefotaxime** (2 g IV q8h), should be started for empiric coverage for gram-negative organisms.
- If *Pseudomonas aeruginosa* is considered to be a possible pathogen, **cefepime** (1 g IV q8h) or ceftazidime with an aminoglycoside such as gentamicin (3–5 mg/kg daily in two to three divided doses) should be initiated.
- When available, culture results and antimicrobial sensitivities should guide treatment.
- Atypical or resistant organisms may require consultation from infectious diseases to tailor antimicrobial therapy.
- Most cases of infectious arthritis require **2 to 4 weeks of intravenous antibiotics.** Once a pathogen has been established as causative, this course can often be completed as an outpatient.

Gonococcal Arthritis

- If gonococcal arthritis is suspected, empiric therapy for disseminated gonococci infection should be initiated.
- **Ceftriaxone** 1 g IV q24h should be continued for 24 to 48 hours after clinical improvement. This can then be switched to oral cefixime 400 mg PO q12h, ciprofloxacin 500 mg PO q12h, or ofloxacin 400 mg PO q12h for 1 week.

Non-bacterial arthritis

- Arthralgias and non-bacterial infectious arthritis are common with many viral infections.
- Viral arthritis tends to present with symmetric polyarthralgias or polyarthritis and may be accompanied by a typical viral exanthem.
- Supportive treatment with rest and nonsteroidal antiinflammatory drugs (**NSAIDs**) is usually effective and sufficient.

Surgical Management

- Surgical or arthroscopic drainage is often necessary in cases of septic hip joints, septic arthritis with concurrent osteomyelitis, septic arthritis in a prosthetic joint, persistent infections, complex anatomy, or loculated effusions.

- Most joints can be adequately drained by arthrocentesis or closed needle aspiration. Daily aspiration is generally necessary, as certain joints (e.g., the knee) may accumulate fluid for up to ten days. Serial cell counts and cultures document response to antibiotic therapy.
- Open drainage, arthroscopy, and joint replacement are options for severe and refractory cases.
- Patients with suspected infections involving prosthetic joints warrant prompt orthopedic surgery consultation.

REFERRAL

Complicated joint infections often require a multidisciplinary approach, most often involving orthopedic surgery, infectious diseases, physical therapy, and occupational therapy.

MONITORING/FOLLOW-UP

- Patients should be followed closely with frequent joint examinations for the first few weeks of treatment with antibiotics.
- Repeated arthrocentesis should confirm sterilization of synovial fluid and decreasing WBC count.
- Failure to improve may warrant alteration in antibiotic regimen or surgical consultation.
- Early rehabilitation should include physical therapy with joint mobilization to prevent loss of joint range of motion.
- Patients should be monitored for side effects from antimicrobials with complete blood counts (CBC), comprehensive metabolic panels (CMP), and drug levels, as appropriate.
- ESR and CRP are helpful to follow serially to confirm that inflammation is resolving.

REFERENCES

1. Matthews CJ, Weston VC, Jones A, et al. Bacterial septic arthritis in adults. *Lancet.* 2010; 375:846.
2. Armstrong RW, Bolding F, Joseph R. Septic arthritis following arthroscopy: Clinical syndromes and analysis of risk factors. *Arthroscopy.* 1992;8:213–223.
3. Margaretten ME, Kohlwes J, Moore D, et al. Does this adult patient have septic arthritis? *JAMA.* 2007;297:1478–1488.

Lyme Disease

33

Rebecca Brinker and Prabha Ranganathan

GENERAL PRINCIPLES

- Lyme disease is a multisystem illness caused by the spirochete *Borrelia burgdorferi*. *B. burgdorferi* is the only species found in the United States while all the three species (*B. burgdorferi, B. afzelii,* and *B. garinii*) are found in Europe. Clinical manifestations and severity of disease may vary with the infecting species. Only *B. burgdorferi* manifestations will be addressed in this chapter.
- **Lyme disease is the most common tick borne illness in the United States** and is transmitted by the *Ixodes* tick (blacklegged tick or deer tick).
- It was initially described in 1977 as "Lyme arthritis" after an outbreak of suspected juvenile rheumatoid arthritis, which was in reality Lyme arthritis, in Old Lyme, Connecticut.
- The incidence of Lyme disease in the United States has continued to increase since its identification. This is thought to be secondary to the **increased deer population and consequent increase in *Ixodes* ticks.**
- According to the Centers for Disease Control and Prevention (CDC) there were approximately 30,000 confirmed cases of Lyme disease in the United States in 2009.
- When a case of Lyme disease is identified, it should be reported to the CDC.

Epidemiology

- Lyme disease is transmitted to humans by the *Ixodes* tick. The tick has four developmental stages: egg, larva, nymph, and adult. **Only ticks in nymph and sometimes larva stage transmit Lyme disease to humans.**
- The *Ixodes* tick life cycle:
  - ○ The egg hatches into larva in the spring. The larvae feed on small rodents (e.g., white-footed mouse) and acquire the spirochete infection from these asymptomatic carriers.
  - ○ In the fall the larvae become dormant for the winter, but molt into nymphs the next spring.
  - ○ The small nymphs feed on rodents, rabbits, and humans. When the nymph feeds, the spirochete is incidentally transmitted to the host during periods of extended attachment.
  - ○ By fall the nymph matures into an adult. The adult transmits the spirochete less often because it is larger, less likely to go unnoticed during attachment and not present during peak hiking season.
- Deer are important in the life cycle of the *Ixodes* tick as they act as blood meal for the adults, thus perpetuating the tick's life cycle.

Etiology

- *B. burgdorferi* is a spirochete, a motile corkscrew-shaped bacterium, with an outer and an inner membrane and flagella.
- The tick **must be attached for 48 hours or more** to transmit the spirochete.

Pathophysiology

- The pathophysiology of Lyme disease is not completely understood, but disease manifestations are thought to be from infection with the spirochete itself as well as the host's immune response to the infection.
- A few pertinent observations include[1]:
  - Patients with HLA-DR4 and HLA-DR2 are more likely to develop chronic arthritis that may be erosive.
  - Spirochetes have been isolated from all affected tissues, except the peripheral nerves.
  - Optimum control of the infection requires an intact innate and adaptive immune response.
  - *B. burgdorferi* does not produce toxins or destructive proteases to harm the host.

Risk Factors

- There is a bimodal incidence of infection, ages 5 to 9 and 55 to 59.
- Greater than 50% of cases occur in males.
- Residence in the upper Midwest of the United States and entry into heavily forested areas.
- The location of tick bite on the body is important. Less visualized areas allow for longer tick attachment time and therefore increase the possibility of spirochete transmission.
- The most active season for infection is **May to July,** with the highest infection rate in June. Clinical peak of disease manifestations lags 2 to 3 weeks behind inoculation.

Prevention

- Remove ticks promptly.
- Wear insect repellent when in endemic areas.
- Rodent management.

DIAGNOSIS

The diagnosis is clinical, manifestations may vary by stage and laboratory data is only supportive.

Clinical Presentation

History

- Patients may or may not recall a **tick bite** or **erythema migrans** (EM).
- They may complain of constitutional or organ-specific symptoms based on the stage of disease at presentation.
- Constitutional symptoms may include fever, fatigue, myalgias, arthralgias, and headache.

Physical Examination

- EM lesions are usually warm, itchy, and nonpainful. They expand slowly over days to weeks and may reach a diameter of 20 cm or more.
- The lesion **may develop a central clearing,** classically known as the "bull's-eye" lesion. This is usually only seen in large lesions that have been present for days.
- Lesions are typically found in the intertriginous areas, popliteal fossa, and belt line.
- In one study of 118 microbiologically confirmed cases, EM lesions appeared in these patterns[2]:
  - Homogenous erythema (59%)
  - Central erythema (32%)
  - Central clearing (9%)
  - Vesicular or ulcerated (7%)
  - Central purpura (2%)

Stage I, Early Localized Disease

- Characterized by the appearance of EM.
  - This rash is an expanding annular red macule or papule at the site of the tick bite and is a sign of spirochetemia.
  - This rash occurs within 3 days to one month after infection and resolves within 3 to 4 weeks.
  - **The rash occurs in 60% to 80% of patients,** but may go unnoticed secondary to its location.
- Patients may report malaise, headache, fever, neck stiffness, arthralgias, myalgias, localized lymphadenopathy, and fatigue.

Stage II, Early Disseminated Disease

- **Multiple EM lesions** (in locations other than the primary bite) result from hematogenous spread of the spirochete. These lesions are seen days to weeks after the primary infection.
- **Systemic symptoms** of fever, malaise, headache, arthralgias, and myalgias become more severe. These symptoms may be constant or intermittent.
- **Cardiac involvement** occurs weeks to months after primary infection and may be the sole manifestation of disseminated disease.
  - Cardiac disease is rare in patients infected with *B. burgdorferi* but occurs more commonly with other species of *Borrelia.*
  - Symptoms include palpitations, lightheadedness, syncope, chest pain, and shortness of breath.
  - Most common manifestations are **varying degrees of heart block.**
  - **Myocarditis and pericarditis** are less common, often self-limited and frequently clinically silent. Myocarditis may result in transient cardiomegaly and pericarditis is associated with mild pericardial effusions.
  - No confirmed cases of valvular damage or chronic cardiomyopathy secondary to Lyme disease have occurred in the United States.
- **Neurologic involvement** occurs weeks to months after primary infection and may affect up to 20% of untreated patients.
  - The most common manifestation is cranial neuropathy, especially unilateral or bilateral **Bell's palsy.**
  - **Meningoencephalitis** may also occur.
- **Articular involvement** occurs 6 or more months after infection and affects about 60% of untreated patients.

- Arthritis is oligoarticular with lower extremity predominance, particularly the knee, and is associated with large inflammatory effusions.
- Few patients have persistent arthritis even after antibiotic treatment and are classified as having antibiotic-refractory Lyme arthritis.

Stage III, Late Lyme Disease

- Occurs months to years after the primary infection and does not have to be preceded by manifestations of stage I or II disease.
- The most common manifestation is episodic, lower extremity predominant oligoarthritis.
- Chronic neurologic sequelae such as radiculopathy, axonal polyneuropathy, or encephalomyelitis may rarely occur.

Differential Diagnosis

- Cellulitis
- Meningitis
- Dementia
- Multiple sclerosis
- Amyotrophic lateral sclerosis
- Radiculopathy
- Depression
- Ehrlichiosis
- Babesiosis
- Rocky mountain spotted fever
- Reactive arthritis
- Rheumatoid arthritis
- Fibromyalgia

Diagnostic Testing

Laboratory

- Confirmatory laboratory testing is not necessary for diagnosis, especially if the patient has an EM rash. A seropositive test alone is not adequate to establish the diagnosis.
- The spirochete is difficult to culture as it grows under microaerophilic or anaerobic conditions. The highest yield for culture is a skin biopsy from the border of the primary EM rash in an untreated patient. Spirochetes may be found in blood and cerebrospinal fluid (CSF) and very rarely in the synovial fluid. Cultures may take up to 12 weeks to reveal the spirochete.
- The CDC recommends two-step serum testing.
  - Enzyme-linked immunosorbent assay (ELISA) or immunofluorescence assay (IFA) as the screening test is designed to be very sensitive. If positive or equivocal, the same serum should be evaluated with Western blot. If the ELISA or IFA is negative, it is highly unlikely the patient has Lyme disease or the testing has occurred too early after primary infection (less than 6 weeks).
  - Western blot is a more specific test and only run if the ELISA or IFA is positive.[3] If the IgM antibody is positive, the patient should be retested in 4 to 6 weeks as they may have early infection. If IgG antibody is positive, the patient is considered to have infection.
    - IgM antibodies usually appear 1 to 2 weeks after infection.
    - IgG antibodies usually appear 2 to 6 weeks after infection.

- ○ **After successful treatment, antibody levels may remain positive but titers should fall over time.** Titer level and rate of resolution do not correlate with disease severity, chronicity, or treatment.
  - ○ **Seropositivity occurs in less than 40% of patients with early skin disease** but more often in patients with early disseminated extracutaneous disease. Patients with late Lyme disease are almost always IgG positive.
- • A lumbar puncture is recommended in patients with neurologic manifestations in an effort to rule out other causes and potentially support the diagnosis.
  - ○ IgG and IgM antibodies in the CSF help confirm the diagnosis, but are not mandatory.
  - ○ Polymerase chain reaction (PCR) testing of CSF has low sensitivity.
- • Synovial fluid is inflammatory with an average white blood cell (WBC) count of about 25,000/mm³ and polymorphonuclear leukocytes predominate.
- • Mild elevations in transaminases have been observed.
- • Although offered by some health departments, testing of ticks removed from a patient is not recommended as presence of the spirochete does not guarantee human infection.

Electrocardiography
- • Electrocardiographic abnormalities are only seen in disseminated infection.
- • Sustained or intermittent first-, second-, or third-degree **heart block** occurs depending on the location of conduction system dysfunction.
- • Variable bundle branch blocks may also be seen.
- • Pericarditis can manifest as diffuse ST and T wave elevations.

Imaging
- • MRI of the brain may be helpful to rule out other pathology. There are no specific MRI findings in Lyme disease.
- • Transthoracic echocardiogram is used to evaluate for the presence of myocarditis and pericarditis.

Diagnostic Procedures
- • Diagnostic procedures are generally not necessary and often not recommended. If performed, it is frequently in an effort to rule out other diagnoses. Such procedures may include:
  - ○ Skin biopsy
  - ○ Myocardial biopsy
  - ○ Lumbar puncture
  - ○ Electromyography and nerve conduction studies

TREATMENT

Medications

Early Lyme Disease
- • Early Lyme disease manifested as only EM may be treated with **doxycycline, amoxicillin, or cefuroxime,** all of which have equivalent effectiveness.
- • Dosing guidelines in adults are as follows[4,5]:
  - ○ Doxycycline 100 mg PO bid for 10 to 21 days.
  - ○ Amoxicillin 500 mg PO tid for 14 to 21 days.
  - ○ Cefuroxime axetil 500 mg PO bid for 14 to 21 days.
  - ○ Macrolides are not recommended.

- **Doxycycline is generally preferred** because it has better central nervous system (CNS) penetration.
- Doxycycline also covers the possibility of coincident *Anaplasma phagocytophilum* infection which is also transmitted by the *Ixodes* tick.

Early Disseminated Lyme Disease

- **IV antibiotics are recommended if there is CNS involvement** (except isolated facial palsy).[4,5]
  - IV ceftriaxone, cefotaxime, or penicillin may be used. Duration of therapy is usually between 10 and 28 days.
  - Isolate Lyme disease with facial palsy can be treated with a 14 to 21 day course of oral doxycycline.
  - Recovery of neurologic symptoms may lag behind clearance of the spirochete and therefore cannot be used to guide length of therapy.
- **For cardiac involvement, IV ceftriaxone, cefotaxime, or penicillin** is given until resolution of heart block. After cardiac recovery, the patient may be switched to oral therapy to complete a total 21-day course of antibiotics.[4,5]

Late Lyme Disease

- This is mainly manifested by arthritis and often treated successfully with one month of oral doxycycline, amoxicillin, or cefuroxime axetil.[4,5]
- If this fails, another 4-week oral course or 2 to 4 weeks of IV antibiotics may be given.[4,5]
- The existence of chronic symptomatic *B. burgdorferi* infection after appropriate antibiotic treatment is rather controversial. The Infectious Disease Society of America does not recommend extended antibiotic treatment for patient with ≥6 months of subjective symptoms.[4–6]

Lifestyle/Risk Modification

- Monitor for tick bites.
- Use insect repellent when in endemic areas.

SPECIAL CONSIDERATIONS

- Must rule out other diseases in differential diagnosis as seropositivity is not adequate for diagnosis.
- Pregnant women should not be treated with tetracyclines. Nor should doxycycline be given to young (<8 years old) children.

COMPLICATIONS

- Complications depend on the stage of infection and may include:
  - Acute or chronic arthritis.
  - Cardiomyopathy, arrhythmia, pericarditis.
  - Neuropathy, radiculopathy, encephalopathy.
  - Cognitive dysfunction, dementia.
  - Conjunctivitis.

PATIENT EDUCATION

- Tick Management Handbook from the CDC.
- CDC website: www.cdc.gov/lyme (last access 2/5/12).

MONITORING/FOLLOW-UP

- If seropositive at diagnosis, **repeat testing is not recommended** as titers do not reflect efficacy of treatment.
- The best evaluation of improvement is to monitor the patient's symptoms and resolution of organ dysfunction.

OUTCOME/PROGNOSIS

- Children and patients treated at earlier stages of infection have a better acute and long-term prognosis.
- Infection is rarely fatal.
- Arthritis may take months to resolve or be chronic.
- Cardiac damage and dysfunction is rarely long term.
- Cranial palsies usually resolve after treatment.
- Myocarditis and pericarditis usually resolve after treatment.

REFERENCES

1. Ilipoulou BP, Huber BT. Infectious arthritis and immune dysregulation: lessons from Lyme disease. *Curr Opin Rheumatol.* 2010;22:451–455.
2. Smith RP, Schoen RT, Rahn DW, et al. Clinical characteristics and treatment outcome of early Lyme disease in patients with microbiologically confirmed erythema migrans. *Ann Intern Med.* 2002;136:421–428.
3. Murray TS, Shapiro ED. Lyme disease. *Clin Lab Med.* 2010;30:311–328.
4. Wormser GP, Dattwyler RJ, Shapiro ED, et al. The clinical assessment, treatment, and prevention of Lyme disease, human granulocytic anaplasmosis, and babesiosis: clinical practice guidelines by the Infectious Diseases Society of America. *Clin Infect Dis.* 2006;43: 1089–1134.
5. Lantos PM, Charini WA, Medoff G, et al. Final report of the Lyme disease review panel of the Infectious Diseases Society of America. *Clin Infect Dis.* 2010;51:1–5.
6. Klempner MS, Hu LT, Schmid CH, et al. Two controlled trials of antibiotic treatment in patients with persistent symptoms and a history of Lyme disease. *N Engl J Med.* 2001;345: 85–92.

Acute Rheumatic Fever

34

Jeffrey Sparks and Prabha Ranganathan

GENERAL PRINCIPLES

- Acute rheumatic fever is characterized by arthritis, carditis, chorea, erythema marginatum, and subcutaneous nodules occurring after a group A streptococcal pharyngeal infection.
- Early treatment and long-term prophylaxis with antibiotics are important measures to prevent long-term sequelae such as valvular heart disease.

Definition

- Acute rheumatic fever (ARF) is a **delayed reaction to a group A β-hemolytic streptococcal pharyngeal infection**, occurring 2 to 3 weeks after the initial infection.
- Diagnosis is based on the revised Jones criteria (see Table 34-1).[1]

Epidemiology

- ARF occurs almost **exclusively in children and adolescents.**
- ARF was associated with significant morbidity and mortality until the late 1800s. There was a dramatic decline in cases after this period which has been attributed to changes in living conditions and bacterial virulence.
- The introduction of antibiotics in the twentieth century significantly reduced the incidence of ARF. By 1962, the incidence had declined to 100/100,000 in many European countries.
- ARF presently continues unabated in developing countries and there are nearly 400,000 new cases each year. The estimated prevalence rate of rheumatic heart disease is over 15 million, which, depending on the screening method, may be an underestimate.[2–4]
- The incidence of disease in the United States ranges from 0.5 to 1.88 per 100,000 children. Some areas of the United States have experienced an unexplained recent increase in disease incidence.[5]

Pathophysiology

- The pathogenesis of ARF is not clearly understood. Group A streptococcal pharyngeal infection, either clinical or subclinical, is necessary for the development of ARF.
- Cellulitis, impetigo, and glomerulonephritis, also caused by group A streptococci, do not cause ARF.
- Some studies suggest that only a few M serotypes of group A streptococcus cause ARF, which are referred to as **rheumatogenic strains.**
- **Genetic susceptibility** and **molecular mimicry**, involving the cross-reaction between group A streptococcal antigens and host antigens, likely play a role in the pathogenesis of ARF.

TABLE 34-1	REVISED JONES CRITERIA FOR DIAGNOSIS OF ACUTE RHEUMATIC FEVER

A high probability of acute rheumatic fever is indicated by the presence of two major criteria or one major plus two minor criteria, if accompanied by evidence of a preceding group A streptococcal infection.[a]

Major Manifestations	Minor Manifestations
Carditis	Arthralgias
Polyarthritis	Fever (usually at least 39°C)
Chorea	Elevated CRP or ESR
Erythema marginatum	Prolonged PR interval on ECG[b]
Subcutaneous nodules	

[a]Positive throat culture or rapid streptococcal antigen test, elevated or rising streptococcal antibody titer (e.g., anti-streptolysin O, anti-DNase B).

[b]Because PR prolongation is nonspecific and common, alone it is an insufficient criterion for carditis.

CRP, C-reactive protein; ESR, erythrocyte sedimentation rate.

Adapted from: Gerber MA, Baltimore RS, Eaton CB, et al. Prevention of rheumatic fever and diagnosis and treatment of acute Streptococcal pharyngitis: A scientific statement from the American Heart Association Rheumatic Fever, Endocarditis, and Kawasaki Disease Committee of the Council on Cardiovascular Disease in the Young, the Interdisciplinary Council on Functional Genomics and Translational Biology, and the Interdisciplinary Council on Quality of Care and Outcomes Research: Endorsed by the American Academy of Pediatrics. *Circulation.* 2009;119:1541–1551.

Prevention

- Primary prevention of ARF consists of recognition of acute group A streptococcal pharyngitis and appropriate antibiotic treatment.
- **Penicillin remains the treatment of choice.**[6,7]
  - ○ Penicillin V 500 mg bid to tid PO for 10 days. For children under 60 pounds, the dose is 250 mg.
  - ○ Benzathine penicillin G 1.2 million units IM once. For children under 60 pounds, the dose is 600,000 units.
- For penicillin allergic patients, appropriate oral alternatives are clindamycin, azithromycin, and clarithromycin.[6,7]

DIAGNOSIS

Clinical Presentation

- ARF is characterized by a constellation of symptoms that arises **2 to 4 weeks after pharyngeal infection.**
- The classic manifestations include **arthritis, carditis, neurologic involvement, and rash.**

- **Arthritis** is usually the first symptom of ARF.
  - It is a **migratory polyarthritis of the larger joints,** (e.g., knees, elbows, ankles, and wrists) and usually starts on the lower extremity. Typically, 6 to 16 joints are affected.
  - The involved joints become tender without evidence of inflammation.
  - Joints may only be involved for a week before other joints become affected and the initial joint involvement subsides.
  - The synovial fluid is generally inflammatory but sterile.
- **Carditis** is an important manifestation of ARF, as it often results in long-term damage.
  - ARF can involve any area of the heart, including pericardium, epicardium, myocardium, endocardium, and valvular structures.
  - **There may be no symptoms despite cardiac involvement** or patients may experience chest discomfort and dyspnea.
  - Physical examination may elicit a **new murmur.**
  - **Mitral valvulitis** associated with ARF classically causes mitral stenosis, and a low-pitched early diastolic murmur at the apex (Carey Coombs murmur). Chronic mitral valve destruction can progress to mitral regurgitation, with a holosystolic apical murmur.
  - **Aortic valvulitis** leads to aortic stenosis, with a high-pitched decrescendo murmur along the left sternal border, heard best with the patient leaning forward. Chronic aortic valve destruction can lead to aortic insufficiency, with a late decrescendo systolic murmur and early diastolic murmur at the right upper sternal border.
  - On examination, one may also find evidence of **pericarditis, heart failure, or cardiomyopathy.**
- The best known neurologic manifestation of ARF is known as **Sydenham's chorea,** also called chorea minor and the St. Vitus dance.
  - Chorea is characterized by nonrhythmic involuntary abrupt movements and muscle weakness. Usually the movements are more distinct on one side. Muscle weakness is rhythmic, with the strength increasing and decreasing on exertion.
  - Frequently, emotional instability (e.g., crying, agitation, and inappropriate behavior) accompanies the chorea.
- **Skin manifestations** of ARF include erythema marginatum and subcutaneous nodules.
  - **Erythema marginatum** is a faint, pink, nonpruritic rash that erupts across the trunk, upper arms, and legs; facial involvement does not occur.
    - The lesion begins with a central area of normal skin and extends outward to a distinct border.
    - The rash is transient, coming and going within hours and worsened by hot conditions (e.g., baths and showers).
    - The rash usually occurs at the onset of disease, but it may recur at any time, including convalescence.
  - **Subcutaneous nodule**s are firm, nontender nodules under non-inflamed skin that occur on bony prominences and near tendons.
    - They may be solitary or occur in groups. They are symmetric, typically occur on the extensor surfaces, and usually resolve within 4 weeks.
    - The subcutaneous nodules of ARF differ from those of RA in that they are smaller, more transient, are typically found on the olecranon and sometimes on the back.[8]

- ○ Both erythema marginatum and subcutaneous nodules usually occur only in the presence of carditis.
- Other symptoms may include abdominal pain, persistent tachycardia, malaise, anemia, epistaxis, and chest pain.[1]

Diagnostic Criteria

- The diagnosis of ARF is clinical and based on the revised Jones criteria (Table 34-1).[1]
- A diagnosis can be made in the setting of recent streptococcal pharyngeal infection if:
  - ○ Two major criteria are present.
  - ○ One major and two minor criteria are present.
- **Exceptions** to the Jones criteria:
  - ○ Sydenham's chorea may be delayed and, therefore, it can be difficult to demonstrate evidence of a preceding group A streptococcal infection.
  - ○ Indolent carditis.
  - ○ Prior history of ARF.

Differential Diagnosis

The differential diagnosis of ARF includes bacterial infections (e.g., septic arthritis, osteomyelitis, and bacterial endocarditis), viral infections (e.g., infectious mononucleosis and Coxsackie virus), rheumatoid arthritis, systemic lupus erythematosus, and malignancies (e.g., lymphoma and leukemia).

Diagnostic Testing

Laboratories

- Evidence of recent streptococcal infection
  - ○ **Increased titers of streptococcal antibodies in serum** (e.g., antistreptolysin O, DNase B, hyaluronidase, or streptokinase).
  - ○ **Positive throat culture** for Group A beta-hemolytic streptococci.
- Markers of inflammation, including white blood cell (WBC) count, C-reactive protein (CRP) and erythrocyte sedimentation rate (ESR), may be elevated.

Electrocardiography

- ECG classically shows prolonged PR interval in acute rheumatic fever but this is a nonspecific finding.
- Other nonspecific ECG changes include T wave flattening, ST segment and repolarization abnormalities, and P wave abnormalities.

Imaging

Echocardiography is useful to characterize possible cardiac involvement, including valvulopathy and cardiomyopathy.

TREATMENT

Treatment of ARF should include **symptom relief, antibiotic treatment, and prophylaxis.**

Medications

- **Nonsteroidal antiinflammatory drugs (NSAIDs), especially aspirin,** are useful for symptomatic relief.
  - ○ Aspirin 4 to 8 g/day for adults.
  - ○ NSAIDs can be continued until patient is asymptomatic and markers of inflammation normalize.
- Treatment of chorea includes the use of antiepileptic drugs such as phenobarbital, phenytoin, and diazepam.
- **Penicillin** is the treatment of choice for ARF, either IM or PO.[6]
  - ○ Benzathine penicillin G 1.2 million units IM once. For children under 60 pounds the dose is 600,000 units.
  - ○ Penicillin V 500 mg PO bid to tid for 10 days. For children under 60 pounds the dose is 250 mg.
  - ○ If a penicillin allergy is present, azithromycin or clindamycin can be used.
  - ○ **Family members and close contacts** should have throat culture and treatment if the culture is positive for beta-hemolytic streptococci.

Prophylaxis

- Prophylaxis for **recurrent ARF** (secondary prevention) is important as symptoms can return, most commonly within 2 years.
  - ○ Penicillin or erythromycin should be begun immediately after the initial 10-day antibiotic treatment course: Penicillin V 250 mg PO bid or erythromycin 250 mg PO bid if a penicillin allergy is present.[6]
  - ○ Benzathine penicillin G 1.2 million units IM every 4 weeks is preferred prophylaxis for high risk individuals.[6]
  - ○ Duration of prophylaxis is controversial, but a 5- to 10-year course is usually recommended.[6]

COMPLICATIONS

Cardiac involvement with valvular damage is the most common and serious long-term sequela of ARF.

MONITORING/FOLLOW-UP

- Cardiac involvement is the most serious sequela of ARF. **Patients may develop significant valvular abnormalities and heart failure even decades after the initial event.**
- ARF requires long-term prophylaxis and sometimes monthly antibiotic injections for years.
- After the planned course for secondary prophylaxis, the risk for group A streptococcal re-exposure and valvular disease should be assessed.

REFERENCES

1. Guidelines for the diagnosis of rheumatic fever. Jones Criteria, 1992 update. Special Writing Group of the Committee on Rheumatic Fever, Endocarditis, and Kawasaki Disease of the Council on Cardiovascular Disease in the Young of the American Heart Association. *JAMA.* 1992;268:2069–2073.

2. Carapetis JR. Rheumatic heart disease in developing countries. *N Engl J Med.* 2007;357:439–441.
3. Carapetis JR, Steer AC, Mulholland EK, et al. The global burden of group A streptococcal diseases. *Lancet Infect Dis.* 2005;5:685–694.
4. Marijon E, Ou P, Celermajer DS, et al. Prevalence of rheumatic heart disease detected by echocardiographic screening. *N Engl J Med.* 2007;357:470–476.
5. Bisno AL, Shulman ST, Dajani AS. The rise and fall (and rise?) of rheumatic fever. *JAMA.* 1988;259:728–729.
6. Gerber MA, Baltimore RS, Eaton CB, et al. Prevention of rheumatic fever and diagnosis and treatment of acute Streptococcal pharyngitis: A scientific statement from the American Heart Association Rheumatic Fever, Endocarditis, and Kawasaki Disease Committee of the Council on Cardiovascular Disease in the Young, the Interdisciplinary Council on Functional Genomics and Translational Biology, and the Interdisciplinary Council on Quality of Care and Outcomes Research: Endorsed by the American Academy of Pediatrics. *Circulation.* 2009;119:1541–1551.
7. Bisno AL. Acute pharyngitis. *N Engl J Med.* 2001;344:205–211.
8. Evangelisto A, Werth V, Schmacher HR. What is that nodule? A diagnostic approach to evaluating subcutaneous and cutaneous nodules. *J Clin Rheumatol.* 2006;12:230–240.

Inflammatory Myopathies

Hyon Ju Park and Prabha Ranganathan

GENERAL PRINCIPLES

The inflammatory myopathies (IM) are a heterogeneous group of disorders characterized by **muscle weakness** and inflammation of skeletal muscles **(myositis)**.

Classification

- The three major distinct IM are **polymyositis** (PM), **dermatomyositis** (DM), and **inclusion body myositis** (IBM).
- Other IM include juvenile DM, malignancy-associated myositis, eosinophilic myositis, granulomatous myositis, and myositis in overlap with other connective tissue diseases (Table 35-1) but this chapter will focus on the three major distinct types mentioned above.[1]

Epidemiology

- IM are rare, systemic, connective tissues diseases with an estimated incidence of 1 in 100,000.
- PM and DM have a bimodal distribution of prevalence: one in childhood (ages 5–15) and the other in midlife (ages 30–50). IBM peaks after the age of 50.
- Females are affected more often (3:1) in DM and PM. IBM affects more men than women (3:1).
- African Americans are at increased risk for IM and when they have the disease, tend to have poorer outcomes.

Etiology

- Etiology is unknown but is likely a result of environmental influences that trigger chronic immune activation in genetically susceptible individuals.
  - Genetic factors: Several alleles in the MHC locus have been identified to confer a genetic risk for IM while others have been found to be protective. The DRB1*0301-DQA1*0501 haplotype confers the strongest risk while HLA DQA1*0201 seems protective for all forms of IM.[2]
  - Autoimmunity: About 50% of patients have myositis-specific, while another 25% have myositis-associated antibodies.
  - Environmental influences: Infections with group A streptococcus and influenza have the strongest evidence of association with onset of IM. Reports of temporal, seasonal, and even geographic clustering of cases also suggest strong environmental influences.

TABLE 35-1	MYOSITIS-ASSOCIATED AUTOANTIBODIES	
Autoantibody	Antigenic Target	Clinical Features
PM-Scl	Exosome proteins	Overlap with limited SSc Mild myositis
U1 RNP	U1 small nuclear ribonucleoprotein	MCTD overlap
Ku	DNA binding complex	PM-SSc overlap
Ro/SSA	Ro60 and Ro52	Sjögren's overlap

MCTD, mixed connective tissue disease; PM, polymyositis; SSc, systemic sclerosis.
Adapted from: Oddis CV. Idiopathic inflammatory myopathies: Treatment and assessment. In: Klippel JH, Stone JH, Crofford LJ, eds. Primer on the Rheumatic Diseases. 13th ed. New York, NY: Springer Science and Business Media, 2008:378.

Pathophysiology

- The IM are idiopathic but are believed to be immune mediated.
- Each subgroup of myositis has unique pathologic features (described below) but as a group, they demonstrate inflammation of endomysium, perimysium, and perivascular areas with infiltration of lymphocytes, plasma cells, dendritic cells, and macrophages.
- Furthermore, although it is unclear whether they are pathogenic, **myositis-specific autoantibodies** define groups of patients with similar clinical features and prognosis (Table 35-2).

TABLE 35-2	MYOSITIS-SPECIFIC AUTOANTIBODIES	
Autoantibody	Clinical Features	Treatment Response
Antisynthetase (anti-Jo-1 is the most common)	Relatively acute onset of polymyositis or dermatomyositis Interstitial lung disease Fever Arthritis Mechanic's hands	Moderate
Anti-SRP	Polymyositis with very acute onset Severe weakness Palpitations	Poor
Anti-Mi2	Dermatomyositis with typical cutaneous findings	Good

SRP, signal recognition particle.

Associated Conditions

- IM can precede other signs and symptoms of **malignancies** up to 2 years.
- Relative risk for cancer is three- to six-fold in DM and about two-fold in PM and IBM.
  - Types of cancers seen are similar to normal populations except for an increased incidence of ovarian cancer.
  - Asian patients with DM have a several-fold increased risk of nasopharyngeal carcinoma.
- Workup of myositis has to include **age- and risk-appropriate cancer screenings.** When patients with IM do not respond to therapies, more invasive testing such as endoscopy to look for occult malignancies like gastric or pancreatic carcinomas should be considered.

DIAGNOSIS

- The diagnosis of IM is based on history, physical examination, and selected tests. Clinical presentation, muscle biopsy results, and serologies differ amongst the three subgroups and will be discussed below.
- Note that **extramuscular manifestations** of IM can present at any time.

Polymyositis

- **History:** Patients develop insidious but progressive, typically painless symmetric muscle weakness involving the shoulder and pelvic girdle muscles. Usual presentation is about 3 to 6 months after the first onset of symptoms. Fatigue and anorexia can accompany weakness. Dyspnea is the most common complaint after weakness. Dysphagia can occur as a result of weakness of oropharyngeal skeletal muscles.
- **Examination:** This is notable most for patients having difficulty getting up from a chair. Reflexes are normal except in muscles with significant atrophy. Sensation to gross touch, pinprick, and temperatures along with proprioception remain intact. Dyspnea can be due to muscle weakness (rare) of diaphragmatic and intercostal muscles which would be evidenced by a decreased peak inspiratory flow. Fine crackles on lung examination indicate interstitial lung disease (ILD), which develops in 10% of patients. Some patients develop cardiac arrhythmias as well.
- **Muscle biopsy:** Characteristic changes include degeneration and regeneration of muscle fibers and CD8+ T lymphocytes in the endomysial region with rare B cells.
- **Diagnostic criteria:** Table 35-3 demonstrates the original criteria for PM and DM.[3]
  - Multiple diseases must be excluded for these criteria to be applied, including neuropathies, muscular dystrophies, infections, drugs and toxins, rhabdomyolysis, metabolic myopathies, and endocrinopathies.
  - However, these criteria do not account for more recent developments in serologies and MRI findings. No new criteria have been developed but it is important to keep in mind that MRIs demonstrating symmetric focal muscle inflammation and the presence of myositis-specific antibodies can aid in the diagnosis of IM.

TABLE 35-3	BOHAN AND PETER'S CRITERIA FOR THE DIAGNOSIS OF POLYMYOSITIS AND DERMATOMYOSITIS

Definite polymyositis requires four criteria (without rash).
Definite dermatomyositis requires three criteria (any three plus rash).

1. Symmetric proximal weakness.
2. Elevation of muscle enzymes (2- to 100-fold increase).
3. Electromyography: Short, small, polyphasic motor unit potentials; fibrillations, positive sharp waves, insertional irritability; bizarre high-frequency repetitive discharges.
4. Muscle biopsy: Degeneration, regeneration, necrosis, atrophy, inflammatory infiltrates.
5. Typical skin findings of dermatomyositis.

———

Adapted from: Bohan A, Peter JB. Polymyositis and dermatomyositis. *N Engl J Med.* 1975; 292:344–347,403–407.

Dermatomyositis

- Clinical manifestations of DM can be thought of as PM with cutaneous manifestations. Rashes often precede muscle weakness. The most common cutaneous findings are listed.
  - **Gottron's papules:** Lilac papules found on the dorsal aspect of metacarpophalangeals (MCPs), proximal interphalangeals (PIPs), elbows, or knees.
  - **Heliotrope rash:** Purplish discoloration of the upper eyelids, often associated with periorbital edema.
  - **Shawl sign:** Erythematous rash seen on the upper chest (in the shape of a V) and back and shoulders which may worsen with UV light exposure.
  - **Mechanic's hands:** Periungual telangiectasias, irregular and thickened cuticles, and darkened horizontal lines across the lateral and palmar aspects of fingers and hands.
  - **Subcutaneous calcifications** are often seen and their persistent development generally indicates that DM is not sufficiently controlled.
- **Diagnostic criteria:** Presented in Table 35-3.[3]
- Patients with classic cutaneous findings of DM but no clinical evidence of muscle disease are said to have **amyopathic DM.**
- **Muscle biopsy:** Characteristic findings include CD4+ and CD8+ T lymphocytes along with macrophages and B cells invading predominantly perimysial and perivascular regions in the setting of perifascicular atrophy.

Inclusion Body Myositis

- IBM is the most common myositis found in elderly people.
- **History:** Onset of weakness is even more insidious and evolves over anywhere from 1 to 10 years prior to diagnosis. Distribution of weakness is more asymmetric and can involve distal muscles. Unlike PM and DM, IBM can cause neuropathic symptoms as well.
- **Examination:** Decreased grip strength or asymmetric foot drops along with asymmetric proximal muscle weakness are the most common findings. Cutaneous manifestations are not seen. IBM is typically not associated with ILD.

- **Muscle biopsy:** Characteristic findings include the presence of lined or rimmed vacuoles and triangulated cells with fiber-type grouping. Note that the presence of vacuoles on muscle biopsy does not mean that the patient has IBM as similar vacuoles are seen in muscular dystrophies and drug-induced myopathies.

Differential Diagnosis

- **Neuropathies:** One of the first steps in diagnosing IM is to evaluate for a neuropathy being the cause of the weakness. Electromyography (EMG) and muscle biopsies are the most useful in helping to differentiate between a neuropathy and a myopathy.
- **Muscular dystrophies:**
  - **Limb-girdle muscular dystrophies** (LGMD) include a number of disorders with muscular dystrophy in a pelvic and shoulder girdle distribution.
  - Unfortunately the age at presentation is highly variable and patients can present even late in adult life.
  - Even in mild cases, however, there is a preferential weakness and atrophy of the biceps muscle.
  - Creatine kinase (CK) levels can be dramatically elevated and cannot be used to differentiate between dystrophies and IM.
  - MRIs are highly useful as active IM shows edema on short tau inversion recovery (STIR) imaging indicative of inflammation but LGMD shows extensive fatty replacement.
  - Muscle biopsies do not demonstrate significant inflammation but degeneration and regeneration of muscles.
  - Diagnosis is performed by genetic testing, serum protein testing, and if negative, immunohistochemical testing of muscle biopsy.
- **Metabolic myopathies:**
  - These **rare diseases of muscle energy metabolism** may present with muscle weakness, elevated CK, and myopathic changes on EMG.
  - Patients with glycogen metabolism abnormalities or with myoadenylate deaminase deficiency (the most common metabolic myopathy) have exercise intolerance and may be asymptomatic at rest.
  - The forearm ischemic exercise test is a standardized test that involves checking ammonia and lactate levels before and after vigorous forearm exercise with a blood pressure cuff inflated above systolic pressure; it is a useful screening test.
  - Metabolic myopathies should be suspected in patients who are young, have a family history of myopathy, or fail to respond to therapy.
- **Mitochondrial myopathies:**
  - Mitochondrial disorders can present with isolated proximal muscle weakness but symptoms tend to be mild or exercise-related.
  - Checking lactate levels before and after vigorous exercise could be helpful in the diagnosis.
  - The classic hallmark of mitochondrial disease is subsarcolemmal and intermyofibrillar accumulations visualized on Gomori trichrome staining due to compensatory proliferation of mitochondria, also known as "ragged red fibers."
  - Staining for various enzymes associated with mitochondria to look for proliferation is also helpful but requires a specialized lab.

- **Drug- or toxin-induced myopathies:**
  - Procainamide and penicillamine can cause an immune-mediated myopathy.
  - Statins and other lipid-lowering agents may cause mitochondrial dysfunction.
  - Chronic ethanol use is associated with painless proximal muscle weakness and atrophy with normal CK.
  - Zidovudine-induced myopathy can have inflammatory infiltrates much like IM but it is reversible over several months if medication is stopped.
- **Endocrine myopathies: Corticosteroid myopathy** is common and usually occurs after months of use; CK level are normal. **Hypothyroid myopathy** can present like PM with progressive symmetric proximal muscle weakness, but can be found simply by checking a serum thyroid stimulating hormone (TSH); CK may be moderately elevated.

Diagnostic Testing

The tests below can aid in the diagnosis of IM but **no one test can confirm the diagnosis.** When patients do not respond to appropriate therapy, the first step should always be a reevaluation of the diagnosis.

Laboratories

- Evaluation of enzymes that leak from injured skeletal muscle: **CK, aldolase, aspartate transaminase (AST), alanine transaminase (ALT), and lactate dehydrogenase (LDH)** are helpful.
  - Isolated normal enzyme levels do not rule out IM.
  - CK has to be elevated at some point in the disease.
  - Unfortunately, an **elevated CK does not necessarily indicate active inflammation** and hence, using this to track disease activity is variable between patients (some do not track at all).
  - Muscle enzymes should be assessed at the time of diagnosis and correlated with patient's symptoms and muscle strength examination to look for a pattern.
  - The level of muscle enzyme elevation at diagnosis can also be helpful as levels less than twice the upper limit of normal or greater than a 100 times the upper limit of normal should make one think of alternative diagnoses.
- Inflammatory markers like erythrocyte sedimentation rate (ESR) and C-reactive protein (CRP) can also be used to track disease if elevated at onset of disease.
- **Myositis-specific antibodies** (Table 35-2) can be checked to aid in diagnosis as they are specific, but note that sensitivity is only about 50%. They may help differentiate subsets of myositis, and define prognosis.
- If there is a suspicion of myositis in association with other connective tissue diseases, based on clinical history and examination, one could send off myositis-associated autoantibodies (Table 35-1) as well.

Electrocardiography

Cardiac involvement is common, usually manifesting as **arrhythmias** and can be detected on ECG but **results are variable and nonspecific.**

Imaging

- **MRI** is becoming more popular as it can help distinguish active inflammation (edema) from previously damaged muscles with chronic changes on STIR images. IM is a patchy disease and can easily be missed on muscle biopsy. **MRI**

has become very useful in guiding biopsy sites and increasing the yield of biopsies.[4]
- **Ultrasound and CT** are much less sensitive in detection of muscular inflammation but are cheaper, more convenient, and more readily available in some areas and have been used to guide biopsy sites as well.
- **High resolution CT of the lungs** can be used to detect early signs of ILD.[5]

Diagnostic Procedures
- **Electromyography:** EMG allows **differentiation between neuropathic and myopathic conditions** and should always be done.
  - ○ EMG is abnormal in greater than 90% of patients with IM but only half of them show the classic findings of inflammation described in Bohan's and Peter's criteria (Table 35-3).[3]
  - ○ Needle insertion can damage muscle fibers for biopsy and hence, EMGs and muscle biopsies cannot be performed on the same side.
- **Muscle biopsy:**
  - ○ Subgroups have different characteristic findings (see above under PM/DM/IBM) but only a minority of patients will demonstrate all of the characteristic findings.
  - ○ Usually, the biopsy report will contain various features of different subgroups and it is important to remember that **a negative biopsy does not rule out IM.**
  - ○ Also, note that a pathology report is only as good as the lab and the pathologist. If results are questionable or if a patient is not improving as he should, it may be prudent to refer the patient and have the pathology reviewed at a center with more experience.
- **Pulmonary function tests:** Testing for extramuscular manifestations should be guided by patient's symptoms except for lung disease in myositis, as it needs to be treated aggressively early on to decrease morbidity.[5]

TREATMENT

Medications
Corticosteroids
- High doses of prednisone at 1 to 2 mg/kg PO daily are used as first line therapy.
- In patients with severe disease and respiratory compromise, IV methylprednisolone 1 g daily for 3 to 5 days should be used.
- High doses should be maintained for 2 to 3 months with a taper of 10 mg/month if patient's CK and strength have normalized.
- Most PM/DM patients respond to steroids whereas **IBM patients do not respond to steroids** or other commonly used immunosuppressive agents.

Steroid-Sparing Agents
- The following immunosuppressive agents should only be used in patients who have responded to corticosteroids but cannot be weaned off without a flare of disease:
  - ○ **Methotrexate or azathioprine** are used alone or even in combination in PM/DM patients.[6,7]
  - ○ **Cyclosporine** has efficacy in both childhood and adult disease.[8]

○ Case reports of patients with myositis and ILD successfully treated with **tacrolimus** have been published.[9]

○ **Mycophenolate mofetil** has successfully been used in PM/DM with ILD as well.[10]

Intravenous Immune Globulin

• Mechanism of action is unclear but several prospective trials of intravenous immunoglobulin (IVIG) have shown the efficacy of IVIG in PM/DM/IBM. It is administered for two consecutive days per month for 3 to 6 months in addition to other steroid sparing agents like methotrexate and azathioprine.[11]

• IVIG cannot be continued indefinitely without a steroid-sparing agent. Currently, recommendations are to use it only as a bridge therapy.

Other Non-Pharmacologic Therapies

Physical therapy is essential to preserve muscle function and prevent joint contractures. In IBM, this is the therapy currently known to be beneficial.

OUTCOME/PROGNOSIS

• Clinical outcome is variable between patients. Patients who develop myositis in association with a connective tissue disease tend to have brief illnesses followed by remission that requires no further treatment.

• PM and DM are generally steroid responsive.

• IBM has not been shown to be responsive to any medications except IVIG. There are no clear guidelines regarding duration of therapy especially since this disease is characterized by a very slow but progressive decline.

• Poor prognostic factors include older age, fever and dysphagia at diagnosis, extramuscular involvement of cardiac and pulmonary systems, delay to diagnosis and treatment, and positive anti-synthetase or anti-SRP antibodies.

REFERENCES

1. Oddis CV. Idiopathic inflammatory myopathies: Treatment and assessment. In: Klippel JH, Stone JH, Crofford LJ, eds. *Primer on the Rheumatic Diseases.* 13th ed. New York, NY: Springer Science and Business Media; 2008:378.

2. Rider LG, Miller FW. Deciphering the clinical presentations, pathogenesis, and treatment of the idiopathic inflammatory myopathies. *JAMA.* 2011;305:183–190.

3. Bohan A, Peter JB. Polymyositis and dermatomyositis. *N Engl J Med.* 1975;292:344–347,403–407.

4. Garcia J. MRI in inflammatory myopathies. *Skeletal Radiol.* 2000;29:425–438.

5. Fathi M, Lundberg IE. Interstitial lung disease in polymyositis and dermatomyositis. *Curr Opin Rheumatol.* 2005;17:701–706.

6. Newman ED, Scott DW. The use of low-dose oral methotrexate in the treatment of polymyositis and dermatomyositis. *J Clin Rheumatol.* 1995;1:99–102.

7. Bunch TW, Worthington JW, Combs JJ, et al. Azathioprine with prednisone for polymyositis. A controlled, clinical trial. *Ann Intern Med.* 1980;92:365–369.

8. Wilkes MR, Sereika SM, Fertig N, et al. Treatment of antisynthetase-associated interstitial lung disease with tacrolimus. *Arthritis Rheum.* 2005;52:2439–2446.

9. Qushmag KA, Chalmers A, Esdaile JM. Cyclosporin A in the treatment of refractory adult polymyositis/dermatomyositis: population based experience in 6 patients and literature review. *J Rheumatol.* 2000;27:2855–2859.

10. Majithia V, Harisdangkul V. Mycophenolate mofetil (CellCept): an alternative therapy for autoimmune inflammatory myopathy. *Rheumatology (Oxford).* 2005;44:386–389.

11. Cherin P, Pelletier S, Teixeira A, et al. Results and long-term followup of intravenous immunoglobulin infusions in chronic, refractory polymyositis: an open study with thirty-five adult patients. *Arthritis Rheum.* 2002;46:467–474.

Fibromyalgia Syndrome

36

Lesley Davila and Amy Joseph

GENERAL PRINCIPLES

Definition

- Fibromyalgia syndrome (FMS) is a chronic pain syndrome of unknown etiology that is characterized by otherwise unexplained diffuse pain, as well as tender points, fatigue, and sleep disturbance.
- Whether this is a rheumatologic condition is controversial but it is a condition seen by rheumatologists because patients present with musculoskeletal pain.

Epidemiology

- Studies in the 1980s estimated a prevalence of 2% to 5%, with a female to male ratio of 8:1.
- The mean age of patients is 30 to 60 years, but FMS may be present in children and the elderly.
- Posttraumatic stress disorder (PTSD) is seen significantly more frequently in patients with FMS than in the general population.

Pathophysiology

- The pathophysiology of fibromyalgia is poorly understood.
- FMS is a disorder of **heightened pain response,** characterized by both hyperalgesia, defined as increased pain sensitivity, and allodynia, defined as pain experienced in response to nonpainful stimuli.
- FMS may be a result of neuroendocrine axis alterations with subsequent **disturbances in mood, sleep, and pain perception.**
- Abnormalities of the muscle or soft tissue have not been identified in FMS patients.
- Studies show that patients often have low serum serotonin, growth hormone, and cortisol levels and elevated cerebrospinal fluid (CSF) substance P concentrations. Substance P, regulated by serotonin, can cause exaggerated perception of normal sensory stimuli.
- Functional MRI studies have demonstrated that the pain centers in the brains of FMS patients are activated by low level stimuli in a very similar way to how the pain centers in normals react to more intense stimuli.[1]
- FMS patients have sleep disturbances, with decreased sleep efficiency, increased arousals, and increased non-REM sleep resulting in nonrestorative sleep and daytime sleepiness. It is unknown if pain disturbs sleep, the disturbed sleep causes pain, or both.[2]

Associated Conditions

- Comorbid conditions found in patients with FMS include headache, chronic fatigue syndrome, irritable bowel syndrome, sleep disturbances, anxiety and/or depression, and obesity/metabolic syndrome.
- Patients with rheumatologic disorders, such as rheumatoid arthritis (RA), Sjögren's syndrome (SS), and systemic lupus erythematosus (SLE), can have concomitant FMS.

DIAGNOSIS

Clinical Presentation

- **The cardinal feature of FMS is diffuse soft tissue pain.** Often described as burning, tingling, or gnawing, the pain may be located in the neck, back, chest, arms, or legs. Usually patients have pain on both sides of the body as well as above and below the waist.
- In addition, patients may complain of **morning stiffness, fatigue, sleep disturbances, or headaches.** The symptoms of pain and fatigue are worsened by inactivity but also after seemingly minor activity.
- **The physical examination is normal except for the presence of tenderness.** Be sure to do a complete joint examination to look for synovitis so you do not miss a concomitant inflammatory arthritis.

Diagnostic Criteria

The American College of Rheumatology recently published preliminary criteria for the diagnosis and measurement of symptom severity of FMS.[3] These criteria are outlined in Table 36-1.

Differential Diagnosis

Other diagnoses to consider include hypothyroidism, drug-induced myopathies (e.g., HMG-CoA inhibitors), polymyalgia rheumatica (PMR), myofascial pain syndrome, Lyme disease, sciatica, multiple sclerosis, metabolic myopathy, depression, temporomandibular joint syndrome, and rheumatologic disorders (e.g., RA, SLE, SS, ankylosing spondylitis [AS]).

Diagnostic Testing

- The diagnosis of FMS is made clinically.
- Lab tests and radiologic studies often are unrevealing but are helpful in excluding other diseases.
- Perform a careful sleep history and consider **sleep studies** in obese patients and in males with fibromyalgia.
- **Screen patients for coexistent depression,** which commonly occurs in patients with chronic pain regardless of the source.

Laboratories

- Initial tests should include a complete blood count (CBC), an erythrocyte sedimentation rate (ESR), standard chemistries, and thyroid function studies.
- Due to the number of false positives, reserve testing for rheumatoid factor (RF), antinuclear antibodies (ANAs), and Lyme antibodies for patients in whom clinical suspicion is high.

TABLE 36-1	THE AMERICAN COLLEGE OF RHEUMATOLOGY 2010 FIBROMYALGIA DIAGNOSTIC CRITERIA

A patient satisfies diagnostic criteria for fibromyalgia if the following three conditions are met:

1. Widespread pain index (WPI) ≥7 and symptom severity (SS) scale score ≥5 OR WPI 3–6 and SS scale score ≥9.
2. Symptoms have been present at a similar level for at least 3 months.
3. The patient does not have a disorder that would otherwise explain the pain.

WPI: Quantify the number of areas in which the patient has had pain over the last week. Score will be between 0 and 19.

Shoulder girdle, left	Hip (buttock, trochanter), left	Jaw, left	Upper back
Shoulder girdle, right	Hip (buttock, trochanter), right	Jaw, right	Lower back
Upper arm, left	Upper leg, left	Chest	Neck
Upper arm, right	Upper leg, right	Abdomen	
Lower arm, left	Lower leg, left		
Lower arm, right	Lower leg, right		

SS Scale Score: The sum of the severity of the three symptoms (fatigue, waking unrefreshed, cognitive symptoms) plus the extent (severity) of somatic symptoms in general. The final score is between 0 and 12.

For each of the three symptoms below, indicate the level of severity over the past week using the following scale:

Fatigue	0 = no problem
Waking unrefreshed	1 = slight or mild problems, generally mild or intermittent
Cognitive symptoms	2 = moderate, considerable problems, often present and/or at a moderate level
	3 = severe, pervasive, continuous, life-disturbing problems

Considering somatic symptoms in general, indicate whether the patient has:[a]

0 = no symptoms
1 = few symptoms
2 = a moderate number of symptoms
3 = a great deal of symptoms

---

[a]Somatic symptoms to consider: fatigue, muscle pain/weakness, irritable bowel syndrome, abdominal pain/cramps, nausea, vomiting, constipation, diarrhea, dry mouth, heartburn, oral ulcers, loss of/change in taste, loss of appetite, thinking problems, memory problems, headache, numbness/tingling, dizziness, blurred vision, hearing problems, tinnitus, seizures, insomnia, depression, nervousness, shortness of breath, wheezing, chest pain, urinary frequency, dysuria and bladder spasms, itching, Raynaud's phenomenon, hives, dry eyes, rash, sun sensitivity, easy bruising, hair loss.

Adapted from: Wolfe F, Clauw DJ, Fitzcharles M, et al. The American College of Rheumatology preliminary diagnostic criteria for fibromyalgia and measurement of symptom severity. *Arth Care Res.* 2010;62:600–610.

Imaging

Radiologic studies may be ordered for patients with evidence of arthritis or radiculopathy.

TREATMENT

Both pharmacologic and nonpharmacologic therapies should be included when tailoring a treatment plan to an individual patient.

Medications

- Pharmacologic therapies with proven effectiveness include antidepressants, antiepileptics, and analgesics.
- Antidepressants, including tricyclic antidepressants (TCAs), monoamine oxidase inhibitors (MAOIs), selective serotonin reuptake inhibitors (SSRIs), and serotonin and norepinephrine reuptake inhibitors (SNRIs) have been shown to be effective in decreasing symptoms of fibromyalgia.[4]
- Two SNRI antidepressants, **duloxetine and milnacipran,** have been approved by the FDA for FMS. They affect pain and sleep disturbance in FMS, but this is thought to be independent of their effect on mood.[5,6]
  - ○ Duloxetine is usually started at 30 mg daily and increased to 60 or 120 mg daily.
  - ○ Milnacipran is titrated slowly to 50 mg twice daily (maximum 200 mg daily).
- The TCA amitriptyline has been shown to reduce pain, sleep disturbance, and fatigue in FMS patients.
- The MAOIs and SSRIs have been shown to diminish pain in FMS patients.
- Antiepileptic medications such as **pregabalin and gabapentin** have been studied in fibromyalgia and pregabalin has been approved by the FDA for treatment of FMS after being shown to significantly reduce pain and fatigue and to improve sleep and health related quality of life.[7–9]
  - ○ Pregabalin is initiated at 150 mg daily and titrated to 300 to 450 mg/day in divided doses.
  - ○ Gabapentin is dosed at 300 to 1800 mg daily in divided doses.
- **Medications that target sleep patterns** by promoting stage 4 sleep and providing analgesic effects include the following:
  - ○ Amitriptyline is usually dosed 10 to 50 mg PO once at bedtime.
- The "muscle relaxant" **cyclobenzaprine** has been studied several times and a meta-analysis suggests that it is beneficial in FMS (global assessment, sleep, and pain). It is usually dosed 10 to 40 mg daily in divided doses.[10] The actual mechanism of action is unclear but its structure is related to TCAs and cyproheptadine.
- Analgesics that are helpful include the following:
  - ○ Tramadol in doses of 50 to 400 mg daily.
  - ○ Acetaminophen.
  - ○ Nonsteroidal antiinflammatory drugs (NSAIDs) may also be used, but given the absence of tissue inflammation, they may not be better than placebo in treating patients with FMS.
  - ○ Topical agents (e.g., capsaicin cream and topical lidocaine) may be used as adjunctive therapies.
  - ○ **Opioids generally are not recommended** because FMS patients have been found to have diminished response to them, perhaps because they have decreased availability of central opioid receptors.[11]

Non-Pharmacologic Therapies

- There is strong evidence to support the use of exercise and cognitive behavioral psychotherapy (CBT) in the treatment of FMS.[12]
  - Physical activity helps maintain function in patients. Aerobic activity should be performed for at least 20 minutes daily, 2 to 3 times a week at a moderate intensity. It can be split into two 10-minute periods. Strength training should be performed 2 to 3 times per week with 8 to 12 repetitions per exercise.
  - Behavioral therapy, CBT, and biofeedback combined with relaxation and movement therapy have been proven effective.
  - Acupuncture and balneotherapy can also be of benefit.
- Patient education is an important component of therapy for FMS. Support groups are also available for these patients.
- Establishing a close patient–physician relationship with frequent visits often helps patients cope with their disease.

REFERENCES

1. Gracely RH, Petzke F, Wolf JM, et al. Functional magnetic resonance imaging evidence of augmented pain processing in fibromyalgia. *Arthritis Rheum.* 2002;46:1333–1343.
2. Abad VC, Sarinas PSA, Guilleminault C. Sleep and rheumatologic disorders. *Sleep Med Rev.* 2008;12:211–228.
3. Wolfe F, Clauw DJ, Fitzcharles M, et al. The American College of Rheumatology preliminary diagnostic criteria for fibromyalgia and measurement of symptom severity. *Arthritis Care Res (Hoboken).* 2010;62:600–610.
4. Hauser W, Bernardy K, Uceyler N, et al. Treatment of fibromyalgia syndrome with antidepressants: A meta-analysis. *JAMA.* 2009;301:198–209.
5. Mease PJ, Smith TR, Kajdasz DK, et al. Efficacy and safety of duloxetine for treatment of fibromyalgia in patients with or without major depressive disorder: Results from a 6-month, randomized, double-blind, placebo-controlled, fixed-dose trial. *Pain.* 2008;136:432–444.
6. Mease PJ, Clauw DJ, Gendreau RM, et al. The efficacy and safety of milnacipran for treatment of fibromyalgia. A randomized, double-blind, placebo-controlled trial. *J Rheumatol.* 2009;36:398–409.
7. Arnold LM, Goldenberg DL, Stanford SB, et al. Gabapentin in the treatment of fibromyalgia: A randomized, double-blind, placebo-controlled, multicenter trial. *Arthritis Rheum.* 2007;56:1336–1344.
8. Mease PJ, Russell IJ, Arnold LM, et al. A randomized, double-blind, placebo-controlled, phase III trial of pregabalin in the treatment of patients with fibromyalgia. *J Rheumatol.* 2008;35:502–514.
9. Russell IJ, Crofford LJ, Leon T, et al. The effects of pregabalin on sleep disturbance symptoms among individuals with fibromyalgia syndrome. *Sleep Med.* 2009;10:604–610.
10. Harris RE, Clauw DJ, Scott DJ, et al. Decreased central mu-opioid receptor availability in fibromyalgia. *J Neurosci.* 2007;27:10000–10006.
11. Tofferi JK, Jackson JL, O'Malley PG. Treatment of fibromyalgia with cyclobenzaprine: A meta-analysis. *Arthritis Rheum.* 2004;51:9–13.
12. Busch AJ, Barber KA, Overend TJ, et al. Exercise for treating fibromyalgia syndrome. *Cochrane Database Syst Rev.* 2007;4:CD003786.

Sjögren's Syndrome

37

Maria C. Gonzalez-Mayda and Amy Joseph

GENERAL PRINCIPLES

- Sjögren's syndrome (SS) is one of the more prevalent autoimmune diseases and its most common features are **dry eyes and dry mouth.**
- Treatment should be aimed at symptomatic relief by keeping mucous membranes moist.

Definition

- SS is a chronic inflammatory disorder characterized by **lymphocytic infiltration and autoimmune destruction of exocrine glands.**
- The **salivary and lacrimal glands** are commonly affected, leading to symptoms of dry mouth (xerostomia) and dry eyes (keratoconjunctivitis sicca). There may also be nasal and vaginal dryness.

Epidemiology

- Of the autoimmune conditions, SS is **one of the more prevalent,** affecting approximately 0.5 to 3 million persons in the United States. The incidence of SS in the general population is estimated to range between 1/1000 and 1/100 new cases per year, depending on the diagnostic criteria used.
- SS most often occurs in women (female to male ratio, 9:1) in their fourth and fifth decades of life.

Pathophysiology

- The primary pathologic mechanism of SS consists of focal infiltration of lymphocytes into glandular tissue.
- SS most commonly affects salivary and lacrimal glands but may occur in any exocrine glandular tissue.
- Antibodies against nuclear antigens **SSA/Ro and SSB/La** are commonly associated with SS, but it is not known if they are pathogenic.
- Although the exact pathophysiologic mechanisms of SS are not completely understood, several different hypotheses have been formulated.
  - A combination of genetic, hormonal and environmental factors are thought to play a role in the initiation and progression of SS.[1]
  - Certain HLA-DR and HLA-DQ alleles are associated with SS.
  - Viral infections, including Epstein–Barr virus, retroviruses, and hepatitis C, might predispose patients to SS by indirectly altering immune response to favor autoimmune glandular destruction.
  - Glandular epithelial cells become activated and assist in the attraction of B cells, T cells, and dendritic cells to the exocrine glands and promote the release of inflammatory cytokines.[1]

- The inflammation becomes chronic because of immune dysregulation, resulting in cell-mediated glandular destruction leading to decreased exocrine secretions.
- The end effect of ocular discomfort in SS is mediated by inadequate tearing, causing increased friction between mucosal surfaces. This results in distortion of epithelial cells during the blinking process, leading to **corneal irritation and abrasions.** A localized inflammatory response is precipitated. In addition, the loss of the nutritive effects of tears delays healing.
- Similar pathologic processes affect the oral cavity. Inflammatory destruction of salivary glands leads to quantitative and qualitative changes in saliva production. The normal bacterial flora is altered by changes in salivation, leading to an **increased frequency of dental caries, oral candidiasis, and periodontal diseases.**

Associated Conditions

- SS may occur as a primary disease.
- However, it **commonly occurs in patients with other systemic autoimmune diseases** (e.g., rheumatoid arthritis [RA], systemic lupus erythematosus [SLE], scleroderma [SSc], mixed connective tissue disease [MCTD], inflammatory myopathies, and autoimmune liver and thyroid diseases).

DIAGNOSIS

Clinical Presentation

History

- Symptoms of SS develop insidiously, commonly over several years.
- Mucosal dehydration, manifested as **dry eyes and dry mouth,** is the most common complaint associated with SS.
- Symptoms of dry eyes include a foreign body sensation, itching, light sensitivity worse in the evening, and thick, crusting film present on awakening. Symptoms are commonly aggravated by airline travel, dry windy conditions, and use of contact lenses.
- Dry mouth often manifests as increased thirst and difficulty swallowing dry foods. Rapidly progressive dental caries, recurrent oral and gingival infections, and discomfort wearing dentures may all be associated with SS.
- **Additional features of exocrine gland dysfunction** include symptoms of dry skin (xerosis), vaginal dryness, upper airway dryness creating a dry cough, and recurrent upper respiratory infections.
- Extraglandular involvement of SS may also occur.
  - **Fatigue and arthralgias** (sometimes arthritis) are common complaints with SS.
  - **Skin lesions** include palpable purpura, urticaria, annular lesions, xerosis, and Raynaud's phenomenon.
  - **Respiratory involvement** includes increased frequency of sinusitis, bronchitis, pneumonia, and pleural effusions. More severe complications include development of **interstitial pneumonitis and pulmonary fibrosis.**
  - **Cardiac involvement** may include pericardial effusions or autonomic dysfunction.
  - **Neurologic complications** may include cognitive dysfunction, demyelinating disease similar to multiple sclerosis, myasthenia gravis, and peripheral neuropathies.

○ **Renal involvement** may manifest as renal tubular acidosis, renal insufficiency, or chronic interstitial nephritis.

○ **Gastrointestinal manifestations** include dysphagia, esophageal dysmotility, nausea, dyspepsia, atrophic gastritis, and hepatic abnormalities.

Physical Examination
- Salivary gland enlargement occurs in up to half of the affected patients.
- The glands are usually diffusely firm and nontender. Painful episodic swelling is common and may be either unilateral or bilateral.
- A hard, nodular gland may suggest a neoplasm. This distinction is clinically significant, as there is an **increased incidence of B-cell lymphomas** in salivary glands affected with SS.

Diagnostic Criteria

Table 37-1 presents the revised international classification criteria for SS proposed by the American-European Consensus Group.[2]

Differential Diagnosis

The differential diagnosis of SS includes any disease process that leads to symptoms of dry eyes and dry mouth, including the following:

- **Infiltrative diseases** (e.g., sarcoidosis, amyloidosis, hemochromatosis, and lymphoma).
- **Infectious diseases** (e.g., viral infections [HIV, hepatitis B and C, mumps, influenza, coxsackie A, cytomegalovirus], syphilis, trachoma, tuberculosis, and bacterial infection).
- **Fat deposition** from diabetes, alcoholism, pancreatitis, cirrhosis, and hypertriglyceridemia.
- **Anticholinergic side effects** from medicines (e.g., antidepressants, neuroleptics, antihypertensives, antihistamines, and decongestants).
- **Endocrine dysfunction** including acromegaly and gonadal hypofunction.

Diagnostic Testing

Laboratories

A general diagnostic workup for SS should include the following laboratory tests:

- Complete blood count (CBC), erythrocyte sedimentation rate (ESR) or C-reactive protein (CRP), rheumatoid factor (RF), antinuclear antibodies (ANA), and serum protein electrophoresis.
- ANA is positive in about 80% and RF is positive in up to 30% of SS patients.
- If the ANA is positive, obtain autoantibodies **SSA/Ro and SSB/La.** SSA/Ro is positive in about 75% and SSB/La in about 40% of patients.
- Most patients have mild anemia and increased ESR or CRP, and polyclonal hypergammaglobulinemia is also common.

Diagnostic Procedures
- Functional studies may include **Schirmer's test** for tear secretion.
- Rose bengal or fluorescein staining with **slit-lamp examination** is used to detect damaged corneal epithelium.
- **Sialometry, sialography, or scintigraphy** can be performed to measure salivary gland function.

| TABLE 37-1 | REVISED INTERNATIONAL CLASSIFICATION CRITERIA FOR SJÖGREN'S SYNDROME[a] |

For primary Sjögren's syndrome without any potentially associated disease:
The presence of any 4 of the 6 items as long as either item 4 or 6 is present.
The presence of any 3 of the 4 objective criteria (i.e., items 3, 4, 5, or 6).

For secondary Sjögren's syndrome:
In patients with a potentially associated disease, the presence of item 1 or 2 plus any 2 from among items 3, 4, or 5.

Criteria	Clinical Findings
1. Ocular symptoms: At least one	Daily, persistent, troublesome dry eyes for more than 3 months Recurrent sensation of sand or gravel in the eyes Use tear substitutes more than 3 times/day
2. Oral symptoms: At least one	Daily feeling of dry mouth for more than 3 months Recurrent or persistently swollen salivary glands as an adult Frequently drink liquids to aid in swallowing dry foods
3. Ocular signs: At least one	Schirmer's I test (≤5 mm in 5 minutes) Rose bengal or other ocular dye score (≥4, according to the van Bijsterveld scoring system)
4. Histopathology	Focal lymphocytic sialadenitis of minor salivary glands with a focus score ≥1 (number of lymphocytic foci [adjacent to normal-appearing mucous acini containing >50 lymphocytes] per 4 mm^2 of glandular tissue)
5. Salivary gland signs: At least one	Unstimulated whole salivary flow ≤1.5 mL in 15 minutes Parotid sialography showing the presence of diffuse sialectasias, without evidence of obstruction in the major ducts Salivary scintigraphy showing delayed uptake, reduced concentration and/or delayed excretion of tracer
6. Autoantibodies	SSA/Ro SSB/La Both

[a]Exclusion criteria: Past head and neck radiation, hepatitis C virus infection, HIV infection with AIDS, preexisting lymphoma, sarcoidosis, graft versus host disease, use of anticholinergic drugs within a time equal to four fold the half life of the drug.

Adapted from: Vitali C, Bombardieri S, Jonsson R, et al. Classification criteria for Sjögren's syndrome: a revised version of the European criteria proposed by the American-European Consensus Group. *Ann Rheum Dis.* 2002;61:554–558.

- Confirmation of SS can be obtained by performing a **minor salivary gland biopsy,** most often obtained from minor salivary glands in the lower lip. Pathologic findings of **focal lymphocyte aggregates, plasma cells, and macrophages** support the diagnosis.

TREATMENT

- Most patients with SS can be managed with education and simple symptomatic relief measures designed to keep mucous membranes moist.
- For dry eyes, patients should use **artificial tears** on a regular basis. Numerous brands are available, and patients are encouraged to try various formulas to find the most suitable one. In general, preservative-free solutions are better tolerated.
  - Some patients may benefit from **punctual occlusion** to prolong the efficacy of artificial tears.
  - **Topical 0.05% cyclosporine** twice daily for patients with moderate to severe dry eye disease has been shown to give the best results in terms of symptomatic relief.[3,4]
  - In cases where ocular symptoms are severe and refractory, refer to an ophthalmologist for initiation of topical steroids or nonsteroidal antiinflammatory drugs (NSAIDs) under their monitoring.
- For dry mouth, patients are encouraged to **drink water frequently.**
  - Stimulation of salivary glands with sugar-free gum or candy may also be useful.
  - Patients should avoid dry foods as well as alcohol and smoking.
  - Artificial saliva products are available.
  - Some patients may benefit from treatment with the **muscarinic agonists pilocarpine,** 5 mg PO qid, or **cevimeline,** 30 mg PO tid; however, many patients experience side effects of increased urination and defecation, sweating, abdominal cramping, and flushing. [3,5]
  - Patients with xerostomia are at increased risk of dental caries and should be followed closely by a dentist. **Topical fluoride treatments** may help prevent tooth decay. Meticulous daily dental hygiene is of utmost importance.
- Dry skin can be managed with moisturizing lotions.
- Vaginal dryness is improved with lubricants.
- Arthralgias and other musculoskeletal complaints are often remedied with NSAIDs.
- Hydroxchloroquine, azathioprine, methotrexate, leflunomide, and tumor necrosis factor (TNF) antagonists have all failed to show conclusive efficacy in SS.[3]
- In those patients with severe progressive disease manifestations of vasculitis, nephritis, interstitial lung involvement, or neuropathy a combination of steroids and IV cyclophosphamide can be considered. Rituximab may also be considered in life-threatening circumstances.[3,6]

COMPLICATIONS

- SS has been associated with the development of **lymphoma** with a lifetime risk between 5% and 10%. This is thought to arise because of unregulated B- and T-cell stimulation.
- Factors associated with an increased risk of lymphoma include lymphadenopathy, splenomegaly, low CD4 count, parotid gland enlargement, cryoglobulinemia, low complement levels, and purpura/vasculitis.[7–9]

REFERRAL

Patients with sicca symptoms should be followed closely by a **rheumatologist** and should be referred to both a **dentist** and an **ophthalmologist** given their increased risk of developing caries and corneal abrasions, respectively.

PATIENT EDUCATION

- Patients with SS should be advised to keep mucous membranes moist for symptomatic relief.
- Encourage patients to avoid dry environments, wind, cigarette smoke, and medications with anticholinergic side effects.
- Humidifiers can counter low-humidity indoor environments, especially in winter months when centralized heating leads to dry air.

OUTCOME/PROGNOSIS

In patients with primary SS without transformation to lymphoma there does not appear to be an increase in all-cause mortality when compared with the general population; those with lymphoma have a higher mortality rate.

REFERENCES

1. Voulgarelis M, Tzioufas A. Pathogenetic mechanisms in the initiation and perpetuation of Sjögren's syndrome. *Nat Rev Rheumatol.* 2010;9:529–537.
2. Vitali C, Bombardieri S, Jonsson R, et al. Classification criteria for Sjögren's syndrome: a revised version of the European criteria proposed by the American-European Consensus Group. *Ann Rheum Dis.* 2002;61:554–558.
3. Ramos-Casals M, Tzioufas A, Stone J, et al. Treatment of primary Sjögren syndrome: a systematic review. *JAMA.* 2010;304:452–460.
4. Sall K, Stevenson OD, Mundorf TK, et al. Two multicenter, randomized studies of the efficacy and safety of cyclosporine ophthalmic emulsion in moderate to severe dry eye disease. CsA Phase 3 Study Group. *Ophthalmology.* 2000;107:631–639.
5. Petrone D, Condemi JJ, Fife R, et al. A double-blind, randomized, placebo-controlled study of cevimeline in Sjögren's syndrome patients with xerostomia and keratoconjunctivitis sicca. *Arthritis Rheum.* 2002;46:748–754.
6. Ramos-Casals M, Brito-Zerón P, Muñoz S, et al; BIOGEAS STUDY Group. A systematic review of the off-label use of biological therapies in systemic autoimmune diseases. *Medicine (Baltimore).* 2008;87:345–364.
7. Theander R, Henriksson G, Ljungberg O, et al. Lymphoma and other malignancies in primary Sjögren's syndrome: a cohort study on cancer incidence and lymphoma predictors. *Ann Rheum Dis.* 2006;65:796–803.
8. Baimpa E, Dahabreh IJ, Voulgarelis M, et al. Hematologic manifestations and predictors of lymphoma development in primary Sjögren syndrome: clinical and pathophysiologic aspects. *Medicine (Baltimore).* 2009;88:284–293.
9. Solans-Laqué R, López-Hernandez A, Angel Bosch-Gil J, et al. Risk, Predictors, and Clinical Characteristics of Lymphoma Development in Primary Sjögren's Syndrome. *Semin Arthritis Rheum.* 2011 Jun 10. [Epub ahead of print]

Scleroderma

38

Hyon Ju Park and Amy Joseph

GENERAL PRINCIPLES

- Scleroderma is a connective tissue disease characterized by skin thickening and tightening. It is divided into two main forms: localized and systemic.
- **Localized scleroderma only involves the skin** with, at most, some atrophy of the subcutaneous tissue underlying the lesions.
  - Localized scleroderma includes **morphea** (patches of thickened skin), **linear scleroderma** (a line of thickened skin on one or more extremities), and **scleroderma en coup de sabre** (linear disease affecting only one side of the face and scalp).
  - Patients with localized scleroderma are generally managed by dermatologists as they have no internal organ involvement.
  - They may have low titer antinuclear antibody (ANA) tests.
- The rest of this chapter will focus on **systemic scleroderma, also known as systemic sclerosis (SSc).**

Definition

SSc is a complex multiorgan disease thought to be the result of autoimmunity, inflammation, vasculopathy, and progressive fibrosis of the skin and visceral organs.

Classification

- SSc is divided further into **limited cutaneous disease (lcSSc, formerly known as CREST** syndrome: calcinosis, Raynaud's phenomenon [RP], esophageal dysmotility, sclerodactyly, and telangiectasias), **diffuse cutaneous disease (dcSSc)**, and **scleroderma sine scleroderma** on the basis of the extent of skin involvement.
- Skin involvement in lcSSc is limited to the face, the upper extremities distal to the elbows and the lower extremities distal to the knees; while dcSSc involves skin proximal to the elbows and knees. This distinction is important in its prognostic implications. The rare case with visceral organ involvement but no skin changes is known as scleroderma sine scleroderma.

Epidemiology

- Estimated annual incidence of SSc in the United States is 1.9/100,000. Prevalence rate is estimated at 28/100,000.[1]
- SSc is about three to five times more common in women than men, with decline of predominance after menopause. The most common age of onset is between 30 and 50 years.
- Having a first degree relative with disease confers a relative risk of about 13 but rates between monozygotic and dizygotic twins are similar.

- Blacks have a higher incidence and have earlier disease onset than whites. Blacks are more likely to have diffuse cutaneous involvement with aggressive interstitial lung disease (ILD) and pulmonary hypertension.

Etiology

- Etiology is unknown and there are no animal models that simulate all the features of SSc.
- A two-hit process has been hypothesized, where this inflammatory and vasculopathic disease is triggered by an environmental or infectious agent in people who have a loss of function mutation in the antifibrotic pathways.

Pathophysiology

- There are four distinct but interrelated pathogenic processes of autoimmunity, inflammation, vasculopathy, and fibrosis.
- It is thought that **autoimmunity with vascular reactivity** precedes development of SSc, as patients usually have autoantibodies and RP prior to the development of other organ involvement. Autoantibodies against components of the extracellular matrix found in 50% of SSc patients can activate fibroblasts, induce collagen production, and prevent collagen degradation, resulting in tissue fibrosis.[2]
- Endothelial injury appears to occur early in the course of SSc, but the trigger for the damage has not been identified. Injury results in endothelial cells becoming activated, producing adhesion molecules and inflammatory cytokines, which can lead to endothelial damage, resulting in tissue hypoxemia.
- Hypoxemia stimulates production of angiogenesis factors like vascular endothelial growth factor (VEGF), tumor (or transforming) growth factor (TGF) β and endothelin-1 (ET-1), which results in vasoconstriction without angiogenesis in SSc patients.

DIAGNOSIS

Clinical Presentation

History

- **RP** is almost universally present in SSc. It is **usually the first manifestation of SSc** and may precede the development of other features by months to years. Patients report episodic, bilateral color changes precipitated by the cold or by emotional stress. Digits, nose, and ears turn white when vasospasm occurs as a result of sympathetic hyperactivation. As oxygen supply is depleted, they turn blue and, upon rewarming, they become red as reperfusion occurs.
- **Skin changes** occur in three phases: edematous, fibrotic, and atrophic. Often the first complaint specific for scleroderma is swelling or "puffiness" of the fingers or hands corresponding to the edematous phase. Patients may also complain of pruritus, dry skin, tightening and decreased flexibility, and skin ulcerations.
- The extent of skin involvement often correlates with overall clinical course.
  ○ lcSSc typically begins with RP followed by thickening of skin of the fingers, progressing to hands and forearms with possible later features of pulmonary fibrosis and pulmonary arterial hypertension (PAH).

- ○ dcSSc has a more rapid course, with skin changes occurring shortly after the development of RP, progressing over the first 1 to 5 years, and then stabilizing thereafter. Unfortunately, internal organ involvement in dcSSc often occurs in the first 2 years and does not parallel the skin findings.
- Other complaints depend on visceral organ involvement. **Gastrointestinal (GI) complaints are common,** with involvement anywhere along the alimentary tract. **Gastroesophageal reflux** is the most common complaint. Patients may also note dry mouth, dysphagia, dyspepsia, nausea, early satiety, cramping abdominal pain, diarrhea, and weight loss. Intestinal pseudo-obstruction may occur secondary to hypomotility.
- With **pulmonary involvement,** patients may complain of dyspnea on exertion or nonproductive cough.
- Chest pain may occur due to esophagitis, pleurisy, pericarditis, costochondritis, coronary vasospasms, and fibrosis of the chest wall.
- **Musculoskeletal complaints** are nonspecific. Patients often experience generalized arthralgias with stiffness of the joints under the fibrotic skin.

Physical Examination
- Affected skin is thickened and leathery or hide-bound; **sclerodactyly** refers to such skin changes affecting the fingers. Fingertips can appear tapered from ischemic loss of the digital pulp.
- Since RP is a transient phenomenon, it usually is not seen on examination, but **fingertip ulcerations** resulting from chronic hypoxia can be seen. Examination of a patient's nailfold capillary bed can be beneficial for early diagnosis.
  - ○ Using a hand-held ophthalmoscope with power <20 diopters, nailfold capillaries are visualized through a water-soluble gel.
  - ○ In cases of secondary RP (associated with scleroderma or inflammatory myopathies), the examination reveals enlarged capillary loops, loss of normal capillary beds, and occasional capillary hemorrhages.
- A tight "purse-lip" appearance associated with **decreased oral aperture** is attributed to increased fibrotic activity within the perioral skin.
- **Telangiectasias** may be appreciated over the face, oropharyngeal mucosa and hands.
- Hyper- and hypopigmentary changes may lead to a "salt-and-pepper" appearance of the skin.
- Subcutaneous **calcinosis** can also be seen.
- Other findings depend on organ involvement.
  - ○ Crackles can be heard in patients with pulmonary fibrosis.
  - ○ Signs of right heart failure can be seen in the setting of PAH.
  - ○ Arrhythmias from conduction system fibrosis, pericardial rubs from pericarditis, or signs of congestive heart failure from myocardial fibrosis can be seen with cardiac involvement.
  - ○ When inflammation and fibrosis of tendon sheaths is significant, coarse friction rubs can be heard with joint movement.
  - ○ Hypertension with microangiopathic hemolytic anemia is seen in **scleroderma renal crisis,** a few patients with scleroderma renal crisis are normotensive.

Diagnostic Criteria
- The American College of Rheumatology classification criteria for SSc are presented in Table 38-1.

TABLE 38-1	AMERICAN COLLEGE OF RHEUMATOLOGY CLASSIFICATION CRITERIA FOR SYSTEMIC SCLEROSIS

Diagnosis of systemic sclerosis requires the presence of either the major criterion or two minor criteria.[a]

Major criterion:
- Proximal scleroderma (thickening, tightening, and induration proximal to the MCP/MTP joints)

Minor criteria:
- Sclerodactyly (localized thickening, tightening, and induration of only the fingers or toes)
- Permanent digital pitting scars or loss of substance of the digital finger pads (due to ischemia)
- Bibasilar pulmonary fibrosis

---

[a]Raynaud's phenomenon is observed in 90% to 98% of systemic sclerosis patients.

MCP, metacarpophalangeal; MTP, metatarsophalangeal.

Adapted from: Subcommittee for Scleroderma Criteria of the American Rheumatism Association Diagnostic and Therapeutic Criteria Committee: preliminary criteria for the classification of systemic sclerosis (scleroderma). *Arthritis Rheum*. 1980;23:581–590.

- Although this diagnostic strategy is purported to have a sensitivity of 97% and specificity of 98%, individuals with CREST features would not necessarily fulfill these criteria, but they are considered to have lcSSc.[3]

Differential Diagnosis

- Skin thickening as that in scleroderma but with some distinguishing features can be seen in other disorders. Keep in mind that **patients with these other diseases do not have RP or digital ulcerations.**
- **Nephrogenic systemic fibrosis (NSF)**, affecting mostly dialysis patients, tends to affect lower extremities more than upper extremities and generally spares the hands.
- Three syndromes with **paraproteinemia** have scleroderma-like skin changes:
  - **Scleredema,** complication of long-standing diabetes or paraproteinemia, causes thickening of the skin in the neck, shoulder girdle, proximal upper extremities, and back, and is characterized by mucin deposition on skin biopsy.
  - **Scleromyxedema,** which can involve the hands, but involved skin tends to be more folded and pendulous rather than tight and thickened.
  - **POEMS syndrome** (polyneuropathy, organomegaly, endocrinopathy, monoclonal gammopathy, and scleroderma-like skin changes).
- **Eosinophilic fasciitis** can have a rapid onset of skin thickening with early development of flexion contractures due to fascial thickening. Skin tends to be more puckered appearing, but a deep biopsy will demonstrate eosinophilic infiltration, separating it from SSc. Eosinophilia is common, and eosinophilic infiltrates are usually seen on biopsy.
- Other conditions with scleroderma-like skin thickening include diabetic digital sclerosis, chronic graft-versus-host disease, vinyl chloride exposure, vibratory

injury, bleomycin toxicity, complex regional pain syndrome/reflex sympathetic dystrophy, amyloidosis, porphyria cutanea tarda, and carcinoid syndrome.
- Diseases with similar organ involvement include primary pulmonary hypertension, ILD, primary biliary cirrhosis, intestinal hypomotility, and collagenous colitis.
- Diseases that may present in a similar fashion to scleroderma include systemic lupus erythematosus (SLE), mixed connective tissue disease (MCTD), rheumatoid arthritis (RA), and inflammatory myopathies.

Diagnostic Testing

Diagnosis is on the basis of clinical findings described above. The following can be helpful in making the diagnosis or in delineating the extent of organ involvement.

Laboratories

- 95% of patients with scleroderma will have a positive **ANA,** with the anticentromere staining pattern of the ANA being specific (but not sensitive) for limited scleroderma. **Anti–Scl-70 (anti–topoisomerase-I)** antibodies are specific (but not sensitive) for diffuse scleroderma, and are associated with risk for ILD.
- Less commonly assayed antibodies associated with scleroderma include **anti-RNA polymerase I, II, and III and U3-ribonucleoprotein (RNP).** RNP is associated with risk for pulmonary hypertension. Anti–U1-RNP antibodies are found in MCTD, and anti–PM-Scl antibodies may be present in overlap syndromes.

Electrocardiography

ECG findings are highly variable, depending on which area of the heart is involved and the extent of involvement.

Imaging

- Transthoracic echocardiography can be used to evaluate for pulmonary hypertension or pericardial effusion.
- Patients with ILD will have interstitial infiltrates on high-resolution CT and a restrictive pattern on pulmonary function testing.

Diagnostic Procedures

- Reflux, dysphagia, and odynophagia are frequent complaints related to esophageal dysmotility, which can be evaluated with barium esophagram or esophageal manometry.
- Patients with elevated pulmonary pressures on echocardiography or those with dyspnea unexplained by other causes should undergo a right heart catheterization, as echocardiography can under- or over-estimate pulmonary pressures in about 10% of patients.[4]

TREATMENT

SSc has the highest mortality rate among the connective tissue disorders. There is no treatment for the underlying disease process and, hence, treatment is targeted at specific organ complications and/or patient symptoms.

Medications

- **Skin involvement:** No effective antifibrotic therapy has been discovered to date.
  - Autologous hematopoietic stem cell transplant for severe dSSc has shown promise in reversing cutaneous disease, improving quality of life, and maintaining internal organ function. Randomized trials are in progress.[5]
- **RP:** Nonpharmacologic measures for treating RP include smoking cessation and avoiding cold exposure.
  - **Diltiazem and dihydropyridine calcium-channel blockers** (CCBs) like amlodipine, nifedipine, and felodipine have been shown to be effective in RP.[6]
  - Other medications that have been shown to have some efficacy in RP include the angiotensin II inhibitors, α-antagonists, selective serotonin reuptake inhibitors, nitrates, phosphodiesterase inhibitors such as sildenafil, and, in severe disease, prostacyclins.[6] All of these agents are more effective in primary RP than in RP associated with scleroderma.
- **Digital ulcers:** Ulcers are extremely painful and, because they result from ischemia, are difficult to heal. Analgesics and local wound care can be helpful.
  - Case series have demonstrated the benefit of **sildenafil and tadalafil** in facilitating healing and preventing new ulcer formation.[7]
  - **Bosentan** has been shown to reduce the development of new ulcers but without any effect on existing ulcers. **Iloprost** has been shown to help heal ulcers and prevent new ones, but only epoprostenol is available in the United States and it must be administered via a central line with close monitoring.[6]
  - Sympathectomies, sympathetic blocks, and intra-arterial injections of vasodilators have been reported to help but responses have been inconsistent.
- Scleroderma renal crisis used to be the number one cause of death in SSc patients but that has changed with the advent of **angiotensin-converting enzyme (ACE) inhibitors.**[8]
  - Early institution of ACE inhibitors now makes this a rare cause of death.
  - An ACE inhibitor should be started even in the setting of an elevated creatinine, and a renal specialist consulted.
  - Patients with early, active, inflammatory diffuse scleroderma are at highest risk and should be educated about warning signs and encouraged to monitor their pressure weekly.
- **Cyclophosphamide** has been used for SSc **ILD** for many years but randomized, controlled trials have demonstrated only modest benefit in forced vital capacity, fibrosis, and dyspnea.[9]
  - Small open case series demonstrating benefit of **mycophenolate mofetil** (MMF) have been published but MMF has not been rigorously studied.
  - A small randomized controlled study demonstrated improvement in skin and ILD with **rituximab** therapy.[10]
- The **prostaglandins** epoprostenol, treprostinil, and iloprost; endothelin receptor antagonist **bosentan;** and the **phosphodiesterase inhibitors** sildenafil and tadalafil have shown benefit in the treatment of **PAH.**[6]
- GI: Reflux symptoms can be controlled with **proton pump inhibitors,** but it may be necessary to use up to three times the usual dose.[6]
  - **Esophageal strictures** are treated with dilatation when necessary.
  - **Gastric antral venous ectasia** is the most common cause of GI bleeding in scleroderma and can be treated with endoscopic laser photocoagulation.

○ **Prokinetic agents** like metoclopramide can be for aperistaltic symptoms. Intestinal pseudo-obstruction can be managed with octreotide.[6]

○ Patients who develop symptoms of small bowel **bacterial overgrowth** can be managed with alternating doses of ciprofloxacin and metronidazole.[6]

Other Non-Pharmacologic Therapies

- Avoiding excess bathing and using proper moisturizing creams can aid in skin care.
- Aggressive occupational and physical therapy may be helpful early in the course of disease to minimize contractures.

Surgical Management

Post-operative healing can be difficult in SSc patients. However, digital ulcers can become infected and may need debridement. Amputations may be necessary for deeper infections.

SPECIAL CONSIDERATIONS

Patients with scleroderma are at increased risk for depression and despair. Support groups may be beneficial. Fear of losing functionality and of increasing pain is a common emotion but is amenable to intervention by early recognition, patient education, and encouragement.

OUTCOME/PROGNOSIS

- The diagnoses of dcSSc and lcSSc have different prognostic implications.
- dcSSc has widely variable but overall poor prognosis with survival of 40% to 60% at 10 years from the onset of the first non-RP scleroderma sign or symptom.
- lcSSc has a relatively good prognosis with survival greater than 70% at 10 years.
- Prognosis of scleroderma sine scleroderma is generally poor but difficult to estimate because it is so rare.
- Most patients with SSc die from pulmonary disease or from infectious complications.

REFERENCES

1. Chifflot H, Fautrel B, Sordet C, et al. Incidence and prevalence of systemic sclerosis: a systematic literature review. *Semin Arthritis Rheum.* 2008;37:223–235.
2. Abraham DJ, Krieg T, Distler J, et al. Overview of pathogenesis of systemic sclerosis. *Rheumatology (Oxford).* 2009;48:iii3–iii7.
3. Subcommittee for Scleroderma Criteria of the American Rheumatism Association Diagnostic and Therapeutic Criteria Committee: preliminary criteria for the classification of systemic sclerosis (scleroderma). *Arthritis Rheum.* 1980;23:581–590.
4. Matucci-Cerinic M, Steen V, Hachulla E. The complexity of managing systemic sclerosis: screening and diagnosis. *Rheumatology (Oxford).* 2009;48:iii8–iii13.
5. Burt RK, Milanetti F. Hematopoietic stem cell transplantation for systemic sclerosis: history and current status. *Curr Opin Rheumatol.* 2011;23(6):519–529.

6. Kowal-Bielecka O, Landewe R, Avouac J, et al. EULAR recommendations for the treatment of systemic sclerosis: a report from the EULAR Scleroderma Trials and Research group (EUSTAR). *Ann Rheum Dis.* 2009;68:620–628.

7. Brueckner CS, Becker MO, Kroencke T, et al. Effect of sildenafil on digital ulcers in systemic sclerosis: analysis from a single centre pilot study. *Ann Rheum Dis.* 2010;69:1475–1478.

8. Penn H, Denton CP. Diagnosis, management and prevention of scleroderma renal disease. *Curr Opin Rheumatol.* 2008;20:692–696.

9. Khanna D, Seibold JR, Wells A, et al. Systemic sclerosis-associated interstitial lung disease: lessons from clinical trials, outcome measures, and future study design. *Curr Rheumatol Rev.* 2010;6:138–144.

10. Daoussis D, Liossis SN, Tsamandas AC, et al. Experience with rituximab in scleroderma: results from a 1 year, proof of principle study. *Rheumatology (Oxford).* 2010;49:271–280.

Antiphospholipid Syndrome

39

Lesley Davila and Amy Joseph

GENERAL PRINCIPLES

Definition

Antiphospholipid syndrome (APS) is a **hypercoagulable disorder** manifested by recurrent arterial and venous thromboses and adverse outcomes in pregnancy that is associated with antiphospholipid (aPL) antibodies.

Classification

- APS may be **primary** (with no concomitant disorder) or **secondary** when associated with another systemic disease (e.g., systemic lupus erythematosus [SLE]).
- **Catastrophic APS** is a variant of APS characterized by acute thrombotic microangiopathy that results in multiorgan failure and a high mortality rate.

Epidemiology

- The syndrome most commonly occurs in young females; however, both sexes and all ages may be affected.
- While aPL occurs in 1% to 6% of the general population, the prevalence of primary APS is thought to be less than 0.5%.
- In patients with SLE, 10% to 44% will develop aPL and of those, about half will eventually develop secondary APS. Among patients with APS, 37% have SLE.[1] Catastrophic APS occurs in less than 1% of patients with APS.

Pathophysiology

- The pathophysiology of APS is poorly understood, although aPL is implicated in the disorder.
- aPL affects coagulation and thrombosis in different ways.[2-4]
  - These antibodies may bind to platelets, upregulating production of thromboxane A2 and expression of glycoprotein 2b-3a; to endothelial cells and monocytes which increases production of tissue factors; or to endothelial cells resulting in an increase in adhesion molecules. These interactions favor thrombosis.
  - The binding of aPL also activates complement, which can initiate an inflammatory cascade resulting in thrombosis. Complement activation has also been linked to fetal loss in APS.
  - Some authors propose that coagulation may result from disruption of proteins that regulate thrombosis, such as protein C, by aPL. Also, antibodies against β-2-glycoprotein I (β-2gpI), a naturally occurring anticoagulant, may induce a prothrombotic state.
  - Cardiovascular risk factors such as smoking and estrogen use can help promote thrombosis in APS.

- The importance of these antibodies in the pathogenesis of disease has been supported by animal studies that have shown that passive transfer of anticardiolipin (aCL) antibodies may induce thrombocytopenia and fetal resorption.

Associated Conditions

- Secondary APS has been associated with various rheumatologic conditions, most commonly SLE, but also Sjögren's syndrome, rheumatoid arthritis, scleroderma, and systemic vasculitis.
- aPL in the absence of APS has also been found in patients with infections, neoplasms, medication exposure and other diseases. These aPL are usually IgM antibodies at low titers and are usually transient and rarely associated with thrombosis.[1]

DIAGNOSIS

- APS should be suspected in patients presenting with **venous or arterial thromboembolism** (deep venous thrombosis or pulmonary embolism, stroke, myocardial infarction, or other presentation) or **pregnancy losses** (miscarriage, preeclampsia, or placental insufficiency).
- Consider APS when a patient has unexplained or recurrent thromboses or thrombotic events at **unusual sites** (e.g., adrenal veins), when thrombosis occurs in **young patients,** and when recurrent pregnancy losses occur in the **second and third trimesters.**

Clinical Presentation

- Clinical presentation of APS varies on the basis of the affected blood vessel. Patients typically present in one of four ways:
  ○ Venous thrombosis
  ○ Arterial thrombosis
  ○ Pregnancy loss
  ○ Thrombocytopenia
- Other manifestations can include livedo reticularis, Raynaud's phenomenon, dementia, premature atherosclerotic lesions, renal insufficiency, and pulmonary hypertension (Table 39-1).
- Catastrophic APS presents with **multiorgan failure** as a result of multiple-vessel occlusion occurring over a short time period. This carries a mortality rate of 50% even with treatment.
- Dermatologic symptoms such as **livedo reticularis** and **Raynaud's phenomenon** occur in 10% to 30% of patients and may provide a clue to diagnosis.

Diagnostic Criteria

- The updated International Consensus Statement on classification criteria for definite APS states that the diagnosis of APS should be considered when at least one clinical criterion and one lab criterion are met (Table 39-2).[5]
- The clinical criteria include vascular thrombosis and pregnancy morbidity, and the laboratory criteria include the presence of aCL antibody, anti–β-2gpI antibody, and the lupus anticoagulant (LAC).

Differential Diagnosis

- Diagnoses of **other prothrombotic conditions** must be entertained: Protein C or S deficiency, antithrombin III deficiency, factor V Leiden mutation,

TABLE 39-1	CLINICAL MANIFESTATIONS OF ANTIPHOSPHOLIPID SYNDROME

Cardiovascular: Myocardial infarction, angina, premature atherosclerotic valvular lesions, pseudoinfective endocarditis, intracardiac thrombosis
Dermatologic: Livedo reticularis, splinter hemorrhages, skin infarcts, leg ulcers, superficial thrombophlebitis, blue toe syndrome, Raynaud's phenomenon, necrotizing purpura
Endocrine: Adrenal insufficiency
Gastrointestinal: Hepatic infarction, Budd–Chiari syndrome
Hematologic: Thrombocytopenia, leukopenia, hemolytic anemia, positive Coomb's test
Musculoskeletal: Deep venous thrombosis, avascular necrosis
Neurologic: Cerebrovascular accidents, transient ischemic attacks, migraines, chorea, multi-infarct dementia, pseudotumor cerebri, peripheral neuropathy, myasthenia gravis, seizures, transverse myelopathy
Obstetric: Eclampsia/preeclampsia; fetal wastage: Intrauterine growth retardation: Hemolysis, elevated liver enzymes, and low platelet count (HELLP) syndrome; oligohydramnios; chorea gravidarum; postpartum syndrome
Pulmonary: Pulmonary embolus, nonthromboembolic pulmonary hypertension
Renal: Renal artery/vein thrombosis, hypertension, glomerular thrombosis, renal insufficiency

---

dysfibrinogenemias, hyperhomocysteinuria, Behçet's syndrome, malignancies, thrombotic thrombocytopenic purpura, nephrotic syndrome, severe diabetes, paroxysmal nocturnal hemoglobinuria, pregnancy, smoking, estrogen therapy, and prolonged bed rest.

- Although often associated with thromboses, aPLs sometimes can be found in a healthy person or in those with lymphoproliferative disorders, viral infections (e.g., HIV), or malignancies. These individuals may not necessarily have APS. The prevalence of aCL antibodies in healthy populations is 1% to 6%.

Diagnostic Testing

- Three types of assays are available to detect aPL:
  ○ The **LAC** is a misnomer; it was characterized by in vitro prolongation of clotting, but it confers a hypercoagulable state in vivo. It is not a specific analyte but a lab phenomenon, which may be found in conditions other than SLE (see Chapter 5, Laboratory Evaluation of Rheumatic Diseases). Assays for the LAC include the **dilute Russell viper venom time, activated partial thromboplastin time (aPTT), kaolin clotting time, and tissue thromboplastin inhibition;** none has a >70% sensitivity to detect all LAC antibodies. Mixing normal platelet-poor plasma with the patient's plasma will not correct an LAC-associated prolonged aPTT, as it would in a patient with a factor deficiency, but addition of excess phospholipids will.
  ○ The **aCL and anti–β-2gpI antibodies** are measured by enzyme-linked immunosorbent assay (ELISA) and reported by isotypes (IgG, IgA, IgM) and titers.

TABLE 39-2	REVISED CLASSIFICATION CRITERIA FOR DIAGNOSIS OF ANTIPHOSPHOLIPID SYNDROME

Definite antiphospholipid syndrome is considered to be present if at least one of the clinical criteria and one of the laboratory criteria are met.[a]

Clinical criteria:

- **Vascular thrombosis:** ≥1 clinical episodes of venous, arterial, or small-vessel thrombosis in any tissue or organ, which must be confirmed by imaging or Doppler studies or by histopathology, with the exception of superficial venous thrombosis; or histopathologic confirmation, thrombosis should be present without significant evidence of inflammation in the vessel wall.

Pregnancy morbidity:

- ≥1 unexplained deaths of a morphologically normal fetus at or beyond the 10th week of gestation, with normal fetal morphology documented by ultrasound or by direct examination of the fetus, or
- ≥1 premature births of a morphologically normal neonate at or before the 34th week of gestation because of severe preeclampsia or eclampsia or severe placental insufficiency, or
- ≥3 unexplained consecutive spontaneous abortions before the 10th week of gestation, with maternal anatomic or hormonal abnormalities and paternal and maternal chromosomal causes excluded.

Laboratory criteria:

- **Lupus anticoagulant** present in plasma, on ≥2 occasions at least 12 weeks apart, detected according to the guidelines of the International Society on Thrombosis and Haemostasis.
- **Anticardiolipin antibody** of IgG and/or IgM isotype in blood, present in medium or high titer, on ≥2 occasions, at least 12 weeks apart, measured by a standardized enzyme-linked immunosorbent assay.
- **Anti–β2 glycoprotein-I** antibody of IgG and/or IgM isotype in blood, present in titer >99th percentile), on ≥2 occasions, at least 12 weeks apart, measured by a standardized enzyme-linked immunosorbent assay.

---

[a]Classification of APS should be avoided if less than 12 weeks or more than 5 months separate the positive aPL test and clinical manifestation.

Adapted from: Miyakis S, Lockshin MD, Atsumi T, et al. International consensus statement on an update of the classification criteria for definite antiphospholipid syndrome (APS). *J Thromb and Haemost.* 2006;4;295–306.

IgG and IgM antibodies are clinically significant at high titer (>99th percentile) and have high specificity for the diagnosis of APS.

- The diagnostic criteria require the presence of the LAC or medium- to high-titer aCL antibodies or high-titer anti–β-2gpI antibodies to be present on at least two occasions, at least 12 weeks apart. **False positive syphilis serology** also represents aPL antibody, but is not included in the criteria.
- Other lab tests to consider in the evaluation of the patient include complete blood count (CBC) and blood chemistries, to evaluate for renal and liver dysfunction. Radiologic studies (CT/MRI) are helpful to assess damage and guide management.

TREATMENT

Prevention of thrombosis is a major goal of therapy in patients with aPL antibodies. Therapy is divided into two clinical settings: Primary prophylaxis (aPL carriers without previous thrombosis) and secondary prophylaxis (patients with APS who have already had a thrombotic event).

Medications

Primary Prophylaxis

- Primary prophylaxis can be considered in purely asymptomatic individuals (who had testing done for unclear reasons), patients with SLE, or women with obstetric APS.
- Healthy patients with high aPL titers but no manifestation of thromboses are advised to take **aspirin** (325 mg PO daily) as prophylaxis. While it is not currently known if this benefits patients with aPL but no underlying autoimmune disease, studies have shown a protective effect in patients with SLE and aPL.[6,7]
- On the basis of data from animal models and indirect evidence from human studies, **hydroxychloroquine** 400 mg PO daily, has been found to be protective against future thrombosis by decreasing the titers of aPL; more studies are needed to determine whether this should be recommended for healthy patients with aPL.[8]

Secondary Prophylaxis

- For patients with documented thrombotic events, long-term intensive anticoagulation is recommended on the basis of the type of thrombotic event.
- **Venous event:** Unfractionated IV **heparin followed by warfarin,** with a goal international normalized ratio (INR) of 2.5 (range 2.0–3.0) is the treatment of choice for patients presenting with a first venous event.[1,2,9]
  - The optimal duration of anticoagulation for prevention of recurrent thrombosis is unknown, but the risk of recurrence appears to be highest in the 6-month period after discontinuing anticoagulant drugs. To date, **the general consensus is to treat indefinitely with anticoagulation.**[2,9]
  - **Recurrent venous thrombosis** has been reported from 3% to 24% per year. If recurrent thrombosis occurs despite adequate anticoagulation, high intensity anticoagulation is recommended (INR range 3.0–4.0), or warfarin (INR 2.0–3.0) plus aspirin, or, if unstable INR, switching to low–molecular weight heparin is recommended.
- **Arterial event:** Arterial events most commonly involve the cerebral circulation (i.e., transient ischemic attack, stroke) and less commonly myocardial infarction or other arterial thrombosis. Evidence for treatment of these groups is controversial and lacks prospective randomized control trials. Current therapy includes **aspirin** only (325 mg/day) or **warfarin** therapy at moderate (goal INR 2.0–3.0) or high (goal INR 3.0–4.0) dose.[2,9–11]
- **Pregnancy morbidity prevention:** The optimal treatment of pregnant women with aPL and recurrent fetal loss without thrombosis is controversial. Current recommendations suggest that combination aspirin and heparin therapy increases the chance of a successful pregnancy in women with aPL and recurrent fetal loss.[10]
  - **Aspirin** (81 mg/day) should be started when attempting conception and heparin should be started when intrauterine pregnancy is confirmed. Both should be discontinued late in the third trimester.

- ○ **Heparin** can be dosed as either **unfractionated** (5000–10,000 units q12h) or **low molecular weight** as enoxaparin 1 mg/kg or 40–80 mg, dalteparin 5000 units, or nadroparin 3800 units all administered once daily during pregnancy.
  - ○ Historically, pregnant patients were treated with prednisone, but due to significant side effects of hyperglycemia, preeclampsia, diabetes, and infection, as well as lack of compelling benefit, this is no longer recommended.
- **Catastrophic APS** is a distinct clinical entity manifesting as multisystem organ failure with clinical evidence of vessel occlusion developing simultaneously or in <1week. Histopathology confirms small-vessel occlusion in at least one organ or tissue. Laboratory tests show presence of aPL. The mortality rate is high (30%–50%) and recent guidelines recommend combination therapy with the following:[12]
  - ○ Treatment of precipitating factors (e.g., infection, underlying SLE flare, etc).
  - ○ Effective anticoagulation with IV **heparin** for 7 to 10 days or longer, depending on patient response.
  - ○ **High-dose steroids** (methylprednisolone 1000 mg IV daily) for 3 or more days.
  - ○ **IV immune globulin** (0.4 gm/kg body weight daily for 4–5 days) and/or plasma exchange (removal of 2–3 liters of plasma for at least 3–5 days) are used, with the goal of removing aPL and replenishing natural clotting factors through fresh frozen plasma (FFP) replacement with exchange. Of note, thrombosis with intravenous immunoglobulin use has been reported, so it needs to be cautiously given, especially when delivered rapidly or when anticoagulation needs to be interrupted.
  - ○ If ineffective, alternative therapies for catastrophic APS with reported success include cyclophosphamide (in patients with SLE, not patients with primary APS) and rituximab (in patients with thrombocytopenia or autoimmune hemolytic anemia).[12]

Lifestyle/Risk Modification

- Lifestyle modifications are recommended in both patients with APS and patients with asymptomatic aPL. This includes **smoking cessation, avoidance of supplemental estrogens, and controlling hypertension and diabetes.**
- The greatest morbidity and mortality are seen in women with a history of arterial thrombotic events who become pregnant, so such patients should be **advised not to become pregnant.**

REFERENCES

1. Cohen D, Berger SP, Steup-Beekman GM, et al. Diagnosis and management of the antiphospholipid syndrome. *BMJ.* 2010;340:1125–1132.
2. Ruiz-Irastorza G, Crowther M, Branch W, et al. Antiphospholipid syndrome. *Lancet.* 2010;376:1498–1509.
3. Matsuura E, Shen L, Matsunami Y, et al. Pathophysiology of B2-glycoprotein I in antiphospholipid syndrome. *Lupus.* 2010;19:379–384.
4. Chen PP, Giles I. Antibodies to serine proteases in the antiphospholipid syndrome. *Curr Rheumatol Rep.* 2010;12:45–52.
5. Miyakis S, Lockshin MD, Atsumi T, et al. International consensus statement on an update of the classification criteria for definite antiphospholipid syndrome (APS). *J Thromb Haemost.* 2006;4:295–306.

6. Hereng T, Lambert M, Hachulla E, et al. Influence of aspirin on the clinical outcomes of 103 anti-phospholipid antibodies-positive patients. *Lupus.* 2008;17:11–15.

7. Erkan D, Harrison MJ, Levy R, et al. Aspirin for primary thrombosis prevention in the antiphospholipid syndrome: a randomized double-blind, placebo-controlled trial in asymptomatic antiphospholipid antibody-positive individuals. *Arthritis Rheum.* 2007;56:2382–2391.

8. Petri M. Hydroxychloroquine use in the Baltimore lupus cohort: effects on lipids, glucose, and thrombosis. *Lupus.* 1996;5:S16–S22.

9. Finazzi G, Marchioli R, Brancaccio V, et al. A randomized clinical trial of high intensity warfarin vs. conventional antithrombotic therapy for the prevention of recurrent thrombosis in patients with the antiphospholipid syndrome (WAPS). *J Thromb Haemost.* 2005;3:848–853.

10. Lim W, Crowther M, Eikelboom JW. Management of antiphospholipid antibody syndrome: a systematic review. *JAMA.* 2006;295:1050–1057.

11. Derksen R, de Groot PG. Towards evidence-based treatment of thrombotic antiphospholipid syndrome. *Lupus.* 2010;19:470–474.

12. Cervera R. Update on the diagnosis, treatment, and prognosis of the catastrophic antiphospholipid syndrome. *Curr Rheumatol Rep.* 2010;12:70–76.

Mixed Connective Tissue Disease

40

Reeti Joshi and Amy Joseph

GENERAL PRINCIPLES

Definition

- Mixed connective tissue disease (MCTD) is a unique connective tissue disease with **overlapping features of systemic sclerosis (SSc), systemic lupus erythematosus (SLE), and polymyositis (PM)**, along with the presence of **antibodies to U1 ribonucleoprotein (RNP)**.
- It was first described by Sharp and colleagues in 1972 in a subset of 25 patients with these overlapping features.
- Initially it was thought to have a benign nature and steroid responsiveness. Subsequent longitudinal studies have shown that in some patients it may not be a benign disease.

Epidemiology and Risk Factors

- Prevalence of MCTD is thought to be 10/100,000 with a female to male ratio of 10:1. It does not show the relative preponderance in African-Americans that is seen in SLE.
- Occupational exposure to vinyl chloride has been described as a risk factor.
- It is associated with HLA-DR4, DR1, and less prominently DR2.

Pathogenesis

- The *sine qua non* of MCTD is an antibody against U1-RNP, one of the major components of the spliceosome.
- The pathogenicity of anti–U1-RNP has not been confirmed, but high-titer anti–U1-RNP is present in most MCTD patients. U1-RNP antibodies in MCTD are directed against a 70 kD polypeptide linked noncovalently to U1-RNA in the spliceosome.
- Anti–U1-RNP antibodies are thought to induce cytokine and adhesion molecule production by binding to endothelial cells. This could lead to vascular disease pathogenesis, such as Raynaud's phenomenon (RP), puffy hands, sclerodactyly, pulmonary hypertension, and possibly interstitial lung disease (ILD) and esophageal dysmotility.[1]
- Alternatively, U1-RNP antibodies could form immune complexes which activate complement to induce myositis, arthritis, and perhaps ILD.
- T cells appear to have a central role in the pathogenesis of MCTD and activation of the innate immune system via Toll-like receptor signaling, autoantibody production, and autoantigen presentation. CD4 T lymphocytes provide differentiation factors that induce B-cell isotype gene switching, and mediate tissue injury via cytokines.[1]

DIAGNOSIS

Clinical Features

- Patients have clinical features of SLE, SSc, and PM, although the features of each might occur at different times over the course of the disease.
- **Polyarthritis** affects most patients with MCTD and is often a presenting feature. Fifty to seventy percent are rheumatoid factor (RF) positive and some have erosive disease.
- **Myalgias and myositis** range from mild to severe and can be histologically indistinguishable from PM or SLE.
- **Swollen or puffy fingers,** acrosclerosis, or sclerodactyly can be seen.
- **RP** is seen in MCTD, with findings on nailfold capillaroscopy similar to those seen in scleroderma.
- **Pulmonary hypertension is the leading cause of death** in MCTD. Blood vessels have intimal hyperplasia (plexiform lesion) and smooth muscle hypertrophy.[2]
- Other pulmonary manifestations of MCTD include **ILD,** pleural effusion, alveolar hemorrhage, diaphragmatic dysfunction, pulmonary vasculitis, and thromboembolic disease.
- **Gastroesophageal reflux disease (GERD)** and **esophageal dysmotility** occur in MCTD, similar to that of scleroderma.
- Additional features may include malar or discoid rash, hemolytic anemia, leukopenia, thrombocytopenia, secondary Sjögren's syndrome trigeminal neuralgia, pericarditis, renovascular hypertension, and glomerulonephritis.

Diagnostic Criteria

- There is no American College of Rheumatology (ACR) criteria for MCTD.
- The criteria developed by both Alarcon-Segovia and Kahn have moderate sensitivity and good specificity.[3] Their criteria include high-titer U1-RNP antibodies in the appropriate clinical setting.
  - ○ Alarcon-Segovia's clinical criteria require three or more of the following clinical features, one of which must be synovitis or myositis: swollen hands, synovitis, myositis, RP and acrosclerosis.
  - ○ Kahn's clinical criteria require the presence of RP plus at least two of the following: swollen fingers, synovitis, and myositis.

Diagnostic Testing

Characteristic immunologic findings include speckled pattern fluorescent antinuclear antibody (ANA) in high titers and antibodies to U1-RNP in moderate to high titer. Fifty to seventy percent are RF positive.

Differential Diagnosis

The differential diagnosis includes SLE, SSc, PM, and rheumatoid arthritis (RA). Of note, up to 20% of SLE patients also have anti–U1-RNP antibody positivity but these are frequently associated with anti-Sm antibodies.

TREATMENT

The mainstay of therapy remains treatment of underlying organ involvement, on the basis of data extrapolated from SLE, RA, myositis, or SSc and presented in Table 40-1.[4]

TABLE 40-1	THERAPY OF MIXED CONNECTIVE TISSUE DISEASE BY ORGAN SYSTEM	
Organ System	**Clinical Manifestation**	**Treatment**
Mucocutaneous	Rashes and oral ulcers	Photoprotection, topical steroids, emollient, hydroxychloroquine
	Raynaud's phenomenon, digital ulcers	Gloves and warm clothing, smoking cessation, calcium-channel blockers, digital sympathectomy, topical nitroglycerin, low-dose aspirin, pentoxifylline, phosphodiesterase-5 inhibitors, direct arterial vasodilators (bosentan, prostaglandin-infusion therapy)
Gastrointestinal	Gastroesophageal reflex, esophageal dysmotility	H2 antagonists, proton pump inhibitors, prokinetics
	Vasculitis	High-dose glucocorticoids, cyclophosphamide
Respiratory: Arterial	Pulmonary arterial hypertension	Calcium-channel blockers, phosphodiesterase-5 inhibitors, prostacyclin, treprostinil, bosentan
Respiratory: Parenchymal	Interstitial lung disease	High-dose glucocorticoids followed by cyclophosphamide, azathioprine, mycophenolate mofetil
Musculoskeletal	Arthritis	Nonsteroidal anti-inflammatory drugs (NSAIDs), hydroxychloroquine, methotrexate; the use of anti-tumor necrosis factor (TNF) agents is not recommended
	Myositis	Glucocorticoids, hydroxychloroquine, azathioprine
Cardiovascular	Pericarditis	High doses of NSAIDs and varying doses of steroids; cyclophosphamide for severe cases

(continued)

TABLE 40-1	THERAPY OF MIXED CONNECTIVE TISSUE DISEASE BY ORGAN SYSTEM (*Continued*)	
Organ System	**Clinical Manifestation**	**Treatment**
Renal	Glomerulonephritis	Angiotensin-converting enzyme (ACE) inhibitors, glucocorticoids, cyclophosphamide, chlorambucil, or mycophenolate mofetil
	Scleroderma renal crisis	ACE inhibitors
Hematologic	Anemia, leukopenia, thrombocytopenia	Glucocorticoids, danazol, intravenous immunoglobulin, splenectomy
	Thrombotic thrombocytopenia purpura	Plasma exchange, immunosuppressants
Neuropsychiatric	Vascular headaches	Aspirin, NSAIDs, low-dose tricyclic antidepressants
	Transverse myelitis	Pulse glucocorticoids and cyclophosphamide or azathioprine

Adapted from: Kim P, Grossman JM. Treatment of mixed connective tissue disease. *Rheum Dis Clin N Am.* 2005;31:549–565.

PROGNOSIS

The inflammatory features (e.g., arthritis, serositis, myositis) of the disease tend to predominate early in disease course, and fibrotic ones (e.g., esophageal dysmotility, pulmonary hypertension, ILD) later. The overall **prognosis is highly variable.**

REFERENCES

1. Hoffman RW, Maldonado ME. Immune pathogenesis of mixed connective tissue disease: a short analytical review. *Clin Immunol.* 2008;128:8–17.
2. Bull TM, Fagan KA, Badesh DB. Pulmonary vascular manifestations of mixed connective tissue disease. *Rheum Dis Clin North Am.* 2005;31:451–464.
3. Amiques JM, Cantagrel A, Abbal M, et al. Comparative study of 4 diagnosis criteria sets for mixed connective tissue disease in patients with anti-RNP antibodies. Autoimmunity Group of the Hospitals of Toulouse. *J Rheumatol.* 1998;25:393–394.
4. Kim P, Grossman JM. Treatment of mixed connective tissue disease. *Rheum Dis Clin North Am.* 2005;31:549–565.

Undifferentiated Connective Tissue Disease

Rebecca Brinker and Amy Joseph

GENERAL PRINCIPLES

- Undifferentiated connective tissue disease (UCTD) is also known as early lupus, latent lupus, or incomplete lupus.
- 30% of patients develop a definite connective tissue disease (CTD) within the first 3 to 5 years of diagnosis. Transition into a definitive CTD decreases each year from the time of diagnosis.[1]
  - The most common CTD to develop is **systemic lupus erythematosus (SLE).**
  - Patients with predominant skin manifestations, such as discoid lupus, alopecia, and photosensitivity, have a greater chance of evolving into SLE.
- 70% of patients who remain classified as UCTD are considered to have stable UCTD.

Definition

- UCTD is a condition in which a patient possesses clinical manifestations and serologic markers suggestive of an autoimmune process but **fails to fulfill the classification criteria** for a definite CTD.
- This diagnosis is **distinct from overlap syndrome,** which occurs when a patient possesses criteria for more than one rheumatologic diagnosis.

Epidemiology

Few reliable epidemiologic data are available because of lack of criteria for diagnosis but the following have been noted:

- UCTD is significantly more prevalent in females.[1]
- Onset typically occurs between 32 and 44 years of age.[1]

Etiology/Pathophysiology

The cause of UCTD is not well understood but it is thought to be caused by immune dysregulation in a genetically susceptible host.

Risk Factors

Risk factors include female gender and having a family history of autoimmune disease.

DIAGNOSIS

Clinical Presentation

- UCTD physical manifestations are generally mild.
- **Raynaud's phenomenon** is a typical feature of UCTD but nailfold capillaroscopy is normal.

- **Inflammatory arthritis** is often a prominent feature but is nonerosive. No reliable studies have evaluated patients for the presence of synovitis or effusions.
- A **nonspecific rash** may be present and on biopsy this typically shows interface dermatitis.

History
- Fever
- Mild to moderate Raynaud's phenomenon
- Diffuse arthralgias
- Oral or nasal ulcerations
- Nonspecific rash with or without photosensitivity
- Alopecia
- Sicca symptoms
- Chest pain with reclining or deep inhalation

Physical Examination
- Dry oral and nasal mucosa
- Nonspecific rash
- Hair loss
- Mild inflammatory arthritis
- Digital color changes consistent with Raynaud's phenomenon

Diagnostic Criteria

There are no commonly accepted diagnostic criteria but the following are often used to aid in diagnosis:

- Signs and symptoms suggestive of a CTD are present but **without fulfilling any specific CTD criteria** and with a duration of at least 3 years in the setting of **positive antinuclear antibodies** (ANA).[2]
- Proposed exclusion criteria included malar rash, cutaneous lupus, skin sclerosis, heliotrope rash, Gottron's plaques, erosive arthritis, and specific antibodies (anti-double stranded DNA [dsDNA], anti-Sm, anti–Scl-70, anticentromere, anti-SSB/La, anti-Jo1, and anti–Mi-2).[3]
- Neurologic involvement is almost always absent.
- Kidney involvement is almost always absent.
- Leukopenia is often present.
- Arthritis is nonerosive and arthralgias are a prominent feature.

Differential Diagnosis

The differential of UCTD includes: Mixed CTD, SLE, Sjögren's syndrome, scleroderma, rheumatoid arthritis (RA), polymyositis/dermatomyositis, vasculitis, and fibromyalgia.

Diagnostic Testing

Laboratory
- Immunologic:[1]
  - **ANA is positive in approximately 90% of patients.**
  - Anti-SSA/Ro and anti-ribonucleoprotein (RNP) are the most commonly positive specific autoantibodies.
  - Up to 80% of patients have only a single stable autoantibody.

○ Patients with homogenous ANA, anti-dsDNA, anti-SSA/Ro, anti-Sm, or anticardiolipin antibodies are more likely to develop SLE.
- Hematologic findings are rarely severe enough to warrant treatment. The most common finding is **leukopenia** but anemia and thrombocytopenia have also been observed.

Imaging
No imaging is specifically required for diagnosis. However, imaging may be completed to help rule out other diagnoses such as RA.

Diagnostic Procedures
Nailfold capillaroscopy will reveal normal capillaries.

TREATMENT

Medications
Medications are directed against specific manifestations of the disease. There are no formal studies on medications used for the treatment of UCTD but the following are often used.

First Line
- **Nonsteroidal antiinflammatory drugs (NSAIDs)** are the mainstay of therapy. They are used to reduce pain and inflammation, and to treat arthralgias.
- **Hydroxychloroquine** is most commonly used to treat patients with myalgias and arthralgias resistant to NSAID monotherapy and to treat mucocutaneous manifestations.
- **Corticosteroids** may be used for disease resistant to the above treatment or for disease flares. Recommended length of corticosteroid treatment varies. The patient should be treated with the lowest dose for the shortest period of time possible to minimize corticosteroid side effects.

Second Line
Immunosuppressive medications are reserved for rare severe systemic disease with internal organ involvement.

Non-pharmacologic Therapies
- Physical therapy and exercise.
- Decrease sun exposure if photosensitive rash is present.
- Decrease exposure to cold and stress if Raynaud's phenomenon is present.

REFERRAL

Possible referrals depend on the patient's manifestation, but may include rheumatology, dermatology, hematology, and neurology.

MONITORING AND FOLLOW-UP

- Review signs and symptoms of UCTD at each visit in an effort to screen for progression to definite CTD.

- Periodically check complete blood count (CBC), serum chemistries, and urinalysis to monitor for the development of CTD.

PROGNOSIS

- 30% of patients develop definitive CTD and outcomes are then determined by the CTD diagnosis.[1]
- A large number of patients only require intermittent symptomatic treatment.
- Up to 20% of patients have symptoms that subside over time.
- Internal organ involvement is very rare.

REFERENCES

1. Mosca M, Tani C, Talarico R, et al. Undifferentiated connective tissue diseases (UCTD): Simplified systemic autoimmune diseases. *Autoimmun Rev.* 2011;10:256–258.
2. Musca M, Neri R, Bombardieri S. Undifferentiated connective tissue diseases (UCTD): a review of the literature and a proposal for preliminary classification criteria. *Clin Exp Rheumatol.* 1999;17:615–620.
3. Doria A, Mosca M, Gambari PF, et al. Defining unclassifiable connective tissue diseases: incomplete, undifferentiated, or both? *J Rheumatol.* 2005;32:213–215.

Adult-Onset Still's Disease

42

Amy Archer and John P. Atkinson

GENERAL PRINCIPLES

Definition

- Adult-onset Still's disease (AOSD) is a rare inflammatory condition consisting of a constellation of clinical and laboratory findings that are similar to those of systemic juvenile arthritis (Still's disease).
- AOSD is characterized by **spiking fevers, arthritis, and an evanescent rash** that occurs concurrently with the febrile periods.

Epidemiology

- The incidence of AOSD is estimated to be 0.16 to 0.40 new cases per 100,000 patients per year, depending on the population.[1,2]
- It occurs in a bimodal distribution, most commonly between the age of 15 and 25 and 36 and 46. However, cases of AOSD have been reported in patients over 60 years old.
- There is no gender predilection.

Pathophysiology

It is speculated that an immune-mediated mechanism as well as a number of viral and bacterial infections play a role in its pathophysiology.[3]

DIAGNOSIS

AOSD is a diagnosis of exclusion.

Clinical Presentation

History

- Patients can present with myriad symptoms.
- The dominant manifestation is a **spiking fever,** often greater than 39 °C. The fever classically follows a **quotidian** (daily) or **double quotidian** (twice a day) pattern of peaks, often with an afebrile period between spikes. The fevers typically occur in the late afternoon or evening and may follow a regular cycle.
- Coincident with fevers is the appearance of a characteristic **transitory salmon-colored rash.**
- **Arthritis and arthralgias** involving the knees, wrists, ankles, proximal interphalangeal (PIP) joints, elbows, and shoulders are common manifestations of AOSD.[4] However, synovitis may not be present at the onset and patients may never develop inflammatory arthritis.
- Patients can also present primarily with myalgias.

Physical Examination

- The salmon-colored macular or maculopapular rash may be difficult to identify on routine examination given its transient nature. It is usually found on the trunk or extremities and may be precipitated by rubbing (the **Koebner phenomenon**).
- **Oligoarticular joint involvement** is usually gradual in onset and mild in nature but may progress to a more destructive arthritis.
- Additional clinical findings may include **pharyngitis, lymphadenopathy, splenomegaly, hepatomegaly,** and **cardiopulmonary involvement** (pericarditis, pleural effusions, and pulmonary infiltrates).

Diagnostic Criteria

- The diagnosis of AOSD is a diagnosis of exclusion.
- The Yamaguchi criteria for AOSD are presented in Table 42-1.[5]
- These criteria carry an estimated sensitivity of 93% when five of the features are present with at least two from the major criteria.

Differential Diagnosis

The differential diagnosis includes **granulomatous disorders, vasculitis, connective tissue diseases** (systemic lupus erythematous, mixed connective tissue disease), **malignancy** (lymphoma, leukemia), and **infection** (viral or bacterial). The more prolonged the clinical course, in the absence of another definitive diagnosis, the more likely the diagnosis will be AOSD.

Diagnostic Testing

Although laboratory and radiographic abnormalities may lend support to the diagnosis of AOSD, no test alone is specific for the disease.

TABLE 42-1 YAMAGUCHI CRITERIA FOR ADULT STILL'S DISEASE[a]

Definitive diagnosis requires at least two major and three minor criteria.

Major criteria:
- Fever of ≥39 °C for ≥1 week
- Arthralgias or arthritis for ≥2 weeks
- Characteristic rash
- Leukocytosis (>10,000 cells/mm^3) with a predominance of neutrophils

Minor criteria:
- Pharyngitis
- Lymphadenopathy
- Hepatomegaly/splenomegaly
- Abnormal liver tests
- Negative ANA and RF

---

[a]Exclusion criteria: Current infection, malignancy (especially lymphoma), and other active rheumatologic diseases.

ANA, antinuclear antibody; RF, rheumatoid factor.

Adapted from: Yamaguchi M, Ohta A, Tsunematsu T, et al. Preliminary criteria for classification of adult Still's disease. *J Rheumatol.* 1992;19:424–430.

Laboratory

- The complete blood count (CBC) usually reveals a **leukocytosis** with a predominance of neutrophils; a normocytic, normochromic anemia; and thrombocytosis.
- **Erythrocyte sedimentation rate (ESR) and C-reactive protein (CRP) are almost always considerably elevated,** which is consistent with an inflammatory condition.
- Liver enzymes often demonstrate mild elevations of aminotransferases, alkaline phosphatase, and lactate dehydrogenase (LDH).
- **Serum ferritin levels can be markedly elevated.**
  - Elevated ferritin levels usually correlate with disease activity and have been proposed as markers of treatment response.
  - Levels between 3,000 and 30,000 are common and levels greater than 250,000 have been reported.
  - The proportion of **glycosylated ferritin is low** and this may also be a clue to diagnosis.[6,7] Hemophagocytic lymphohistiocytosis is also associated with hyperferritinemia and a low percentage of glycosylation.[8]
- Antinuclear antibodies (ANAs) and rheumatoid factor (RF) are usually negative but may be present in low titers. Anti-cyclic citrullinated protein (CCP) antibodies are almost always negative.[9]

Imaging

- Radiographic findings in AOSD are relatively uncommon.
- A nonerosive **narrowing of the carpometacarpal joints and the intercarpal spaces** within the wrist (with sparing of metacarpophalangeal joints) may be seen, which can lead to ankylosis of the wrist. Other joints may uncommonly be involved.

Diagnostic Procedures

- **Lymph node biopsies** display a large range of nonspecific histologic changes including typical/atypical paracortical hyperplasia, vascular proliferation, histiocyte aggregation, exuberant immunoblastic reaction, and follicular hyperplasia.[10] Clearly, such findings could be confused with lymphoproliferative disorders but immunohistochemistry can be used to differentiate.
- Skin biopsy reveals a nonspecific mild perivascular inflammation of the superficial dermis with infiltration of lymphocytes and histiocytes.
- Joint fluid aspiration shows a leukocytosis with neutrophil predominance.

TREATMENT

Medications

- **Nonsteroidal antiinflammatory drugs (NSAIDs)** are effective in most patients with AOSD for relief of mild to moderate inflammatory symptoms. Indomethacin and naproxen may be more efficacious than salicylates. Monitoring for renal, hepatic, and gastrointestinal (GI) toxicity is recommended.[3,4]
- **Corticosteroids** are indicated for severe inflammatory manifestations. Oral prednisone, dosed at 0.5 to 1 mg/kg daily or IV methylprednisolone followed by oral prednisone, is usually effective.[3,4]
- Small studies suggest that oral **methotrexate** is effective as a steroid-sparing agent. Polyarthritis, in particular, often responds to methotrexate.[3,4,11]

- Observational evidence suggests that hydroxychloroquine, azathioprine, cyclophosphamide, cyclosporine, IV immunoglobulin, etanercept, infliximab,[12] anakinra,[13] abatacept,[14] tocilizumab,[15] and rituximab may be useful in the treatment of AOSD.
- Sulfasalazine has been associated with a high rate of toxicity and should be avoided.[16]

Other Non-pharmacologic Therapies

Local joint injections with steroids may provide symptomatic relief.

COMPLICATIONS

Patients with AOSD have been noted to develop reactive/secondary **hemophagocytic lymphohistiocytosis** (also known as the hemophagocytic syndrome or macrophage activation syndrome),[17] cardiac tamponade, acute hepatic failure, myocarditis, amyloidosis, disseminated intravascular coagulation (DIC), interstitial lung disease and pulmonary hypertension.

REFERRAL

Patients can benefit from the input of physiotherapists, occupational therapists, psychologists and/or arthritis support groups.

OUTCOME/PROGNOSIS

- The course of AOSD is variable. Approximately one-third of patients experiences a complete resolution within a year of onset. One-third will experience a cyclic relapsing and remitting pattern of the disease. The remaining one-third experiences a chronic active disease, which is often associated with destructive arthritis similar to rheumatoid arthritis.
- Factors associated with a poor prognosis include disease refractory to corticosteroids, polyarthritis, and a persistently elevated ferritin.
- Factors associated with a good prognosis are a prompt resolution of clinical and laboratory abnormalities, and lack of a relapse as steroids are reduced (usually over a 2–3 month period).

REFERENCES

1. Magadur-Joly G, Billaud E, Barrier JH, et al. Epidemiology of adult Still's disease: estimate of the incidence by a retrospective study in west France. *Ann Rheum Dis.* 1995;54:587–590.
2. Evensen KJ, Nossent HC. Epidemiology and outcome of adult-onset Still's disease in Northern Norway. *Scand J Rheumatol.* 2006;35:48–51.
3. Efthimiou P, Georgy S. Pathogenesis and management of adult-onset Still's disease. *Semin Arthritis Rheum.* 2006;36:144–152.
4. Efthimiou P, Paik PK, Bielory L. Diagnosis and management of adult onset Still's disease. *Ann Rheum Dis.* 2006;65:564–572.
5. Yamaguchi M, Ohta A, Tsunematsu T, et al. Preliminary criteria for classification of adult Still's disease. *J Rheumatol.* 1992;19:424–430.

6. Vignes S, Le Moël G, Fautrel B, et al. Percentage of glycosylated serum ferritin remains low throughout the course of adult onset Still's disease. *Ann Rheum Dis.* 2000;59:347–350.

7. Fautrel B, Le Moël G, Saint Marcoux B, et al. Diagnostic value of ferritin and glycosylated ferritin in adult onset Still's disease. *J Rheumatol.* 2001;28:322–329.

8. Lamboote O, Cacoub P, Costedoat N, et al. High ferritin and low glycosylated ferritin may also be a marker of excessive macrophage activation. *J Rheumatol.* 2003;30:1027–1028.

9. Riera E, Olivé A, Narváez J, et al. Adult onset Still's disease: review of 41 cases. *Clin Exp Rheumatol.* 2001;29:331–336.

10. Jeon YK, Paik JH, Park SS, et al. Spectrum of lymph node pathology in adult onset Still's disease; analysis of 12 patients with one follow up biopsy. *J Clin Pathol.* 2004;57:1052–1056.

11. Manger B, Rech J, Schett G. Use of methotrexate in adult-onset Still's disease. *Clin Exp Rheumatol.* 2010;28:S168–S171.

12. Fautrel B, Sibilia J, Mariette X, et al. Tumour necrosis factor alpha blocking agents in refractory adult Still's disease: an observational study of 20 cases. *Ann Rheum Dis.* 2005;64:262–266.

13. Laskari K, Tzioufas AG, Moutsopoulos HM. Efficacy and long-term follow-up of IL-1R inhibitor anakinra in adults with Still's disease: a case-series study. *Arthritis Res Ther.* 2011;13:R91.

14. Quartuccio L, Maset M, De Vita S. Efficacy of abatacept in a refractory case of adult-onset Still's disease. *Clin Exp Rheumatol.* 2010;28:265–267.

15. Perdan-Pirkmajer K, Praprotnik S, Tomšič M. A case of refractory adult-onset Still's disease successfully controlled with tocilizumab and a review of the literature. *Clin Rheumatol.* 2010;29:1465–1467.

16. Jung JH, Jun JB, Yoo DH, et al. High toxicity of sulfasalazine in adult-onset Still's disease. *Clin Exp Rheumatol.* 2000;18:245–248.

17. Hot A, Toh ML, Coppéré B, et al. Reactive hemophagocytic syndrome in adult-onset Still disease: clinical features and long-term outcome: a case-control study of 8 patients. *Medicine (Baltimore).* 2010;89:37–46.

Relapsing Polychondritis

43

Lesley Davila and John P. Atkinson

GENERAL PRINCIPLES

Definition

Relapsing polychondritis (RP) is a rare disease characterized by recurrent inflammation of cartilaginous structures, most commonly the outer ear, nose, tracheobronchial tree, and peripheral and axial joints. RP can also affect other proteoglycan-rich structures (e.g., the eye, heart, vessels, and inner ear).

Epidemiology

- RP occurs mostly in Caucasian patients aged 40 to 60 years.
- It tends to occur with equal frequencies in both sexes but, some case series report a female predominance.
- About one-third of cases is associated with either a myelodysplastic syndrome or an autoimmune disease, including primary systemic vasculitides and connective tissue diseases (CTD).[1,2]

Etiology/Pathophysiology

- The etiology of RP is unknown, but strong evidence suggests that RP is caused by an immune-mediated attack on cartilaginous structures. Both humoral and cell-mediated mechanisms are thought to be involved.
- 20% to 50% of patients have serum antibodies to collagen II, which is normally found in large amounts in cartilage. These antibodies are also found in other autoimmune diseases so their detection is not a useful clinical test.
- HLA-DR4 has been associated with increased risk for RP.

Associated Conditions

- RP is also associated with a number of **vasculitides, CTDs** especially rheumatoid arthritis (RA) and systemic lupus erythematosus (SLE), and **hematologic and autoimmune diseases.**
- These include most other rheumatic diseases and CTDs, myelodysplastic syndromes, lymphoma, pernicious anemia, acute leukemias, hypothyroidism, Hashimoto thyroiditis, Graves' disease, ulcerative colitis, myasthenia gravis, primary biliary cirrhosis, and diabetes mellitus.[1,2]

DIAGNOSIS

The main manifestations of RP are otorhinolaryngeal disease, respiratory compromise, arthritis, and ocular inflammation.

Clinical Presentation

- The most common symptom is **auricular chondritis.**
  - ○ It is characterized by the sudden onset of unilateral or bilateral auricular swelling, pain, warmth, and erythema or violaceous discoloration.
  - ○ The inflammation affects the cartilaginous structures of the ear with sparing of the lobes, which do not contain cartilage.
  - ○ The episode usually resolves, with or without treatment, within days or weeks.
  - ○ Recurrent attacks result in soft, nodular, and deformed ears.
- RP causes conductive and/or neurosensory **hearing loss** in approximately 50% of patients.
  - ○ Conductive hearing loss is caused by collapse of auricular cartilage or by swelling of the external auditory canal or Eustachian tubes. Serous or purulent otitis media can also occur.
  - ○ Neurosensory hearing loss is caused by vasculitis of the cochlear branch of the internal auditory artery.
- Vasculitis of the vestibular branch is also common, resulting in **vertigo, ataxia,** nausea, and vomiting.
  - ○ If acute, these symptoms can mimic a posterior circulation stroke.
  - ○ Although the hearing loss is often permanent, vestibular symptoms usually improve.
- **Nasal chondritis** occurs in approximately 50% of patients.
  - ○ It is more common in women and in those <50 years.
  - ○ It presents as nasal pain, a sensation of nasal and adjacent tissue fullness, and, occasionally, epistaxis.
  - ○ Recurrent attacks may result in saddle nose deformity.
- **Respiratory tract involvement** is the main cause of death in some case series.
  - ○ Inflammation of the cartilage in the larynx, trachea, and bronchial tree causes hoarseness, throat pain, difficulty talking, aphonia, dyspnea, cough, stridor, wheezing, and choking.
  - ○ Obstruction can occur in varying degrees and at different levels.
    - ▪ Total obstruction of the upper airways can occur from attempted bronchoscopy, intubation, or tracheostomy.
    - ▪ Involvement of the lower airways is often asymptomatic until detected by radiographs, bronchoscopy, or spirometry.
  - ○ Respiratory infections are common and result from impaired drainage of secretions caused by airway collapse and impaired mucociliary function.
  - ○ Parenchymal pulmonary disease is not a feature of RP.
- **Arthritis** is the second most common manifestation of RP.
  - ○ It is a presenting symptom in 30% of patients and occurs in up to 80% of patients during the course of disease.
  - ○ The arthritis is nondeforming and nonerosive.
  - ○ The most commonly affected joints are the metacarpophalangeal (MCP), proximal interphalangeal (PIP), knee, ankle, wrist, and metatarsophalangeal (MTP).
  - ○ Acute monoarthritis and tenosynovitis can also occur.
- The **eye** is involved in approximately 50% of patients.
  - ○ Eye inflammation is more common in men and is frequently associated with systemic manifestations.
  - ○ Inflammation affects any part of the eye, most commonly as scleritis, episcleritis, keratoconjunctivitis sicca, and peri-orbital edema. Uveitis, keratitis, corneal thinning, proptosis (from inflammation of posterior globe elements) and retinal vasculitis can also occur.

- **Systemic vasculitis** occurs in up to one-quarter of patients with RP. Large, medium, and small vessels may be affected.
  - ○ In some patients, vasculitis appears to be due to the primary disease process and in others it is a separate but associated condition.
  - ○ Described vasculitides include Takayasu's arteritis, polyarteritis nodosa, Henoch–Schönlein purpura, Wegener's granulomatosis, Behçet's syndrome, microscopic polyangiitis, cutaneous vasculitis, and urticarial vasculitis.
  - ○ The overlap between Behçet's syndrome and RP is sometime referred to as "MAGIC" syndrome (mouth and genital ulcers with inflamed cartilage).[3]
- The **kidney** is affected in approximately 15% of patients. The most common histopathologic findings are mild mesangial proliferation and focal segmental necrotizing glomerulonephritis caused by glomerular deposition of C3, IgG, and IgM.
- **Skin** involvement occurs in approximately 20% of cases. Palpable purpura, urticaria, and angioedema are the most common cutaneous manifestations. Livedo reticularis, migratory superficial thrombophlebitis, erythema nodosum, erythema multiforme, and panniculitis are rare.
- **Cardiovascular** involvement includes aortic and mitral inflammation with subsequent aortic root dilatation, valvulitis, papillary muscle dysfunction, valvular regurgitation, cardiomyopathy, and atrioventricular conduction blocks.

Diagnostic Criteria

The original criteria proposed by McAdam et al. for RP with modifications suggested by Damiani et al. are presented in Table 43-1.[2,4]

Differential Diagnosis

- The differential diagnosis depends on manifestations of RP.
- The auricular chondritis resembles infectious cellulitis of bacterial origin. Sparing of the earlobe is a diagnostic clue but biopsy is helpful for culture and histology. Recurrence of relapsing "bacterial infection" of the outer ear should always raise suspicion for RP.

TABLE 43-1	PROPOSED McADAM'S DIAGNOSTIC CRITERIA FOR RELAPSING POLYCHONDRITIS

Diagnosis requires (1) three or more of the following criteria OR (2) one or more of the following with cartilage biopsy compatible with chondritis OR (3) chondritis in two or more separate locations that responds to steroids or dapsone.

- Recurrent bilateral auricular chondritis
- Nonerosive inflammatory polyarthritis
- Nasal chondritis
- Ocular inflammation defined as conjunctivitis, keratitis, scleritis, episcleritis, or uveitis
- Respiratory tract chondritis (laryngeal and/or tracheal cartilage)
- Cochlear and/or vestibular dysfunction (e.g., neurosensory hearing loss, tinnitus and/or vertigo)

Adapted from: McAdam LP, O'Hanlan MA, Bluestone R, et al. Relapsing polychondritis: prospective study of 23 patients and a review of the literature. *Medicine (Baltimore)*. 1976;55:193–215.

- Saddle nose deformity and laryngotracheal chondritis can be mistaken for Wegener's granulomatosis, although RP is confined strictly to cartilaginous portions of the airways. Antineutrophil cytoplasmic antibodies (ANCA) are negative in RP. Trauma, lymphoma, and syphilis should also be considered.
- The arthritis can mimic RA.
- Ocular symptoms and arthritis can be mistaken for some of the seronegative spondyloarthropathies.

Diagnostic Testing

Laboratories

Laboratory findings of RP are nonspecific markers of inflammation: elevated ESR, normochromic normocytic anemia of chronic inflammation, leukocytosis, thrombocytosis, and hypergammaglobulinemia.

Imaging

- ECG or echocardiography should be considered if valve disease is suspected.
- CT or other imaging should be done of the neck and lungs to assess the laryngotracheobronchial tree.

Diagnostic Procedures

Spirometry with inspiratory and expiratory volume curves should be performed and may show various dynamic intrathoracic or extrathoracic obstructive patterns.

TREATMENT

Treatment is aimed at prevention of flares and managing complications of the disease.

Medications

First Line

- Corticosteroids are the main form of therapy for RP.
- Oral prednisone, 1 mg/kg daily, is often necessary to suppress inflammation. The dose can be decreased on the basis of clinical response to the lowest necessary dose.
- Pulse IV methylprednisolone 1000 mg daily for 3 days followed by daily PO prednisone, is used for acute airway closure.

Second Line

- Recommendations for therapy are based on rather limited data and are, therefore, empiric in nature.
- Other immunosuppressants have been tried as steroid-sparing drugs, with methotrexate possibly being the most effective.[5,6]
- Other treatments (e.g., dapsone, colchicine, azathioprine, cyclosporine, penicillamine, and plasma exchange) have been tried and seem to be less effective.
- On the basis of other data and case reports regarding RP patients, focal segmental glomerulonephritis may be successfully treated with steroids and either daily PO or monthly IV cyclophosphamide.[7–10]
- Recently, anti-tumor necrosis factor (anti-TNF) agents such as etanercept, adalimumab, and infliximab have been used with some success for refractory disease.[11–13]
- The interleukin (IL)-1 inhibitor anakinra has also been reported to be effective in refractory disease.[14]

Surgical Management

Surgical management of respiratory tract RP includes tracheostomy or bronchial stent placement. Iatrogenic trauma may cause complete obstruction.

OUTCOME/PROGNOSIS

- Most patients experience intermittent episodes of inflammation and develop some degree of disability (e.g., bilateral deafness, impaired vision, phonation difficulties, or cardiorespiratory problems).
- Follow-up involves clinical assessment of disease activity with careful attention to the pulmonary status.
- Associated conditions such as CTD or hematologic abnormalities may develop at any point in the disease course.

REFERENCES

1. Saif MW, Hopkins JL, Gore SD. Autoimmune phenomena in patients with myelodysplastic syndromes and chronic myelomonocytic leukemia. *Leuk Lymphoma.* 2002;43:2083–2092.
2. McAdam LP, O'Hanlan MA, Bluestone R, et al. Relapsing polychondritis: prospective study of 23 patients and a review of the literature. *Medicine (Baltimore).* 1976;55:193–215.
3. Kötter I, Deuter C, Günaydin I, et al. MAGIC or not MAGIC–does the MAGIC (mouth and genital ulcers with inflamed cartilage) syndrome really exist? A case report and review of the literature. *Clin Exp Rheumatol.* 2006;24:S108–S112.
4. Damiani JM, Levine HL. Relapsing polychondritis—report of ten case. *Laryngoscope.* 1997;89:929–946.
5. Park J, Gowin KM, Schumacher HR Jr. Steroid sparing effect of methotrexate in relapsing polychondritis. *J Rheumatol.* 1996;23:937–938.
6. Trentham DE, Le CH. Relapsing polychondritis. *Ann Intern Med.* 1998;129:114–122.
7. Lahmer T, Treiber M, von Werder A, et al. Relapsing polychondritis: an autoimmune disease with many faces. *Autoimmun Rev.* 2010;9:540–546.
8. Ruhlen JL, Huston KA, Wood WG. Relapsing polychondritis with glomerulonephritis. Improvement with prednisone and cyclophosphamide. *JAMA.* 1981;245:847–848.
9. Rotey A, Navasa M, del Olmo A, et al. Relapsing polychondritis with segmental necrotizing glomerulonephritis. *Am J Nephrol.* 1984;4:375–378.
10. Chang-Miller A, Okamura M, Torres VE, et al. Renal involvement in relapsing polychondritis. *Medicine (Baltimore).* 1987;66:202–217.
11. Richez C, Dumoulin C, Coutouly X, et al. Successful treatment of relapsing polychondritis with infliximab. *Clin Exp Rheumatol.* 2004;22:629–631.
12. Lahmer T, Knoph A, Treiber M, et al. Treatment of relapsing polychondritis with the TNF-alpha antagonist adalimumab. *Clin Rheumatol.* 2010;29:1331–1334.
13. Carter JD. Treatment of relapsing polychondritis with a TNF antagonist. *J Rheumatol.* 2005;32:1413.
14. Vounotrypidis P, Sakellariou GT, Zisopoulos D, et al. Refractory relapsing polychondritis: rapid and sustained response in the treatment with an IL-1 receptor antagonist (anakinra). *Rheumatology.* 2006;45:491–492.

Deposition and Storage Arthropathies

Hyon Ju Park and Zarmeena Ali

44

- Arthropathies can result from deposition of **normal materials like metal ions** or from accumulation of **abnormally processed biochemical intermediates.** Arthropathy is often the initial presentation of storage and deposition diseases.
- Due to storage and deposition arthropathies being relatively rare, they are often mistaken for more common diseases like osteoarthritis (OA) and rheumatoid arthritis (RA).
- Given the systemic nature of these arthropathies, an accurate diagnosis is important to guide appropriate therapy.

HEMOCHROMATOSIS

GENERAL PRINCIPLES

Definition

Hemochromatosis is a disease characterized by **excessive body iron stores** and the visceral **deposition of hemosiderin** in susceptible organs (i.e., liver, adrenal glands, heart, skin, gonads, joints, and pancreas).

Classification

- **Genetic or hereditary hemochromatosis** (HH) is an **autosomal recessive** disorder. More than 90% of patients with HH possess a **C282Y mutation of the HFE gene.** Individuals who are heterozygous for C282Y HFE mutation may have an increased risk for hand OA.
- **Secondary hemochromatosis** occurs in the setting of prolonged excessive iron ingestion or repeated blood transfusions in patients with chronic hypoproliferative anemia, sickle cell anemia, and thalassemia. End-organ damage due to secondary hemochromatosis tends to be milder than that of HH.

Epidemiology

- The incidence is fairly common, one in 200 to 300 people.
- HH affects men more than women (10:1) with age of onset delayed in women secondary to regular iron loss through menstruation. Median age of men is about 50, while median age of women is the mid-60s at presentation.
- Patients of European descent are six times more likely to develop HH than blacks.

Pathophysiology

- HFE gene mutation leads to **increased intestinal iron absorption and decreased hepcidin expression** in the liver, resulting in iron deposition in hepatocytes and other viscera.
- The pathogenesis of HH arthropathy is unknown but there is speculation that ionic iron inhibits pyrophosphatase activity leading to pseudogout arthropathy.

Associated Conditions

Patients with HH also have an increased susceptibility to certain infectious diseases caused by siderophilic microorganisms such as *Vibrio, Yersinia, Listeria,* and *Escherichia coli.*

DIAGNOSIS

Clinical Presentation

- Patients with HH can present with **cirrhosis, adrenal insufficiency, heart failure, diabetes, or polyarthropathy.**
- **Chronic progressive arthritis,** mechanical in nature, is a frequent complaint (about 50%) and often predates other symptoms of iron overload.
  - ○ **Second and third metacarpophalangeal (MCP) and proximal interphalangeal (PIP)** joints are the most common joints affected (about 50%) with the **dominant hand** either solely or more severely involved.
  - ○ On examination, joints are not inflamed but are mildly tender with slightly decreased range of motion.
  - ○ Larger joints like shoulders, hips, and knees may also be affected.
  - ○ **Chondrocalcinosis** is a late but characteristic feature of arthropathy seen in HH and can manifest as episodes of acute monoarticular arthritis.

Diagnostic Testing

Laboratories

Diagnosis is based on detection of HFE genotype in the setting of elevated ferritin (300–1000 mg/L) and transferrin saturation greater than 45%.[1]

Imaging

- Radiologic changes resemble OA with **irregular joint space narrowing and sclerotic cyst formation.** HH arthropathy has less osteophytosis and no involvement of carpometacarpal (CMC) joints as classically seen in OA.
- There may be isolated ulnar styloid erosions.
- **Chondrocalcinosis** may be the sole abnormality in about 50% of patients with HH arthropathy.

TREATMENT

- Treatment is aimed at reduction of iron load using **phlebotomy and iron chelators.** However, **reduction in body iron stores has little effect on HH arthropathy.**

- Symptoms are managed much like OA with **acetaminophen, nonsteroidal antiinflammatory drugs (NSAIDs), physical therapy, and local steroid injections.**
- Limiting alcohol and red meat intake while increasing consumption of substances that inhibit iron absorption like high tannin teas may be of benefit.

WILSON'S DISEASE

GENERAL PRINCIPLES

Definition

Wilson's disease, also known as **hepatolenticular degeneration,** is an autosomal recessive disorder resulting in **excess copper accumulation.**

Epidemiology

- Incidence is one in 30,000 to 40,000.
- Age at presentation ranges from 6 to 40 years.

Pathophysiology

- Wilson's disease is caused by mutations in the **ATP7B gene,** which is translated into a **membrane-bound copper-transporting ATPase.**
- Membrane-bound copper-transporting ATPase deficiency leads to **excess copper accumulation affecting liver, kidney, brain, and joints.**
- Pathogenesis of arthropathy is unclear but its severity does not correlate with neurologic, hepatic, or renal disease. By elemental analysis, copper has been found in the synovium of Wilson's disease patients and is thought to contribute to the development of arthropathy.

DIAGNOSIS

Clinical Presentation

- Patients presenting before the age of 20 usually have **progressive hepatic failure.** Patients presenting after their 20s tend to have more **psychiatric or neurologic manifestations.**
- Arthropathy tends to be mild and is present in about 50% of patients.
  - ○ Joint manifestations are **similar to those of OA** with mechanical pain and crepitus.
  - ○ Commonly affected joints include knees, shoulders, ankles, and spine, but feet, wrists, and neck can be involved. Hip and MCP involvement is rare.
- **Kayser–Fleischer rings** are present in more than 99% of patients if neurologic or psychiatric symptoms are present. The presence of Kayser–Fleischer rings on slit-lamp examination supports the diagnosis of Wilson's disease.

Diagnostic Testing

Laboratories
- Although **serum ceruloplasmin** is the cheapest test, it is low only in 90% of Wilson's patients.
- **24-hour urine copper** (>100 μg/day) has greater than 98% sensitivity but can easily be contaminated or collected improperly.
- Genetic testing is currently not useful because of the large number of inactivating mutations.
- The "gold standard" for diagnosis is a **liver biopsy** with quantitative copper assays.

Imaging
- Radiographic changes seen resemble OA with **irregular joint space narrowing, sclerotic cyst** formation, and **marked osteophyte formation** with often calcified loose bodies seen predominately at the wrist.
- Generalized osteoporosis is seen in 50% of patients.

TREATMENT

- Treatment is aimed at reduction of copper load using **chelation therapy.** Penicillamine was previously the chelator of choice but due to its toxicity, it has been supplanted by **zinc and trientine (triethylenetetramine).**[2]
- Avoidance of high copper food items including mushrooms, nuts, chocolate, shellfish, and liver is recommended.
- Arthropathy is managed with local therapy as symptoms are mild. **Acetaminophen and NSAIDs should be used with great caution in patients with liver and possible renal tubular acidosis.**

OCHRONOSIS (ALKAPTONURIA)

GENERAL PRINCIPLES

Definition
Alkaptonuria is a rare autosomal recessive disorder resulting from a **deficiency of homogentisic acid oxidase (HGO).**

Epidemiology
- Incidence is one in 200,000.
- An unusually high incidence has been found in an area of Germany near the Czech border, presumably as a result of consanguineous mating.

Pathophysiology
- A loss of function mutation leading to a complete deficiency of HGO leads to **accumulation of homogentisic acid,** a normal intermediate in tyrosine metabolism.
- **Homogentisic acid deposits as a pigmented polymer in the cartilage, skin, and sclerae.**
- The pigmented polymers penetrate into bone, synovium, and joint cavity, possibly triggering formation of osteochondral bodies.

DIAGNOSIS

Clinical Manifestation

- Diagnosis is suspected in patients who develop **early OA in atypical joints** or in those complaining of passing **dark urine.**
- Patients usually present with **progressive degenerative arthropathy** involving **spine and larger peripheral joints** beginning in their late 30s or early 40s. Hands and wrists are usually spared.[3]
- Stiffness and loss of joint mobility lead to severe disability but arthritis is non-inflammatory and nonerosive in nature.
- Cutaneous manifestations are common later in life and include **slate-blue or gray discoloration of sclerae, pinnae, nose, axillae, and groin.**
- Pigment may also appear in perspiration, staining clothes.
- Prostatic and renal calculi may form. Cardiac valvular pigment deposits are rare but may contribute to degeneration of valves.

Diagnostic Testing

Laboratories

- Diagnosis is supported by **fragments of darkly pigmented cartilage seen as black specks in synovial fluid,** patient's urine turning black upon oxidation or alkalinization, or darkly pigmented synovium seen incidentally during arthroscopy.
- Diagnosis is confirmed by quantification of **homogentisic acid in serum and urine.**
- Genetic testing is available but usually not necessary for diagnosis.

Imaging

- The earliest radiologic changes are **multiple vacuum discs** of the spine. Disease progresses with **calcification of the discs** with narrowing, collapse, and even autofusion of the vertebral discs. Sacroiliac (SI) and apophyseal joints are spared.
- Radiographs of knees, hips, shoulders will show **changes much like OA** with joint space narrowing, marginal osteophytes, and subchondral cysts. Pigmented cartilage is radiolucent.

TREATMENT

- Current available therapy is supportive only. This includes **NSAIDs, physical therapy,** protection of joints from overuse injury and weight reduction.
- **Nitisinone, an agent blocking an earlier step in tyrosine metabolism,** has been shown to decrease urinary excretion of homogentisic acid. In a small trial, six out of seven patients who received nitisinone for more than 1 week reported significant improvement in their joint pain.[4] There is an ongoing larger trial evaluating for long-term safety and efficacy.
- **Arthroplasty** of knees or hips is reserved for the most severe cases.

MULTICENTRIC RETICULOHISTIOCYTOSIS

GENERAL PRINCIPLES

Definition

Multicentric reticulohistiocytosis (MRH) is a rare dermatoarthritis primarily affecting middle-aged women and is characterized by cellular accumulation of **glycolipid-laden histiocytes in joints and in skin.**

Pathophysiology

- Etiology is unknown but is thought to involve an often self-limited inflammatory reaction triggered by autoimmunity, malignancy, and infections.[5]
- Some studies have also demonstrated an increase in tumor necrosis factor (TNF)-α in blood and tissue.
- MRH is **associated with autoimmune diseases** like scleroderma, Sjögren's syndrome, and dermatomyositis in about 10% to 15% of cases.
- At diagnosis, up to 30% of patients were found to have a **concomitant malignancy.**
- Up to 25% of patients were reported to have been exposed to **tuberculosis** in the 6 months before being diagnosed with MRH. Five percent of patients were found to have active tuberculosis at diagnosis.

DIAGNOSIS

Clinical Manifestation

- In 60% of cases, patients present with **arthritis as their initial sign of disease.**[6]
- MRH arthritis is a **severe symmetric, erosive, inflammatory polyarthritis predominately affecting hands, wrists, and knees.**
- Active synovitis is seen on examination and hence, is most often mistaken for aggressive seronegative RA. However, MRH tends to destroy **both the distal interphalangeals (DIPs) and PIPs prior to significant destruction of the MCPs.**
- **Cutaneous manifestations** comprise **papulonodular lesions** ranging from a few millimeters to a centimeter in diameter. The lesions are scattered and isolated well-circumscribed, round, yellow-brown nodules preferentially affecting fingers, nailfolds, and oral and nasal mucosa.

Diagnostic Testing

Diagnosis is made by **skin or synovial biopsy** demonstrating the presence of numerous **multinucleated giant cells and histiocytes** with an abundant eosinophilic, finely granular cytoplasm (glycolipids).

Imaging

Hand radiographs may show articular **punched out lesions** like gouty tophi but these will rapidly progress to severe joint destruction and even **arthritis mutilans.**

TREATMENT

- When not associated with a malignancy, MRH **spontaneously resolves** in an average time period of about 8 years in most patients.
- Systemic steroids, cyclophosphamide, chlorambucil, or methotrexate may prevent further joint destruction and cause skin lesions to regress.
- Antimalarials have also been used.
- TNF antagonists' use is anecdotal.

LYSOSOMAL STORAGE DISEASES

- There are more than 30 different lysosomal storage diseases, which are classified on the basis of their accumulated material.
- Most are diagnosed during infancy and childhood, with **a few milder forms presenting in adulthood.**
- Gaucher's disease and Fabry's disease are two of the more common lysosomal storage diseases with arthritic manifestations. They will be briefly reviewed but further details are beyond the scope of this manual.

GAUCHER'S DISEASE

- Gaucher's disease is an **autosomal recessive** disorder resulting from defective activity of **lysosomal β-glucosidase** leading to accumulation of glucocerebroside in the reticuloendothelial system.[7]
- **Painless splenomegaly** is a common presenting feature.
- Patients have infiltration of bone marrow by lipid-laden macrophages (Gaucher cells), which can lead to **cortical bone destruction, infarction, and necrosis of long bones.**
- Marrow involvement spreads proximal to distally in limbs and may involve the spine causing vertebral collapse.
- Patients can develop acute "bone crises" due to sudden ischemia of infiltrated bone and cause excruciating pain and erythema in the affected area. Fever simulating osteomyelitis or septic arthritis may also be seen. Bone remodeling is also defective leading to **osteoporosis, osteonecrosis, and vertebral compression fractures.**
- Diagnosis is based on leukocyte β-glucosidase levels.
- Treatment of significantly affected patients is with enzyme replacement therapy with modified glucocerebroside. Enzyme replacement is effective in diminishing hematologic findings. Bone pain and disease decrease with enzyme replacement. Bisphosphonates are used as adjunctive therapy for osteoporosis and pain.

FABRY'S DISEASE

- Fabry's disease is an **X-linked** disorder resulting in mutations in the α-**galactosidase** gene leading to accumulation of glycosphingolipids in nerves, viscera, and osteoarticular tissues.
- Disease manifestations include hypohidrosis, corneal and lenticular opacities, acroparesthesia, angiokeratomas, and small vessel disease of kidneys, brain, and heart.

- Patients develop **degenerative polyarthritis** involving shoulders, knees, hips, wrists, and hands with significant flexion contractures of DIPs.
- Enzyme replacement therapy is effective for renal and cardiac disease only at early stages. **Enzyme replacement therapy does not impact joint disease.** Management of joint disease is palliative.

REFERENCES

1. Beutler E, Felitti VJ, Koziol JA, et al. Penetrance of 845G→ A (C282Y) HFE hereditary haemochromatosis mutation in the USA. *Lancet.* 2002;359:211–218.
2. Roberts EA, Schilsky ML; American Association for Study of Liver Diseases (AASLD). Diagnosis and treatment of Wilson disease: an update. *Hepatology.* 2008;47:2089–2011.
3. Yancovitz M, Anolik R, Pomeranz MK. Alkaptonuria. *Dermatol Online J.* 2010;16:6.
4. Suwannarat P, O'Brien K, Perry MB, et al. Use of nitisinone in patients with alkaptonuria. *Metabolism.* 2005;54:719–728.
5. Baghestani S, Khosravi F, Dehghani Zahedani M, et al. Multicentric reticulohistiocytosis presenting with papulonodular skin eruption and polyarthritis. *Eur J Dermatol.* 2005;15:196–200.
6. Santilli D, Lo Monaco A, Cavazzini PL, et al. Multicentric reticulohistiocytosis: a rare cause of erosive arthropathy of the distal interphalangeal finger joints. *Ann Rheum Dis.* 2002;61:485–487.
7. Harmanci O, Bayraktar Y. Gaucher disease: new developments in treatment and etiology. *World J Gastroenterol.* 2008;14:3968–3973.

Sarcoid Arthropathy

45

Lesley Davila and Leslie E. Kahl

GENERAL PRINCIPLES

Definition

- Sarcoidosis is a **granulomatous inflammatory disease** of unknown etiology that can involve any organ, most commonly the lung, skin, eye, and joints.
- The **lung is the most commonly involved organ,** occurring in over 80% of patients. Patients usually present with fatigue and pulmonary symptoms (e.g., cough, dyspnea, and chest pain).
- Extrapulmonary involvement frequently accompanies the pulmonary symptoms. Lymph nodes, liver, and spleen are frequently involved. Heart, kidney, and pancreas are less commonly involved.
- Sarcoidosis of the musculoskeletal system occurs in 15% to 25% of patients.
- This chapter will focus mainly on musculoskeletal manifestations of sarcoidosis.

Classification

- **Acute sarcoid arthritis** occurs most commonly as a **polyarthritis of the ankles, knees, elbows, and wrists.**
  - ○ Erythema, warmth, swelling, and tenderness of joints occur.
  - ○ Involvement is usually **symmetrical,** and **periarticular swelling,** rather than joint effusions, is common.
  - ○ Acute arthritis commonly occurs in the presence of **erythema nodosum and acute uveitis.**
  - ○ Acute arthritis usually lasts several weeks to months and often does not recur.
- **Löfgren's syndrome** is the triad of acute arthritis, erythema nodosum, and bilateral hilar adenopathy. It usually has good prognosis.
- **Chronic sarcoid arthritis** is rare, presenting several months after the onset of disease.
  - ○ It commonly involves the knee but also can involve the ankles and proximal interphalangeal (PIP) joints. This arthritis is not associated with erythema nodosum.
  - ○ Periosteal bone resorption appears as cysts.
  - ○ Joint destruction can occur rarely with shortening and deformity of the phalanges.
- **Muscle and bone involvement** is also common in sarcoidosis.
  - ○ Sarcoidosis affects the muscle in the form of **myopathy, atrophy, myositis, or palpable nodules.** Asymptomatic granulomatous involvement of the muscles is documented frequently at autopsy.
  - ○ Sarcoidosis causes **lytic and sclerotic lesions in the bone,** both of which can be painful. Typically, lesions occur in the hands and feet but can potentially

involve any bone. Along with bone resorption, the lesions contribute to a high risk of fracture in sarcoid patients.

Epidemiology

- The prevalence of sarcoidosis is 10 to 20 cases/100,000 population.
- The incidence is higher among blacks than other races.
- The disease also varies by geographic region and may have a genetic component.
- Sarcoidosis occurs most commonly in patients aged 20 to 40 years.

Etiology

The underlying etiology of sarcoidosis is not known. Evidence exists for genetic, environmental, and infectious associations.[1]

Pathophysiology

- Sarcoidosis is characterized pathologically as the presence of **noncaseating granulomas** in affected organs. This process has been best characterized in the lung.
- The earliest clinical manifestation is a mononuclear infiltration of CD4+ T cells into the organ, which then organizes into noncaseating granulomas.
- Over time the granulomas can heal without sequelae or undergo fibrosis leading to organ dysfunction.

Associated Conditions

Sarcoidosis has been described in association with other autoimmune disorders, including rheumatoid arthritis, systemic lupus erythematosus, Sjögren's syndrome, and psoriatic arthritis.

DIAGNOSIS

Clinical Presentation

- Clinical manifestations of sarcoidosis vary depending on which organ systems are involved. It may be easy to diagnose sarcoidosis in a patient with bilateral hilar adenopathy, pulmonary infiltrates, or characteristic skin and eye involvement, but more difficult if arthritis is the only manifestation.
- A thorough history and physical examination is important to identify any extra-articular manifestations that can lead to the proper diagnosis.
- Löfgren's syndrome (i.e., bilateral hilar adenopathy, erythema nodosum, and acute arthritis) is a common initial clinical presentation of sarcoidosis.
- Bone involvement in chronic arthritis is commonly asymptomatic but pain and soft tissue swelling over affected areas (joints or bones) can occur.
- Skin lesions may be the first manifestation to occur. They most commonly present as papules around the eyelids and nasolabial folds or in old scars. Larger subcutaneous nodules, plaques, or indurated purplish facial lesions (lupus pernio) may also occur.

Differential Diagnosis

- The differential diagnosis will vary depending on the symptoms manifested by individual patients.

- Patients with Löfgren's syndrome have a primarily lower extremity inflammatory arthritis, which may also be seen in reactive arthritis or infectious arthritides (viral, gonococcal). Septic arthritis should always be considered if monoarticular or acute in nature.
- In patients with significant lymphadenopathy, **infections and malignancy** should be excluded.
- Sarcoidosis can also manifest with pulmonary infiltrates, myositis, and vasculitis and rheumatologic causes of those symptoms should be considered as well.

Diagnostic Testing
Laboratories
- Erythrocyte sedimentation rate (ESR) and C-reactive protein (CRP) can be elevated but are not specific for sarcoidosis.
- Serum **angiotensin converting enzyme (ACE) levels** are high in three-fourths of untreated patients; however, false positives occur frequently and **limit diagnostic utility.**
- **Hypercalcemia** and more often **hypercalciuria** occur due to dysregulated calcitriol metabolism.
- 1,25-dihydroxyvitamin D levels may also be elevated.

Imaging
- Chest radiograph findings in sarcoidosis include **bilateral hilar lymphadenopathy, diffuse parenchymal changes,** or a combination of both. CT or MRI can be used to better characterize the lung and mediastinum, especially in a patient with suspected Löfgren's syndrome and a normal chest radiograph.
- Joint radiographs in acute arthritis can be normal or show soft tissue swelling. In patients with chronic arthritis or bone involvement, radiographs can be striking.
  - Characteristic bone involvement involves bilateral metacarpals, metatarsals, and phalanges, although any bone can be affected, even vertebra.
  - Radiographs of affected hands show **subchondral lesions or cysts** that sometimes can extend into joint spaces. The bone itself can have a lacy-reticulated appearance from granulomatous involvement.

Diagnostic Procedures
- **Biopsy** of the affected organ(s) is the most effective way to demonstrate the noncaseating granulomas.
  - Biopsy of lymph nodes, skin, and lacrimal glands often yields diagnostic histology.
  - Biopsy of lung tissue requires fiberoptic bronchoscopy with transbronchial lung biopsy.
  - Biopsy is required for diagnosis if any other diagnoses (e.g., tuberculosis) are being considered, as treatment is vastly different.
  - Synovial biopsy occasionally reveals granulomas but is not often performed.
- **Arthrocentesis** of an involved joint can be performed and is characterized by noninflammatory synovial fluid in both acute and chronic forms of arthritis.

TREATMENT

- The decision to medicate patients for sarcoidosis should be based on clinical assessment of disease activity.

- There is some controversy regarding whom to treat, because **sarcoidosis clears spontaneously in approximately 50% of patients.**
- The choice to use corticosteroids is typically guided by persistence of symptoms for >2 to 3 months, unless there is significant respiratory impairment or worrisome symptoms (e.g., eye involvement, significant heart involvement, neurologic impairment, or severe fevers, fatigue, and weight loss).

Medications

There are no FDA-approved treatments for sarcoidosis or any of its manifestations. Large randomized clinical trials have not been performed and treatments are based on case reports and unblinded case series.

First Line

- Mild joint symptoms often can be controlled with **nonsteroidal antiinflammatory drugs** (NSAIDs).
- **Corticosteroids** are effective for patients with moderate to severe symptoms, including musculoskeletal symptoms. Although corticosteroid therapy clearly reduces inflammation and symptoms attributable to disease, there is a paucity of data regarding the optimal dose and duration of treatment.
  - For severe vital organ dysfunction initial doses of prednisone 1 mg/kg/day PO for 4 to 6 weeks are used, followed by slow tapering.
  - Löfgren's syndrome can be treated with observation, NSAIDs, or low doses of prednisone (10–20 mg/day) depending on severity of symptoms.
  - Disease can often recur after withdrawal of steroids, requiring reinitiation of therapy.
  - In patients who have relapse of disease on prednisone or are unable to taper prednisone to a tolerable dose (5–10 mg/day), second line agents can be considered.

Second Line

- **Methotrexate** has been successfully used to treat pulmonary and extrapulmonary manifestations of sarcoidosis at doses similar to those used in rheumatoid arthritis.
- **Antimalarials** (hydroxychloroquine and chloroquine) have also been used to treat extrapulmonary manifestations successfully.
- There may be a role for other medications such as leflunomide, sulfasalazine, and minocycline.
- The use of **anti-tumor necrosis factor** (TNF) **medications** is controversial. Preliminary evidence suggests that infliximab and adalimumab may be efficacious in pulmonary and extrapulmonary sarcoidosis.[2] However, many case reports and series show that sarcoidosis (pulmonary and extrapulmonary) can develop in patients treated with these medications for other diagnoses.[3]

OUTCOME/PROGNOSIS

- Sarcoidosis **clears spontaneously** in approximately 50% of patients. Relapse of spontaneous remission is rare and most (90%) of the patients have remission with few sequelae.
- In patients with chronic sarcoidosis, morbidity, and mortality are often from sequelae of long-term prednisone use and pulmonary or cardiac involvement.

REFERENCES

1. Sweiss N, Patterson K, Sawaqued R, et al. Rheumatologic manifestations of sarcoidosis. *Semin Respir Crit Care Med.* 2010;31:463–473.
2. Baughman RP, Drent M, Kavuru M, et al. Infliximab therapy in patients with chronic sarcoidosis and pulmonary involvement. *Am J Respir Crit Care Med.* 2006;174:795–802.
3. Clementine RR, Lyman J, Zakem J, et al. Tumor necrosis factor-alpha antagonist-induced sarcoidosis. *J Clin Rheumatol.* 2010;16:274–279.

Amyloidosis and Amyloid Arthropathy

46

Rebecca Brinker and Zarmeena Ali

GENERAL PRINCIPLES

- Amyloidosis is a disorder characterized by deposition of various protein subunits in extracellular tissue.
- Disease manifestations depend on the tissue distribution, concentration of deposits, and specific precursor protein leading to fibril formation.
- There are four classes of **systemic amyloidosis.** However, only primary (AL) and secondary (AA) systemic amyloidosis will be discussed in detail here. Hereditary amyloidosis and hemodialysis-related amyloid β-2-microglobulin (AB2M) are the remaining two types.
- Alzheimer's disease is an example of isolated (brain) amyloidosis and is one of the most common forms of **isolated amyloidosis.**
- At this time, 27 different proteins precursors of amyloid fibrils have been identified. These proteins are not all structurally similar. Therefore, consideration must be given to the role of cofactors, such as glucosaminoglycans, apolipoproteins, and serum amyloid P component (SAP) in the pathologic formation of these fibrils.
- **Amyloid arthropathy** is infrequent but occurs in up to 5% of patients with amyloidosis from multiple myeloma (MM).

Definition/Classification

- Amyloid fibrils are extracellular insoluble polymers comprised of various low molecular weight protein subunits.
- The subunits are composed of soluble precursors which undergo conformational change leading to the formation of predominately **insoluble antiparallel β-pleated sheets** that deposit in tissues.
- Most protein fibrils weigh from 5 to 25kD.
- **Primary amyloidosis:**
  - Also known as **immunoglobulin light chain (AL) amyloidosis.**
  - This group includes all forms of systemic amyloidosis in which the fibrils are derived from **monoclonal light chains.** Causal conditions include to monoclonal gammopathy of undetermined significance (**MGUS**), MM, and **Waldenström's macroglobulinemia (WM).**
  - It may be distinguished from a similar disorder, **light chain deposition disease (LCDD)** by the fact that fibril formation of monoclonal light chains does not occur in LCDD.
- **Secondary amyloidosis:**
  - Also known as serum **amyloid A (AA) amyloidosis.**
  - It is characterized by extracellular tissue deposition of fragments of an **acute phase reactant protein, serum amyloid A.**

Epidemiology

- AL amyloidosis is more common in developed countries and AA amyloiodosis is more common in second and third world countries.
- The increased incidence of AA amyloid in developing countries is thought to be secondary to a higher burden of chronic infections promoting long-standing inflammation.

Pathophysiology

- Except for in Alzheimer's disease, where direct cell cytotoxicity from amyloid is observed, other systemic manifestations and organ dysfunction from amyloidosis are thought to be secondary to mechanical disruption by the plaques.
- **Primary amyloid is a clonal plasma cell proliferative disorder** that results in monoclonal **light chain** fibril deposition in multiple organs. Seventy-five percent are derived from the λ light chain variable region and the remaining 25% are derived from the κ light chain variable region.
- **Secondary amyloid** is characterized by extracellular tissue deposition of fragments of an acute phase reactant protein, serum amyloid A.
- **Hemodialysis related amyloidosis** is a result of β-2-microglobulin deposition.

Risk Factors

- Primary amyloid: blood cell dyscrasias including MGUS, MM, WM, and non-Hodgkin's lymphoma.
- Secondary amyloid: chronic inflammatory states including infection, inflammatory disorders, and autoimmune diseases. Susceptibility to developing the amyloidosis relies on genetic and environmental factors.
- Hereditary amyloid:
  - Most familial mutations are autosomal dominant missense mutations that alter the precursor proteins.
  - Almost all hereditary mutations cause kidney, nervous system, and cardiac disease.
  - A significantly higher prevalence of these diseases is seen in patients of Turkish decent.

Associated Conditions

- Primary amyloid is often associated with **plasma cell dyscrasias.** Most classically, MM. (11;14)(q13;32) translocation is frequently found in MM or MGUS patients.
- Secondary amyloid is associated with **systemic inflammatory conditions.**
  - Chronic Infections: tuberculosis, osteomyelitis, and leprosy.
  - Autoimmune: rheumatoid arthritis, juvenile rheumatoid arthritis, ankylosing spondylitis, familial Mediterranean fever (FMF), psoriatic arthritis, and Sjögren's syndrome.
  - It is less commonly seen as a complication of non-Hodgkins lymphoma, Castleman's disease, intravenous drug abuse, systemic lupus erythematosus, and renal failure requiring chronic dialysis.

DIAGNOSIS

Amyloidosis may often be able to be diagnosed in the appropriate clinical setting, but definitive diagnosis requires tissue biopsy.

Clinical Presentation

- Primary amyloid most classically present with **nephrotic range proteinuria** (from deposition of protein in the glomerulus), **edema, hepatosplenomegaly, right-sided heart failure, and carpal tunnel syndrome.**
  - ○ Central nervous system (CNS) disease is almost never seen, but peripheral nervous system involvement manifested by autonomic instability may occur.
  - ○ **Cardiac involvement** is insidious and often advanced at the time of diagnoses. It may result in **dilated or restrictive cardiomyopathy.**
  - ○ The most common **gastrointestinal (GI) manifestations** are stomach and small intestinal bleeding from ulcers, polyps, or hematomas, and motility disorders such as dysphagia, gastroparesis, constipation, or pseudo-obstruction.
- Secondary amyloid most classically presents with nephrotic range proteinuria, signs of heart failure, and peripheral neuropathy.
- Hemodialysis related amyloid (AB2M) most commonly presents with musculoskeletal complaints such as shoulder pain, tendonitis, and nerve entrapment syndromes. Less commonly it may present with GI predominant symptoms.
- **Amyloid arthropathy is most commonly seen in patients with primary amyloidosis** and usually does not occur in patients with inflammatory arthritis. Massive infiltration of amyloid into the periarticular structures is rare (shoulder pad sign, macroglossia, and hip stiffness) and seen in <2% of cases.

History

The clinical presentation is highly variable, depending on the systems involved. Symptoms may include:

- Constitutional symptoms of fatigue, weight loss, anorexia, early satiety, or halitosis.
- Hematemesis, melena, or bloody stool.
- Shortness of breath, hoarseness, sinus congestion.
- Lower extremity edema (signifying renal or cardiac involvement).
- Increased abdominal girth (signifying renal, cardiac, or hepatic involvement).
- Stiffness and pain with active range of motion about the shoulders and hips.
- Enlarged muscles, especially the deltoids or tongue.
- Symmetrical arthritis with disease concentrated at the **wrists, metacarpophalangeal (MCP) and proximal interphalangeal (PIP) joints,** thus mimicking rheumatoid arthritis.
- Neurologic manifestations including decreased fine touch sensation and nerve entrapment syndromes, most classically **carpal tunnel syndrome.**
- Cutaneous manifestations including waxy skin papules and easy bruising.
- Impaired cognition.
- Hypotension with standing due to autonomic dysfunction.

Physical Examination

Similarly, the physical findings vary with the organ system involved, and may include:

- Physical signs of rapid weight loss.
- Macroglossia with or without waxy papules, dry mouth, papules in the sinus, trachea, or larynx and secondary dysfunction.
- Abnormal heart rate or rhythm, S3, elevated jugular venous distention (JVD) or holosystolic murmur (tricuspid or mitral regurgitation).
- Crackles or decreased breath sounds at the lung bases.
- Increased abdominal girth, hepatomegaly, splenomegaly, and signs of ascites.

TABLE 46-1	DIAGNOSTIC CRITERIA FOR PRIMARY SYSTEMIC AMYLOIDOSIS

All of the following four criteria are required:
- Presence of amyloid-related systemic syndrome (e.g., renal, heart, liver, or peripheral nerve)
- Positive amyloid staining by Congo red from any biopsied tissue (under polarized light amyloid protein glows green after staining with Congo red)
- Immunohistochemical staining or direct sequencing light chain amyloid
- Evidence of monoclonal plasma cell proliferative disorder: Serum or urine electrophoresis with a monoclonal protein, disproportionate light chain ratio (normal total serum κ to λ ratio is approximately 2, normal free serum κ to λ ratio 0.26–1.65), or clonal plasma cells on bone marrow biopsy

Adapted from: Rajkumar SV, Dispenzieri A, Kyle RA. Monoclonal gammopathy of undetermined significance, Waldenström macroglobulinemia, AL amyloidosis, and related plasma cell disorders: diagnosis and treatment. *Mayo Clin Proc.* 2006;81:693–703.

- Enlarged soft tissue structure about the rotator cuff (shoulder pad sign); this is essentially pathognomonic for primary amyloidosis and is most commonly seen with IgG κ deposition.
- Diffuse lymphadenopathy.
- Decreased peripheral sensation, with or without focal weakness.
- Waxy papules most commonly located on the face, neck, groin, armpits, perianal area, tongue, external auditory canals; hair loss.
- Signs of cognitive dysfunction.

Diagnostic Criteria

- **Primary amyloidosis** should be suspected when classic history and physical examination findings occur along with typical organ involvement in the setting of a serum or urine monoclonal protein or free light chains (FLC).[1]
- Diagnostic criteria for systemic AL amyloidosis are presented in Table 46-1.[2]
- **Secondary amyloidosis:** Biopsy staining positive by immunohistochemical and immunoelectron microscopy with anti-AA serum, and absence of AL amyloid. Laboratory testing is of no confirmatory utility but is useful in ruling out AL amyloid and related disorders. Eighty percent of patients have renal disease.
- **Amyloid arthropathy:** Definitive diagnosis is by observing the presence of amyloid in synovial fluid or synovial membrane biopsy.
- **Cardiac amyloid:** Definitive diagnosis is by myocardial biopsy or the presence of amyloid on extracardiac tissue biopsy in a patient with appropriate other cardiac findings.

Diagnostic Testing

Laboratories
- Primary amyloidosis:
  - **Immunofixation** will identify 90% of patients.
    - **Serum protein electrophoresis (SPEP)** will reveal a **monoclonal paraprotein** (M protein).
    - **Urine protein electrophoresis (UPEP)** will reveal **monoclonal light chains.**

○ **Serum free light chain anaylsis** may identify monoclonal FLC in patients who fail to have a positive SPEP or UPEP.[1]
- Secondary amyloidosis:
  ○ No specific serum or urine laboratory testing will reveal the diagnosis.

Electrocardiography

Changes seen in patients with cardiac amyloidosis:

- Most common abnormality is decreased voltage in limb leads.
- Conduction abnormalities (e.g., first-, second-, or third-degree heart block), nonspecific intraventricular conduction delay, atrial fibrillation or flutter, ventricular tachycardia, or pseudoinfarct patterns.[3]

Imaging

- **Radiography** in amyloid arthropathy:
  ○ Radiographic evidence of disease always precedes symptoms.
  ○ Preservation or widening of joint space with no periarticular or cartilage erosions, bone cysts. Amyloid bone erosions are classically extra-articular.[4]
  ○ Soft tissue swelling and bone demineralization.
  ○ Lytic lesions may be seen if arthropathy is associated with MM.
- Transthoracic **echocardiography:**
  ○ Amyloid infiltration into the myocardium causes increased echogenicity resulting in a "**granular sparkling**" appearance to myocardium under echocardiography.
  ○ **Left ventricular wall thickening with diastolic dysfunction** is the most commonly observed abnormality. With advanced disease restrictive cardiomyopahty may be seen with a normal to small left ventricle and biatrial enlargement, right ventricular dilation, and mitral and aortic valve thickening may also occur.
  ○ Intracardiac thrombus is most commonly seen in the atria and may be a complication of disease.

Diagnostic Procedures

- **Tissue biopsy** is required for diagnosis of primary or secondary amyloidosis and amyloid arthropathy.
- Kidney and liver biopsy will be positive in about 90% of patients but is invasive and, therefore, not recommended as first line.
- **Abdominal fat pad biopsy** has a relatively high sensitivity (up to 80%) and specificity (up to 99%) for identifying primary and secondary amyloidosis in patients with multiorgan involvement.
- If the above sites are negative and the diagnosis is still in question, **a rectal, bone marrow, or skin biopsy** may be considered.
- Amyloid fibers stained with **Congo red** and will produce **green birefringence** under polarized light. Fibers stained with thioflavin T will produce yellow–green fluorescence.
- **Immunohistochemical staining and immunofluorescence** microscopy will reveal κ or λ light chains in primary amyloidosis.
- Amino acid sequencing and mass spectroscopy are useful but only available in research labs.
- Scintigraphy with radioisotope labeling of SAP component has a high sensitivity for determining the distribution and amyloid burden in patients with

primary and secondary disease. SAP is derived from donor blood and, therefore, carries infectious risks and does not reliably identify cardiac involvement.[5]

TREATMENT

Regardless of the type of amyloid, the goal of treatment is to decrease fibril production and extracellular deposition.

Medications

First Line

- **Primary amyloidosis:**
  - ○ **Hematopoietic cell transplantation** (HCT) is a possibility and a few patients may have complete remission of disease. Decision making regarding this therapy is complex.[2]
  - ○ In patients who are not candidates for HCT, **melphalan and steroid** is used. Complete remission is very uncommon as bone marrow toxicity of melphalan often limits control of the plasma cell dyscrasia.
- **Secondary amyloidosis:**
  - ○ **Control of the primary inflammatory disease** to stabilize and possibly reduce amyloid burden. Depending on the inflammatory disease, this may be done with immunosuppressive, cytotoxic, or biologic medications. For infectious etiologies, antibiotics, and removal of infected tissue are helpful.
  - ○ **Colchicine** is commonly used in FMF and has shown success. However, use of colchicine for amyloidosis secondary to other etiologies is questionable.[6]

Second Line

- **Primary amyloidosis:**
  - ○ In patients who fail melphalan and prednisone or HCT, **thalidomide** alone or in combination with cyclophosphamide may be used.[7]
- **Secondary amyloidosis:**
  - ○ **Dimethyl sulfoxide** (DMSO) may be effective in patients with chronic inflammatory states; however, literature and experience for this indication is limited.[8]
  - ○ Multiple cytotoxic and immunosuppressive agents have been tried for treatment of AA amyloid. Results are mixed and each case is unique.

Other Non-Pharmacologic Therapies

Physical therapy and occupational therapy are useful in amyloid arthropathy

Surgical Management

- Organ transplantation for failure or complications (kidney, heart, liver).
- Surgical debridement of infected tissue.
- Surgical resection of enlarged tissue (e.g., tongue).
- Carpal tunnel and other peripheral neuropathy releases.
- Joint replacement.

PATIENT EDUCATION

Amyloidosis Foundation (www.amyloidosis.org).

OUTCOME/PROGNOSIS

- Survival in **primary amyloidosis** may be months or years depending on organs affected, bone marrow involvement, and circulating plasma cell percentage.[9]
  - Main causes of death are **cardiac dysfunction, infection, and hepatic failure.**
  - Primary amyloidosis is often diagnosed after identification of the blood cell dyscrasia. Progression to MM after the diagnosis of primary amyloidosis is rare.
- If untreated, **secondary amyloidosis** may lead to cardiac or renal failure, infection, or bowel perforation.

REFERENCES

1. Katzmann JA, Clark RJ, Abraham RS, et al. Serum reference intervals and diagnostic ranges for free kappa and free lambda immunoglobulin light chains: Relative sensitivity for detection of monoclonal light chains. *Clin Chem.* 2002;48:1437–1444.
2. Rajkumar SV, Dispenzieri A, Kyle RA. Monoclonal gammopathy of undetermined significance, Waldenström macroglobulinemia, AL amyloidosis, and related plasma cell disorders: Diagnosis and treatment. *Mayo Clin Proc.* 2006;81:693–703.
3. Panduranga P, Mukhaini M. Catastrophic cardiac amyloidosis. *Cardiol Res Pract.* 2010; 2011:479314.
4. Leonard PA, Clegg DO, Lee RG. Erosive arthritis in a patient with amyloid arthropathy. *Clin Rheumatol.* 2010;4:212–217.
5. Hazenberg BP, van Rijswijk MH, Piers DA, et al. Diagnostic performance of 123I-labeled serum amyloid P component scintigraphy in patients with amyloidosis. *Am J Med.* 2006; 119:355.e15–e24.
6. Wechalekar AD, Hawkins PN, Gillmore JD. Perspectives in treatment of AL amloidosis. *Br J Haematol.* 2008;140:365–377.
7. Palladini G, Perfetti V, Perlini S, et al. The combination of thalidomide and intermediate-dose dexamethasone is an effective but toxic treatment for patients with primary amyloidosis (AL). *Blood.* 2005;105:2949–2951.
8. Amemori S, Iwakiri R, Endo H, et al. Oral dimethyl sulfoxide for systemic amyloid A amyloidosis complication in chronic inflammatory disease: A retrospective patient chart review. *J Gastroenterol.* 2006;41:444–449.
9. Lachmann HJ, Goodman HJ, Gilbertson JA, et al. Natural history and outcome in systemic AA amyloidosis. *N Engl J Med.* 2007;356:2361–2371.

Miscellaneous Skin Conditions

47

Reeti Joshi, Zarmeena Ali, and Leslie E. Kahl

T he skin is often the target organ for autoimmune diseases, and sometimes the first clinical clues to the diagnosis or a systemic inflammatory disorder are found in the dermatological exam.

PALPABLE PURPURA

- Palpable purpura is defined as **nonblanching, violaceous discoloration** of skin due to extravasated red blood cells (RBCs) in the dermis, **representing leukocytoclastic vasculitis.** Smaller lesions are called petechiae and larger ones are called ecchymoses.
- Associated clinical features are related to the underlying cause.
- Histopathology shows leukocytoclastic vasculitis. In Henoch–Schönlein purpura (HSP) immunofluorescence reveals IgA deposits in the dermis.
- The differential diagnosis includes:
  - **Infections:** infective endocarditis, septic emboli, *Neisseria* infections, *Rickettsia* infections (e.g., rocky mountain spotted fever, typhus), acute viral infections (e.g., HIV, hepatitis B and C, herpes simplex virus [HSV], and Epstein–Barr virus [EBV]).
  - **Small vessel cutaneous vasculitis** (see Chapter 20).
  - **Neoplasia** (e.g., myeloma, leukemia, lymphoma, myelodysplastic syndrome).
- Treatment is management of the underlying cause of disease.

ERYTHEMA NODOSUM

- **Clinical features** of erythema nodosum (EN) are **cutaneous nodules** that vary in size from 1 to 10 cm and usually appear acutely over the anterior aspect of the legs and, less commonly, on the thighs and forearms. The nodules are usually **tender** and may be surrounded by erythema and bruising. The lesions of EN may resolve spontaneously in weeks or become chronic.
- Associated causes:
  - **Infections** (e.g., *Streptococcus, M. tuberculosis,* histoplasmosis).
  - **Medications** (e.g., sulfonamides, penicillin, oral contraceptives).
  - **Sarcoidosis** (Löfgren's syndrome is the triad of bilateral hilar lymphadenopathy, EN, and acute polyarthritis seen in acute sarcoidosis).
  - **Inflammatory bowel disease** (IBD) and spondyloarthropathies.
  - **Malignancy.**
- Histopathology includes a lobular, **septal panniculitis,** usually without vasculitis.

- Treatment includes symptomatic relief with **nonsteroidal antiinflammatory drugs (NSAIDs)**. Severe and unresponsive cases may require **oral corticosteroids**. Oral potassium iodide may also be useful.[1]

CHOLESTEROL MICROEMBOLIZATION SYNDROME

- Cholesterol microembolization syndrome (CES), also known as cholesterol emboli or purple/blue toe syndrome, is caused by **embolization of lipid debris from an ulcerated atherosclerotic plaque,** generally from a large artery to smaller arterioles or end-arteries.
- It may be a complication of interventional arterial procedures, bypass surgery, intra-aortic balloon pump therapy, thrombolytics, trauma, post-cardiopulmonary resuscitation (CPR), and warfarin treatment. **Time of onset of embolization varies from hours to days** after these events.
- **Thrombolytic therapy and anticoagulants** may precipitate cholesterol emboli by dissolving protective thrombi and fibrin deposits coating an atheromatous plaque, permitting the release of cholesterol. However, a causal relationship remains uncertain.[2]
- **Clinical features** include symptoms related to **ischemia** of organ(s) distal to the occlusion.
  - Common sites are lower extremities (toes), intestine, pancreas, central nervous system (CNS), kidneys, spleen, liver, and bone marrow.
  - **Acute renal failure (ARF), livedo reticularis,** limb pain, and good peripheral pulses in unaffected areas are also noted. Both cutaneous and renal disease may be progressive due to repeated showers of emboli or secondary vascular inflammation induced by the emboli.
  - Up to 40% of patients have ARF at onset, as a direct result of preglomerular emboli to kidney as well as an inflammatory response to the emboli. Frequently ARF does not resolve and patients who survive often develop chronic renal failure.
- **Laboratory findings** include elevated erythrocyte sedimentation rate (ESR), C-reactive protein (CRP), eosinophilia, urinary eosinophils, proteinuria, and hyaline and granular casts.
- **Histopathology** is the gold standard for diagnosis. Routine staining reveals **biconvex, needle-shaped clefts** with intimal proliferation and a chronic inflammatory infiltrate. Frozen or wet formalin-fixed sections reveal doubly refractile **cholesterol crystals.** In paraffin-fixed sections, the cholesterol crystals are dissolved and leave needle-like clefts.
- **Differential diagnosis** includes small or medium vessel vasculitis, thromboangiitis obliterans, cocaine-induced ischemia, septic shock, and gangrene.
- A high threshold of suspicion is needed for making the diagnosis.
- **Medical treatment is mainly supportive.**
  - There is no clear consensus on the use of aspirin and other antiplatelet agents, pentoxifylline, or low molecular weight dextran.
  - Steroids have a variable rate of response.
  - **Anticoagulation is probably not indicated** and in fact may worsen the outcome.[2]
  - Control of hypertension is indicated. Vasodilators may be used, and some experts advocate use of angiotensin converting enzyme (ACE) inhibitors

for efferent arteriolar vasodilation. Statins have a theoretical advantage and reduce the risk of myocardial infarction from CES.[2]

- **Surgical treatment** includes amputation or resection of gangrenous tissues to prevent infection.
  - Angiographic confirmation of the embolic source is needed prior to removal of atheromatous lesions by endarterectomy, stenting, or bypass.
  - Renal arteries should be protected before manipulation proximal to renal vasculature.
- Prognosis remains guarded with significant mortality rates, limb-threatening consequences, and chronic renal failure.

PYODERMA GANGRENOSUM

- Pyoderma gangrenosum (PG) is an uncommon, diffuse, **neutrophilic dermatitis undermining the adjacent epidermis around a shallow ulceration.**
- Clinical features include onset as an inflammatory nodule or pustule that ulcerates and enlarges. The ulcers appear necrotic with **violaceous, undermined borders,** and may be as large as 20 cm.
- Clinical variants include pustular, bullous, vegetative, peristomal, and drug-induced lesions.
- An important characteristic of PG is **pathergy.** Normal skin of patients with PG that is subjected to trauma may develop the lesions. **Debridement or biopsy may, therefore, worsen the lesions.**
- **Associated conditions** include IBD, seronegative rheumatoid arthritis (RA), hematologic malignancies, and pyogenic arthritis with PG and acne (PAPA syndrome).
- Histopathology may show **marked neutrophilic infiltration** but may also be inconclusive.
- **Treatment** includes management of the associated disorder, which may result in improvement of the PG.
  - Oral **corticosteroids** are the mainstay of treatment for PG lesions.
  - Methotrexate, dapsone, and azathioprine have been used as steroid-sparing agents.
  - Secondary infection must be treated if present.
  - Newer treatment modalities include:
    - **Tumor necrosis factor** (TNF)-α **inhibitors** (e.g., infliximab, adalimumab, efalizumab), particularly in patients with Crohn's disease.[3]
    - **Alefacept,** which reduces T-cell activation, has been successful in reducing severity in a pilot study.[4]
- **Topical tacrolimus** has been used as an off-label treatment for localized, idiopathic PG of recent onset with negative microbiological results.[5]

SWEET'S SYNDROME

- Sweet's syndrome is a rare type of **neutrophilic dermatosis** that may be associated with many different diseases.
- Clinical features include **tender red or purple papules or nodules** with sharply demarcated borders, which appear most commonly over the upper extremities, face, and neck.

- The lesions may mimic EN when they appear on the lower extremities.
- Cutaneous manifestations are **usually accompanied by fever and leukocytosis.**
- Arthralgias, arthritis, CNS, and renal involvement sometimes occur.
- **Associated disorders** may include malignancy (especially acute myelogenous leukemia), bacterial and viral infections, IBD, certain medications (e.g., furosemide, oral contraceptives, trimethoprim–sulfamethoxazole, minocycline, granulocyte colony-stimulating factor), RA, sarcoidosis, Behçet's syndrome, and pregnancy.
- Histopathology shows a dense **neutrophilic infiltrate without evidence of leukocytoclastic vasculitis.**
- Treatment with **prednisone** at doses of up to 60 mg PO daily provides prompt relief of cutaneous and systemic manifestations.
  - Dapsone has been also been used to treat Sweet's syndrome.
  - Treatment of underlying condition is essential.

CALCIPHYLAXIS

- Calciphylaxis is a rare disease causing **deposition of calcium in the media of arterioles,** leading to ischemia and subcutaneous necrosis.
- The pathogenesis of this disorder is poorly understood.
- Associated conditions include:
  - **Endocrine:** primary and secondary hyperparathyroidism, diabetes, obesity, and excess vitamin D.
  - **Renal:** uremia, calcium–phosphate product >70 mg^2/dL^2, serum aluminum >25 ng/mL.[6]
  - **Autoimmune:** RA, systemic lupus erythematosus (SLE), sarcoidosis, Sjögren's syndrome, Crohn's disease, and antiphospholipid syndrome.
  - Other conditions: paraneoplastic, deficiency of protein C or S, alcoholic liver disease.
- Clinical features include **painful ischemic plaque-like lesions which can ulcerate and progress to necrosis or eschar formation,** typically lower limbs and areas of adiposity such as the trunk, gluteal regions, and thighs. Other complications include mesenteric ischemia and gastrointestinal (GI) hemorrhage, and ischemic myopathy.
- The clinical diagnosis is confirmed by biopsy. Histopathology shows **arterial medial calcification, subintimal fibrosis, and arterial occlusion without vasculitis.** Acute and chronic calcifying septal panniculitis may also be seen. Biopsies are complicated by profuse bleeding and secondary infection is common.
- The differential diagnosis is broad and includes:
  - **Vasculitis:** Wegener's granulomatosis, pancreatic panniculitis, polyarteritis nodosa (PAN), hypersensitivity vasculitis, bullous SLE.
  - **Vasculitis mimics:** cholesterol emboli syndrome, cryoglobulinemia, PG, livedoid vasculopathy, warfarin skin necrosis, antiphospholipid syndrome, deficiency of protein C or S.
  - **Infections:** cellulitis, necrotizing fasciitis, brown recluse spider bite, *Vibrio vulnificus* infection, endocarditis, fungal, and atypical mycobacterial infections.
- Treatment includes removing factors that contribute to the development of the disorder, and supportive care. Options include:

- Provide **wound care and pain control.**
- **Elimination of triggers** if possible by discontinuing calcium supplementation, vitamin D supplementation, and parenteral iron therapy.
- **Correction of metabolic abnormalities,** particularly plasma calcium and phosphorous concentrations, with dietary alterations, use of noncalcium, nonaluminum binders, and low-calcium bath dialysis.
- **Sodium thiosulfate** has shown benefit in some patients, usually at a dose of 25 g after each dialysis.[7]
- Some benefit may be achieved with **increasing the frequency or duration of dialysis** sessions.
- Calcimimetics such as **cinacalcet** hydrochloride may be beneficial by controlling secondary hyperparathyroidism.[8]
- **Parathyroidectomy** can be considered in hyperparathyroid patients if conservative management fails. However, a meaningful affect on survival is uncertain.
- Judicious use of **antibiotics and hyperbaric oxygen** may be advantageous.[9]
- **Bisphosphonates** increase osteoprotegerin production and inhibit arterial calcification. Several case reports suggest they may be useful in treating this disorder.[10]
- Early use of systemic **glucocorticoids** may be helpful, unless ulcerated lesions are present, but this approach is controversial.[11]
- **Anticoagulation** is beneficial if there is an underlying hypercoaguable state.[12]

ERYTHROMELALGIA

- Erythromelalgia (EM) is a rare condition characterized by **red hot painful burning feet,** less commonly hands, accompanied by erythema, pallor, or cyanosis, in the presence of palpable pulses.
- The diagnosis is a clinical one. One useful finding is that patients generally seek relief by placing the affected extremities in ice water.
- EM is considered by some to be the opposite of Raynaud's phenomenon.
- The pathogenesis of EM is not well understood.
- As a primary disorder, it can be the result of a disease-specific novel **mutation causing sodium channelopathy** in nociceptive fibers.
- Conditions associated with in **secondary EM** include:
  - **Myeloproliferative disorders:** polycythemia, essential thrombocythemia, pernicious anemia, and myelodysplastic syndrome.
  - **Drug-induced:** cyclosporine, calcium channel blockers, norepinephrine, and influenza vaccine.
  - **Infections:** HIV, hepatitis B, and EBV.
  - Other conditions: SLE, RA, diabetic neuropathy, and multiple sclerosis.
- **Treatment** is mainly supportive and includes:
  - **Avoidance of triggers** that induce vasodilation, such as strenuous exercises, warm climate, or hot baths.
  - Wearing open toed shoes, no socks, keeping a fan by the feet.
  - Although there are no controlled trials, medications which may be useful in individual patients include gabapentin, venlafaxine, diltiazem, sertraline, amitriptyline, imipramine, paroxetine, fluoxetine, and diphenhydramine.

○ Additionally, medications that effect voltage-gated sodium channel such as lidocaine and mexiletine show promise.[13]
○ Treatment of underlying disease.

COCAINE AND LEVAMISOLE-INDUCED VASCULOPATHY

- Cocaine has historically been associated with cardiovascular morbidities due to its vasoconstrictive and platelet activating properties but it has also been implicated in a variety of dermatologic conditions.
- The pathogenesis of these dermatologic lesions is unknown but is **likely related to levamisole**, a veterinary antihelminthic that has been used to cut the cocaine. Levamisole, a known immunomodulator, has been associated with neutropenia and the development of antibodies, including antinuclear antibodies (ANA), antineutrophil cytoplasmic antibodies (ANCA), lupus anticoagulant, and anticardiolipin antibodies.[14]
- The clinical features associated with cocaine and levamisole include non-specific and lichenoid eruptions, a fixed drug eruption, and a very **distinctive cutaneous vasculopathy. Purpura of the ears and cheeks is the most characteristic finding** but ischemic lesions can appear anywhere on the limbs or body.
- **Histopathology** demonstrates a range of reactions including leukocytoclastic vasculitis, a thrombotic vasculitis and, most commonly, bland vascular occlusive disease without a true vasculitis.[14]
- **Treatment** includes abstinence from levamisole-tainted cocaine. The role of steroids and anticoagulation is yet to be determined.

REFERENCES

1. Gilchrist H, Patterson JW. Erythema nodosum and erythema induratum (nodular vasculitis): diagnosis and management. *Dermatol Ther.* 2010;23:320–327.
2. Kronzon I, Saric M. Cholesterol embolization syndrome. *Circulation.* 2010;122:631–641.
3. Juillerat P, Christen-Zäch S, Troillet FX, et al. Infliximab for the treatment of disseminated pyoderma gangrenosum associated with ulcerative colitis. Case report and literature review. *Dermatology.* 2007;215:245–251.
4. Foss CE, Clark AR, Inabinet R, et al. An open-label pilot study of alefacept for the treatment of pyoderma gangrenosum. *J Eur Acad Dermatol Venereol.* 2008;22:943–949.
5. Le Cleach L, Moguelet P, Perrin P, et al. Is topical monotherapy effective for localized pyoderma gangrenosum? *Arch Dermatol.* 2001;147:101–103.
6. Weenig RH, Sewell LD, David MD, et al. Calciphylaxis: natural history, risk factor analysis, and outcome. *J Am Acad Dermatol.* 2007;56:569–579.
7. Noureddine L, Landis M, Patel N, et al. Efficacy of sodium thiosulfate for the treatment for calciphylaxis. *Clin Nephrol.* 2011;75:485–490.
8. Robinson MR, Augustine JJ, Korman NJ. Cinacalcet for the treatment of calciphylaxis. *Arch Dermatol.* 2007;143:152–154.
9. Basile C, Montanaro A, Masi M, et al. Hyperbaric oxygen therapy for calcific uremic arteriolopathy: a case series. *J Nephrol.* 2002;15:676–680.
10. Shiraishi N, Kitamura K, Miyoshi T, et al. Successful treatment of a patient with severe calcific uremic arteriolopathy (calciphylaxis) by etidronate disodium. *Am J Kidney Dis.* 2006;48:151–154.

11. Fine A, Zacharias J. Calciphylaxis is usually non-ulcerating: risk factors, outcome and therapy. *Kidney Int.* 2002;61:2210–2217.

12. Harris RJ, Cropley TG. Possible role of hypercoagulability in calciphylaxis: review of the literature. *J Am Acad Dermatol.* 2011;64:405–412.

13. Davis MD, Sandroni P. Lidocaine patch for pain of erythromelalgia: follow-up of 34 patients. *Arch Dermatol.* 2005;141:1320–1321.

14. Gross RL, Brucker J, Bahce-Altuntas A, et al. A novel cutaneous vasculitis syndrome induced by levamisole-contaminated cocaine. *Clin Rheumatol.* 2011;30:1385–1392.

Osteoporosis

48

Ashwini Komarla, Richa Gupta, and
Zarmeena Ali

GENERAL PRINCIPLES

Definition

- Osteoporosis is the **most common metabolic disorder in the United States** and is generally asymptomatic until complications develop.
- The National Institutes of Health (NIH) 2000 consensus panel describes osteoporosis as a "skeletal disorder characterized by compromised bone strength predisposing a person to an increased risk of fracture."[1]
- The World Health Organization (WHO) defines osteoporosis as a bone density of 2.5 SD or more below the mean for young healthy white women.[2]

Classification

- Osteoporosis can be classified as primary or secondary on the basis of causality.
- In **primary osteoporosis,** the deterioration of bone mass is related to aging or decreased gonadal function. It is typically seen in postmenopausal women and older men, usually over age 70.
- **Secondary osteoporosis** results from chronic conditions or medications, like corticosteroids, that accelerate bone loss.

Epidemiology

- Osteoporosis affects an estimated 10 million people, and an additional 34 million people have low bone mineral density (BMD). Approximately, 1.5 million osteoporosis-related fractures occur each year in the United States. Direct medical costs for these fractures exceed 18 billion dollars.[1,2]
- **White postmenopausal women are most at risk for osteoporosis and related fractures.** This population suffers three-fourths of all hip fractures. Men and black women have lower hip fracture rates, as do Hispanic women and Native Americans. Asians have lower bone mineral densities, but fewer fractures than the white population.
- A 50-year-old white woman has an approximate 50% risk of experiencing an osteoporotic fracture during her lifetime, while a 50-year-old man has an approximate 13% risk.[1]
- Osteoporosis is a **common comorbidity in patients with rheumatologic diseases** because of the increased use of corticosteroids, decreased physical activity, systemic inflammation, and alteration of the normal balance of bone resorption/formation.

Pathophysiology

- Osteoporosis is characterized by **either low bone density or poor bone quality.**
  - Bone quality is determined by architecture, turnover, damage, and mineralization.

- ○ BMD is determined by peak bone mass and the amount of bone lost over time.
- Loss of bone mass occurs during remodeling of bone when resorption, a result of osteoclast activity, occurs more quickly than bone formation, a consequence of osteoblast activity.
  - ○ Crucial regulators of osteoclastic bone resorption include **RANK ligand** (RANKL; a member of the tumor necrosis factor [TNF] ligand family), and **its two receptors, RANK and osteoprotegerin (OPG).**
  - ○ RANK ligand is expressed by osteoblasts. It interacts with its corresponding receptor, RANK, which is expressed by osteoclasts.
  - ○ This interaction promotes osteoclast differentiation, activation, and prolonged survival.
  - ○ OPG, which is secreted by osteoblasts and stromal cells, blocks the interaction of RANK ligand with RANK, thereby regulating bone turnover (see Fig. 48-1).
- After age 40, cortical bone is lost at a rate of 0.3% to 0.5% per year.
  - ○ Trabecular bone loss may begin at an even younger age. This loss of cortical and trabecular bone accelerates after menopause, as **estrogen deficiency results in increased bone turnover and a remodeling imbalance.**
  - ○ The enhanced activity and function of osteoclasts during this period appears to be due to the increased expression of **osteoclastogenic proinflammatory cytokines like interleukin (IL)-1 and TNF,** which are negatively regulated by estrogen.
- Histologically, the bone has decreased cortical thickness and a decreased number and size of trabeculae.
  - ○ Although trabecular or cancellous bone found mainly in the axial skeleton compromises only 20% of bone, and cortical bone found primarily in the diaphyses of long bones compromises 80% of bone, **trabecular bone is the site of the greatest bone turnover** as a result of its greater surface area.
  - ○ Thus, it is more susceptible to imbalances in remodeling and more frequently associated with osteoporotic fractures.

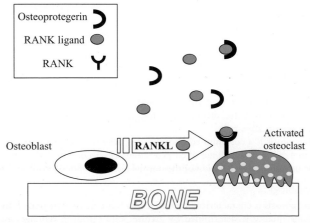

FIGURE 48-1. Pathophysiology of osteoporosis.

○ The most frequent sites of osteoporotic fractures are the spine, hip, and distal radius.

Risk Factors

- Low BMD correlates with an increased risk of primary osteoporosis. **Predictors of low BMD** include female gender, increased age, estrogen deficiency, white or Asian race, low weight and body mass index, family history of osteoporosis, smoking, history of fracture, late menarche, and early menopause.
- Secondary causes of osteoporosis are extensive.
  ○ They involve **diseases of hormone dysregulation** including Cushing's syndrome, primary or secondary amenorrhea, hypogonadism, hyperthyroidism, diabetes mellitus type I, and hyperparathyroidism.
  ○ Malnutrition, malabsorption syndromes, pernicious anemia, parenteral nutrition, and gastrectomy are predisposing factors.
  ○ Severe liver and renal diseases, chronic obstructive pulmonary disease, hemochromatosis, and mastocytosis also place patients at a higher risk for osteoporosis.
  ○ **Rheumatologic diseases** that predispose to osteoporosis include amyloidosis, systemic lupus erythematosus (SLE), ankylosing spondylitis, rheumatoid arthritis (RA), and sarcoidosis.
  ○ **Certain drugs and toxins** (e.g., corticosteroids, anticonvulsants, heparin, lithium, thyroxine, cytotoxic drugs, ethanol use, and tobacco) have also been implicated.

DIAGNOSIS

Clinical Presentation

- Osteoporosis is commonly asymptomatic until fractures occur.
- **Vertebral compression fractures** most commonly occur in the T-11 to L-2 region and may present as loss of height rather than back pain.
- Other common fracture sites are the **distal wrist (Colles' fracture), hip, and pelvis.**
- Physical examination may reveal tenderness along the spine, scoliosis, kyphosis, or dowager's hump.
- Signs and symptoms of secondary causes can be elicited during the history and physical examination (e.g., hypogonadism, evidence of thyroid disease, and cushingoid features).

Diagnostic Criteria

- **In general, women who present with fragility fractures in the absence of trauma should be screened.** The American College of Rheumatology and National Osteoporosis Foundation recommend **screening all women over age 65 and men over age 70, along with any adult with a condition or taking medication associated low bone mass or bone loss.**
- Assessment of BMD is the standard of care in diagnosis and evaluation of adults for osteoporosis. Measuring BMD at any skeletal site has value in predicting fracture risk. Hip BMD, however, is the best predictor of hip fractures

and is also good at predicting fractures at other sites. BMD is expressed as two values:

○ **Z score:** Comparison with the expected BMD for the patient's age and sex.

○ **T score:** Comparison with the average peak BMD for young healthy white adults of the same gender.

- **The T score is more helpful in assessing fracture risk** as most studies use it. The difference between the patient's BMD and the norm is expressed as SD above or below the mean. With central dual energy x-ray absorptiometry (DEXA) BMD testing, a change in T or Z score of 1 SD roughly corresponds to a 10% change in BMD.
- The WHO defines four diagnostic categories based on T score.[2]

○ **Normal:** BMD within 1 SD of the reference mean (T ≥ −1.0).

○ **Osteopenia:** BMD between 1 and 2.5 SDs below the reference mean (−2.5 < T < −1.0).

○ **Osteoporosis:** BMD 2.5 SDs or more below the reference mean (T ≤ −2.5).

○ **Established or severe osteoporosis:** BMD over 2.5 SDs below the reference mean (T ≤ −2.5) and the presence of one or more fragility fractures.

- BMD is an excellent predictor of fracture risk but when it is combined with clinical risk factors, it is a better predictor than either alone. **The Fracture Risk Assessment Tool (FRAX)** estimates the 10-year probability of fracture on the basis of clinical risk factors and BMD at the femoral neck. FRAX is an electronic clinical tool (www.shef.ac.uk/FRAX) and is only helpful in making treatment decisions in patients with osteopenia.

Differential Diagnosis

The differential diagnosis of osteoporosis includes osteomalacia, metastatic malignancy to bone, multiple myeloma, hyperthyroidism, hyperparathyroidism, renal osteodystrophy, malabsorption syndromes, vitamin deficiencies, and Paget's disease.

Diagnostic Testing

Laboratories

- Limited laboratory testing as suggested by history and physical examination (e.g., serum and urine calcium, serum phosphorus, alkaline phosphatase, thyroid hormone levels, serum protein electrophoresis, parathyroid hormones [PTHs], vitamin D level, serum testosterone in men, cortisol, and renal and liver functions) can be helpful in diagnosing secondary causes.
- Markers of bone turnover are not useful in making the diagnosis of osteoporosis.

Imaging

- **Plain radiography** can demonstrate osteopenia and vertebral compression fractures but is a generally unreliable markers of bone mass, as 20% to 50% of bone must be lost before changes are evident on radiographs.
- BMD testing techniques include **DEXA**, single energy x-ray absorptiometry, peripheral DEXA, quantitative CT, and ultrasound densitometry.

○ **Central DEXA is the gold standard and recommended for adults who have had osteoporotic fractures or who are undergoing general screening.**

○ DEXA imaging results in a low level of radiation exposure (one-tenth of a traditional radiograph) and has excellent reproducibility and precision.

○ Bone density testing should be obtained at both the spine and the hip. **In women younger than 65 years, spine imaging may be more helpful,** as bone is apt to be lost more rapidly in the spine, and vertebral fractures are the most common fracture in this age group. **In women older than 65 years, bone density at the hip is more clinically useful** as hip fractures are more of a concern and the spine bone density has a higher chance of false elevations due to vascular calcifications or osteoarthritis of the spine.

○ DEXA can also be used to measure the wrist, but measurements at that site are of limited clinical significance due to lower predictive values and less reproducibility.

○ **Quantitative CT** has a similar ability to predict fractures as central DEXA. Quantitative CT is less affected by superimposed osteoarthritis. However, quantitative CT scans are more expensive and require a larger dose of radiation, so clinically they are not so frequently used.

○ **Peripheral bone density** performed with either DEXA or single energy x-ray absorptiometry can measure forearm, finger, or heel BMD, while peripheral ultrasonography most commonly measures bone mass of the heel. The advantages of peripheral bone density testing and ultrasonography are the portability and the ability of these tests to be performed in primary care offices. However, there are not universally agreed upon diagnostic criteria for the different machines available. In addition, the precision of the machines does not allow for their use in monitoring response to therapy. **Peripheral testing has not been endorsed for use in the diagnosis of osteoporosis,** but if it is performed, abnormal results should be followed up with central DEXA to establish or confirm the diagnosis.

TREATMENT

• The National Osteoporosis Foundation has issued clinical practice guidelines for treating osteoporosis and addresses postmenopausal women and men over the age of 50 years for all ethnic groups in the United States. It is intended for use by clinicians in making decisions in the care of individual patients.

• **The main goal in treatment of osteoporosis is the prevention of fractures.** On average, risk of fracture approximately doubles for each 1 SD decrease in T score. The following are indications to initiate specific therapy for osteoporosis. It is important to be aware that the prospective randomized controlled pharmacologic trials for the treatment of osteoporosis have taken place mainly in the population of white women, so limited data are available on therapeutic benefit of pharmacologic agents in men or minority groups.

○ All adults with osteoporotic fractures of the hip or spine.

○ Adults with a T score ≤ −2 SD who do not have specific risk factors for osteoporosis.

○ Adults with a T score ≤ −1.5 SD who have risk factors for osteoporosis.

○ Women >70 years with multiple risk factors are at high enough risk to begin treatment without BMD testing.

• Adequate intake of **calcium and vitamin D is recommended for all patients.**

○ Daily intake of elemental **calcium** should be at least **1200 mg.** Calcium supplements are mostly available as calcium carbonate or calcium citrate. Foods rich in calcium include dairy products, sardines, and fortified juices.

○ All adults should receive at least **800 to 1000 IU of vitamin D** per day. Foods rich in vitamin D include fortified milk and cereals, egg yolks, and liver.

- Regular **weight-bearing exercise** is also recommended for all patients.
- **Fall prevention:** Most osteoporotic fractures involve falling or low-impact trauma. Patients should be assessed for reversible causes of falls like overmedication, neurologic or vision problems, and poor footwear.
- Avoidance of tobacco use and excessive alcohol intake should be encouraged.
- Other factors that have been suggested to negatively impact the risk of osteoporosis are high intakes of caffeine, protein, and phosphorus.

Medications

First Line

- **Bisphosphonates:** Alendronate, risedronate, ibandronate, and zoledronic acid are generally the best agents currently available for treating osteoporosis.
- Bisphosphonates bind avidly to hydroxyapatite crystals in bone and are resistant to metabolic degradation. They **reduce the ability of osteoclasts to resorb bone and accelerate osteoclast apoptosis.**
- Alendronate (5 mg PO daily or 35 mg PO weekly), risedronate (5 mg PO daily or 35 mg PO weekly), and ibandronate (2.5 mg PO daily) are FDA approved for use in prevention, whereas alendronate (10 mg PO daily or 70 mg PO weekly), risedronate (5 mg PO daily or 35 mg PO weekly), and ibandronate (2.5 mg PO daily or 150 mg PO monthly) are FDA approved for use in treatment of osteoporosis.
- Randomized clinical trials have shown that the benefit in fracture risk has lasted up to 4 years. Sustained benefit in BMD has lasted up to 10 years with alendronate and 7 years with risedronate.
- In clinical practice, **esophageal and gastric side effects** are the most commonly reported and are reduced with weekly or monthly dosing preparations.
- Zoledronic acid is a parenterally administered bisphosphonate dosed annually. Ibandronate is also available for parenteral administration every 3 months and is another alternative for patients who cannot tolerate oral bisphosphonates. Intravenous administration of bisphosphonates can cause an acute phase response type of reaction with symptoms like fever and myalgias.
- **Osteonecrosis of the jaw** has been recognized as a complication of nitrogen containing bisphosphonate therapy. Most cases have been associated with the use of intravenous bisphosphonates in patients with metastatic bone disease.
- **Atypical femur fractures of the subtrochanteric and diaphyseal femoral shaft** that occur with minimal or no trauma have been reported in the setting of long-term use of bisphosphonates. Epidemiologic studies have suggested that these atypical fractures are reduced by increased adherence to bisphosphonate therapy and are more likely to be caused by osteoporosis than by bisphosphonates. The incidence of atypical fractures associated with bisphosphonates is very low, but the new onset of groin or mid-thigh pain in patients taking bisphosphonates for more than 5 to 10 years should require further evaluation.[3]
- Long-term data with alendronate and risedronate have demonstrated efficacy and safety for 10 and 7 years, respectively.
- Stopping therapy after 5 years or a "drug holiday" of a year or two may be reasonable, as there appears to be residual BMD and fracture benefit.

Second Line

- **Raloxifene is a selective estrogen receptor modulator (SERM)** that exhibits proestrogen effects on some tissues and antiestrogen effects on other tissues. It has been shown in trials to decrease the rate of new vertebral fractures by 40% to 50% and improve BMD at the spine and hip. It has not been found to have a significant effect on hip or total nonvertebral fractures. The ideal candidate for raloxifene is a woman who cannot tolerate a bisphosphonate. Typical dose is 60 mg PO daily. On raloxifene, there is an increased risk of stroke or deep vein thrombosis and pulmonary embolism. Other SERMs undergoing clinical trials include bazedoxifene and lasofoxifene.

- **Calcitonin** is an endogenous peptide that enhances BMD by inhibiting osteoclast activity. It is available in both subcutaneous and intranasal forms. Its beneficial effects on the BMD of the spine are less than with other agents. Of note, intranasal calcitonin has been found to be **beneficial in treating the pain of acute vertebral compression fractures.**
- **Teriparatide** is a recombinant formation of the active 34 N-terminal peptide portion of PTH.
  - Although continuous exposure to PTH, as in patients with primary hyperparathyroidism, leads to increased bone resorption, intermittent exposure has been shown to stimulate bone formation.
  - Teriparatide is the first anabolic pharmacologic agent and increases bone formation by stimulating osteoblast activity. It is administered by daily subcutaneous injections for up to 2 years.
  - **The BMD improvement seen with teriparatide is greater than other available agents for osteoporosis.**
  - Due to the significant cost, teriparatide should be reserved for patients with severe or established osteoporosis who cannot take or have unsuccessful results with bisphosphonates. It is contraindicated in patients with preexisting hypercalcemia, metastatic bone disease, and those at increased risk for osteosarcoma, such as patients with Paget's disease, prior radiation treatment to bone, and children.
- **Denosumab** is a humanized monoclonal antibody that specifically binds RANKL and blocks the binding of RANKL to RANK. It thereby reduces the formation, function, and survival of osteoclasts, resulting in decreased bone resorption, increased bone density, and decreased fractures.[4] It is administered as 60 mg subcutaneously every 6 months. Potential adverse effects include hypocalcemia, skin reactions, osteonecrosis of the jaw, and suppression of the immune system, possibly predisposing patients to infections and neoplasms.
- **Strontium ranelate** is a new agent recently approved in Europe but not approved by the FDA. It increases calcium uptake and bone formation, as well as inhibiting bone resorption.[5]
- **Hormone replacement therapy** has been shown to prevent bone loss but it is not used in the treatment of osteoporosis because of an **unfavorable balance of benefits and risks,** like coronary heart disease and thromboembolic events.
- **Combination therapy** with two antiresorptive medicines has not demonstrated a reduction in the fracture risk above what would be found with a single agent. Starting a bisphosphonate after completing 2 years of treatment with teriparatide makes theoretical sense and a recent study found that BMD improvements with 1 year of teriparatide were maintained or improved with subsequent alendronate but lost if therapy was not followed by a bisphosphonate. This sequence is possibly the best combination but more studies are needed to validate this.[6]

SPECIAL CONSIDERATIONS

- **Glucocorticoid therapy** causes bone loss through a number of different mechanisms, including impaired intestinal calcium absorption, increased urinary calcium excretion, decreased bone formation, increased bone resorption through the stimulation of osteoclast activity by macrophage colony-stimulating factor, and suppression of endogenous gonadal steroid production.
- Therapy with glucocorticoids leads to an early and sometimes dramatic loss of trabecular bone with less effect on cortical bone.
- Glucocorticoid use is **the most common form of drug-related osteoporosis** and is often seen in patients with rheumatic diseases.
  - Glucocorticoids should be prescribed at the **lowest effective dose for the shortest duration possible.**
  - Patients who receive glucocorticoids (e.g., prednisone at >5 mg PO/day) for >2 months are considered at high risk for excessive bone loss but there has been some controversy regarding the dose at which an increased risk of fracture occurs.
  - To diagnose and prevent glucocorticoid-induced osteoporosis, **obtain a baseline assessment of BMD of the hip or spine before initiating any long-term (>3 months) therapy.**
- For steroid-induced osteoporosis, randomized controlled studies demonstrate calcium carbonate, 1000 mg PO daily and vitamin D, 500 IU PO daily, to be an effective preventive therapy for some patients receiving prednisone.
- The American College of Rheumatology published guidelines for the prevention and treatment of glucocorticoid-induced osteoporosis in 2010.[7]
  - Postmenopausal women and men over age 50 with an estimated steroid course of at least 3 months were stratified into low, medium, and high risk groups on the basis of T score and age with consideration for other risk factors.
  - Low risk patients should be put on a bisphosphonate for a prednisone dose of ≥7.5 mg/day, while medium and high risk groups should be on bisphosphonates for any dose of steroid.
  - Teriparatide can also be considered for high risk women on steroids for a long period of time.
  - For premenopausal women and men less than age 50, the data are inadequate to make a recommendation. Individual circumstances and childbearing potential in women need to be considered.

COMPLICATIONS

- Possible consequences of fracture due to osteoporosis are acute and chronic pain, depression, deconditioning, dependency, and changes in appearance including loss of height and kyphosis.
- Hip fractures are associated with an up to 20% mortality rate in women and a 30% mortality rate in men within the first year of fracture, most often due to comorbidities. Twenty percent of patients with hospitalization due to a hip fracture require nursing home care and fifty percent of survivors are unable to ambulate independently or have some other permanent disability.

MONITORING/FOLLOW-UP

- Follow-up of patients includes monitoring for complications, side effects, and response to treatment. Continued assessment for modifiable risk factors and fall risk is necessary. Height should be followed to screen for asymptomatic vertebral fractures.
- **BMD should be revaluated every 1 to 2 years to assess response to therapy.** Repeat measurements made sooner than that can be difficult to interpret, as the expected change in BMD over a short period of time may be similar to the precision of the machine. **BMD changes need to be ≥3% to be considered significant.** Repeat measurements need to be made on the same DEXA machine to allow results to be accurately compared. Patients who are being screened for osteoporosis but are not on treatment should wait 2 years before undergoing repeat BMD testing.
- Monitoring with markers of bone turnover is another option. Fasting urinary N-telopeptide (NTX) or serum carboxy-terminal collagen crosslinks (CTX) can be measured before and then 3 to 6 months after initiating bisphosphonate or other antiresorptive therapy. A decrease of greater than 50% in urinary NTX excretion or 30% in serum CTX provides evidence of compliance and drug efficacy.[8] A decrease in markers of less than this amount may not necessarily indicate treatment failure, and noncompliance or poor absorption should be considered.

REFERENCES

1. NIH consensus development panel on osteoporosis prevention, diagnosis, and therapy. Osteoporosis prevention, diagnosis, and therapy. *JAMA*. 2001;285:785–795.
2. World Health Organization. WHO scientific group on the assessment of osteoporosis at a primary health care level. *Summary Meeting Report*. Brussels, Belgium, 2004.
3. Shane E. Evolving Data about subtrochanteric fractures and bisphosphonate. *N Engl J Med*. 2010;362:1825–1827.
4. von Keyserlingk C, Hopkins R, Anastasilakis A, et al. Clinical efficacy and safety of denosumab in postmenopausal women with low bone mineral density and osteoporosis: A meta-analysis. *Semin Arthritis Rheum*. 2011;41:178–186.
5. Kanis JA, Johansson H, Oden A, et al. A meta-analysis of the effect of strontium ranelate on the risk of vertebral and non-vertebral fracture in postmenopausal osteoporosis and the interaction with FRAX. *Osteoporos Int*. 2011;22:2347–2355.
6. Black DM, Bilezikian JP, Ensrud KE, et al. One year of alendronate after one year of parathyroid hormone (1–84) for osteoporosis. *N Engl J Med*. 2005;353:555–565.
7. Grossman JM, Gordon R, Ranganath VK. American college of rheumatology 2010 recommendations for the prevention and treatment of glucocorticoid-induced osteoporosis. *Arthritis Care Res (Hoboken)*. 2010;62:1515–1526.
8. Bonnick SL, Shulman L. Monitoring osteoporosis therapy: Bone mineral density, bone turnover markers, or both? *Am J Med*. 2006;119:S25–S31.

Avascular Necrosis

49

Richa Gupta, Ashwini Komarla, and
Zarmeena Ali

GENERAL PRINCIPLES

Definition
Avascular necrosis (AVN), also known as **osteonecrosis** and **aseptic necrosis,** involves
vascular compromise to bone with subsequent bone death and joint destruction.

Epidemiology
- Incidence is estimated at 15,000 cases annually in the United States, with a
  male to female ratio of 8:1.
- It accounts for about 10% of the 500,000 joint replacements performed
  annually.
- Most of the patients are <50 years, although AVN can affect persons of any age.
- Various bones can be affected, including the femur (femoral head and condyles), tibia (tibial plateau), humerus (humeral head), vertebrae, and small
  bones of the foot, ankle, and hand. **Osteonecrosis of the hip causes the most
  severe and debilitating impairments.**
- AVN develops **bilaterally** in more than 80% of cases.

Pathophysiology
- The pathogenesis of AVN is poorly understood. The **circulatory compromise**
  to the bone is thought to occur by one of these mechanisms:[1]
  ○ Mechanical vascular interruption.
  ○ Thrombosis or embolism.
  ○ Injury to a vessel wall (vasculitis, radiation injury, or spasm).
  ○ Venous occlusion (blood flow is impeded as venous pressure is greater than
    arterial pressure).
  ○ Direct bone cell injury.
  ○ Intraosseous marrow displacement and increased pressure in the bony com-
    partment.
- Any of these events may lead to **medullary infarction** in the fatty marrow,
  resulting in bone death with subsequent cell necrosis.
- Initially there is necrosis of the hematopoietic and fatty bone marrow elements.
  The necrotic zone remains acellular and cannot be repaired or revascularized.
  This ultimately leads to **death of the bone and fibrous scar tissue formation.**

Risk Factors
- The most common risk factors for developing AVN include oral **corticosteroid
  use, alcohol abuse, and cigarette smoking.** For glucocorticoids, doses of >2 g
  of prednisone (or its equivalent) within the last 2 to 3 months are considered
  to increase the risk of AVN.

- **Other risk factors** include systemic lupus erythematosus (SLE), rheumatoid arthritis (RA), trauma, sepsis, renal failure, sickle cell disease, vasculitis, Gaucher's disease, dysbaric conditions (Caisson disease), radiation injury, chemotherapy, organ transplantation, hypersensitivity reactions, coagulation factor deficiencies, cancer, pregnancy, and bisphosphonate use in malignant disease.
- In approximately 15% of patients, the occurrence of AVN may be idiopathic, where no clear cause is identified.
- Genetic factors have been reported, showing an association between AVN and certain polymorphisms involving alcohol-metabolizing enzymes and the drug transport protein P-glycoprotein. Also, a mutation in the type II collagen gene was identified in three families demonstrating autosomal dominant inheritance of AVN.[2]

DIAGNOSIS

Clinical Presentation

History

- Patients commonly present with vague and mild **joint pain** but acute, severe, deep, throbbing pain presentations are also possible.
- Early in the course of the disease, pain is increased with activity, but over time it progresses to pain with rest.
- More severe pain can occur with larger infarcts (most often associated with Gaucher's disease, dysbarism, and hemoglobinopathies).
- Some patients remain relatively asymptomatic despite advanced radiographic changes.
- The time course for AVN varies and may range from months to years between initial symptom onset and the development of end-stage disease with joint dysfunction.
- AVN **usually involves anterolateral femoral head** but can also involve femoral condyles, humeral head, proximal tibia, vertebrae, and small bones of hand and foot.

Physical Examination

- The physical examination is nonspecific but usually patients will have pain, mild swelling, and decreased range of motion of the affected joint.
- Large effusions are sometimes seen when the knee is involved.

Differential Diagnosis

Other diagnoses to consider include infection, fractures, tumors, soft tissue injuries, and exacerbation of existing joint disease.

Diagnostic Testing

Laboratories

Laboratory tests are useful only for finding an underlying cause of AVN or excluding other diseases.

Imaging

- **Radiologic evaluation plays a key role in helping make the diagnosis.** Evaluation may begin with plain radiographs, but early in the disease course these can be normal. Later findings include mild changes in bone density that progress to sclerosis and cyst formation.

- Radiographs may demonstrate a "**crescent sign**" as a result of subchondral collapse, indicating biomechanical compromise of the bone.
- Bone scans that are obtained early in the disease demonstrate a dead central area surrounded by increased activity described as the "**doughnut sign.**" With disease progression, the bone scan shows only a uniformly high level of activity. However, **bone scans are not so sensitive as MRI.**
- **MRI is the most sensitive study available** for evaluation of osteonecrosis. The earliest sign is marrow edema, later followed by marrow necrosis and cortical bone changes. Classically, the "**double-line sign**" is seen. This is a high signal intensity line within two parallel lines of decreased signal intensity on a T2-weighted MRI image.
- AVN is generally staged by plain radiographs. The staging system is used to bring uniformity to clinical trials and treatment strategies. The stages of each system are shown in Table 49-1.[3] These staging techniques are based on disease of the femoral head.

TREATMENT

The goal of therapy is to preserve the native joint for as long as possible.

Medications

- Treatment varies according to site and whether an underlying cause is found. **Cessation of the offending agent** may be beneficial.
- Pharmacologic measures are intended to allow **revascularization and bone growth.** The most common drugs used are vasodilators, lipid-lowering agents, prostacyclin analogs, anticoagulants, and bisphosphonates.[4]

Other Non-Pharmacologic Therapies

- Assisted weight-bearing modalities such as canes or crutches have proven to be unsuccessful. More than 80% of patients treated with these modalities progress to femoral head collapse by 4 years after diagnosis.
- Several other treatment modalities are under study including hyperbaric oxygen treatment, extracorporeal shock wave therapy, and various types of electrical stimulations.

Surgical Management

- Surgical modalities include:
  - "Core decompression," which decreases the intramedullary pressure.
  - Osteotomy, which helps to redistribute forces to healthy bone by moving necrotic tissues away from the areas which are weight bearing.
  - Nonvascularized bone grafting.
  - Vascularized bone grafting (to provide mesenchymal stem cells and vascular supply to necrotic tissue).
  - The purpose of bone grafts is to provide structural support to the subchondral bone and cartilage.
- For advanced cases of AVN, **total joint replacement and resurfacing arthroplasty** remains the standard treatment.

TABLE 49-1	RADIOGRAPHIC CLASSIFICATION OF OSTEONECROSIS OF THE FEMORAL HEAD

Stage	Description
Ficat and Arlet	
I	Normal
II	Sclerotic or cystic lesions, without subchondral fracture
III	Crescent sign (subchondral collapse) and/or step-off in contour of subchondral bone
IV	Osteoarthritis with decreased articular cartilage, osteophytes
University of Pennsylvania System of Staging	
I, II	First two stages are the same as Ficat and Arlet
III	Crescent sign only
IV	Step-off in contour of subchondral bone
V	Joint narrowing or acetabular changes
VI	Advanced degenerative changes Each lesion is divided into A, B, and C depending on the MRI size of the lesion (small, moderate, and large)
ARCO	
0	None
1	X-ray and CT normal; at least one other technique is positive
2	Sclerosis, osteolysis, focal porosis
3	Crescent sign and/or flattening of articular surface
4	Osteoarthritis, acetabular changes, joint destruction
Japanese Investigation Committee	
1	Demarcation line Subdivided by relationship to weight-bearing area (from medial to lateral), 1A, 1B, 1C
2	Early flattening without demarcation line around necrotic area
3	Cystic lesions Subdivided by site in the femoral head, 3A (medial), 3B (lateral)

ARCO, association research circulation osseous.

Adapted from: Mont MA, Marulanda GA, Jones LC, et al. Systemic analysis of classification systems of osteonecrosis of the femoral head. *J Bone Joint Surg Am.* 2006;88(suppl 3): 16–26.

• Young or active patients should be considered as candidates for the procedures that delay total joint arthroplasty, such as bone grafts or bone preserving operations like metal-on-metal resurfacing.

COMPLICATIONS

Complications include incomplete fractures and superimposed degenerative arthritis.

REFERENCES

1. Jones LC, Hungerford DS. Osteonecrosis: Etiology, diagnosis, and treatment. *Curr Opin Rheumatol.* 2004;16:443–449.
2. Liu YF, Chen WM, Lin YF, et al. Type II collagen gene variants and inherited osteonecrosis of the femoral head. *N Engl J Med.* 2005;352:2294–2301.
3. Mont MA, Marulanda GA, Jones LC, et al. Systemic analysis of classification systems of osteonecrosis of the femoral head. *J Bone Joint Surg Am.* 2006;88(suppl 3):16–26.
4. Lai KA, Shen WJ, Ynag CY, et al. The use of alendronate to prevent early collapse of the femoral head in patients with non traumatic osteonecrosis. A randomized clinical study. *J Bone Joint Surg Am.* 2005;87:2155–2159.

Hereditary Periodic Fever Syndromes

50

Hyon Ju Park and John P. Atkinson

- Hereditary periodic fever syndromes are rare diseases characterized by recurrent episodes of dramatic inflammation arising from **mutations of genes regulating aspects of innate immunity.**
- As opposed to autoimmune diseases, there is a lack of high-titer autoantibodies or self-reactive T cells. As a result, they are considered a subgroup of autoinflammatory diseases.[1]
- In most hereditary periodic fever syndromes clinical manifestations usually start during childhood, but diagnosis is often not made until adulthood.
- The major syndromes are:
  - Familial Mediterranean fever (FMF).
  - Tumor necrosis factor (TNF) receptor–associated periodic syndrome (TRAPS).
  - Hyperimmunoglobulinemia D with period fever syndrome (HIDS).
  - Cryopyrinopathies.

FAMILIAL MEDITERRANEAN FEVER

GENERAL PRINCIPLES

Definition

FMF is a **recessively inherited** disease characterized by recurrent attacks of fever and serositis.

Epidemiology

- FMF is the **most common hereditary periodic fever syndrome.**
- FMF is mostly found in people from around the Mediterranean basin (Jewish, Arab, Armenian, Italian, Turkish populations).
- Prevalence of FMF among Sephardic Jews is 100 to 400 per 100,000 but, like the other period fever syndromes, is highly variant depending on geographical location.

Pathophysiology

- FMF is caused by mutations in the *MEFV* gene, with more than 70 mutations that have been described.
- *MEFV* encodes the protein **pyrin that is involved in regulation of interleukin (IL)-1β processing.**
- *MEFV* is highly expressed in neutrophils, activated monocytes, synovial fibroblasts, and peritoneal fibroblasts.

DIAGNOSIS

Clinical Presentation

- Most patients experience their first clinical episode before the age of 20.
- Patients present with seemingly unprovoked episodes of **fever, serositis, mono-articular arthritis, and rash** of 1 to 3 days duration.
  - ○ Serositis involves peritoneum, pleura, and less commonly, pericardium. Repeated bouts of serositis can lead to fibrosis and formation of intra-abdominal adhesions.
  - ○ Monoarticular arthritis typically involves the knee, ankle, or hip. **Arthritis is inflammatory but nonerosive.**
  - ○ The characteristic rash described with FMF is **erysipeloid erythema,** an erythematous, sharply demarcated, tender, swollen area with a predilection for the lower extremity.[2]
- Episodes spontaneously resolve with return to baseline health between febrile episodes. The time between attacks can range from days to years.

Diagnostic Testing

Laboratories

- During attacks, acute phase reactant levels like erythrocyte sedimentation rate (ESR), C-reactive protein (CRP), fibrinogen, and serum amyloid A (SAA) are elevated.
- Genetic testing is not required in patients from high risk groups with typical symptoms who are responsive to colchicine. However, in atypical patients, genetic analysis is recommended.

TREATMENT

- Daily **colchicine** (1.2–1.8 mg/day) is the treatment of choice. Colchicine is effective in preventing acute attacks and the development of amyloidosis. If amyloidosis is already present, some recommend titrating colchicine up to decrease SAA level to 10 mg/L.
- Patients who develop febrile episodes despite daily colchicine therapy may benefit from **TNF antagonist therapy** but evidence for such therapy is anecdotal.

COMPLICATIONS

- **The most serious adverse effect of FMF is amyloidosis.** Repeated elevated levels of SAA can lead to amyloid deposition in kidneys, lungs, intestine, and adrenal glands. Prior to the use of colchicine, renal failure due to amyloidosis was the leading cause of mortality in FMF patients.
- Risk factors for amyloidosis include a family history of amyloidosis, male gender, and M694V genotype and the SAA1 alpha/alpha genotype.

HYPERIMMUNOGLOBULINEMIA D WITH PERIODIC FEVER SYNDROME

GENERAL PRINCIPLES

Definition

HIDS is an **autosomal recessive disorder** characterized by recurrent episodes of fever, rash, abdominal pain, and polyarticular arthritis.

Epidemiology

- Exact prevalence of HIDS is unknown but it is rare.
- HIDS has been described primarily in people of Dutch and northern European origin.

Pathophysiology

- HIDS is caused by mutations in *MVK,* a gene encoding **mevalonate kinase.** Currently, over 50 disease-associated mutations have been described.
- MVK is an enzyme involved in both cholesterol and nonsterol isoprene biosynthesis.
- Although the exact mechanism of disease is unknown, it is hypothesized that the overactivity of the innate immune system is due to a **deficiency in anti-inflammatory isoprenylated products or activation by excess mevalonic acid.**

DIAGNOSIS

Clinical Presentation

- The first clinical episode occurs during infancy.
- Episodes may occur twice a month during childhood but become less frequent and severe during adulthood.
- Likely triggers include **infections, trauma, menstruation, and vaccinations.**
- HIDS episodes often start with **headache and chills** followed by **abdominal pain, rash, polyarticular arthritis,** and often **cervical lymphadenopathy.**
  - ○ Abdominal pain with nausea, vomiting, and diarrhea is a common complaint. Unlike FMF, it is **not due to peritonitis** and etiology of pain is unknown.
  - ○ A wide of variety of rashes have been described with HIDS and, as a result, are nonspecific.
  - ○ Polyarticular arthritis is typically an **inflammatory, symmetric arthritis that involves large joints like the hips and knees.**
  - ○ Although children may get diffuse lymphadenopathy, adults tend to develop only cervical lymphadenopathy.
- Amyloidosis is a rare complication of HIDS.

Diagnostic Testing

Laboratories
- Like other periodic fever syndromes, acute phase reactants are elevated during attacks.

- **Elevated urinary mevalonic acid** levels during attacks are pathognomonic of HIDS.
- Diagnosis of HIDS can be made on the basis of elevated urinary levels of mevalonic acid during attacks or in patients with a typical history, a finding of two mutations in *MVK* on genetic testing.
- Although **elevated serum levels of IgD** are seen in 85% to 90% of patients, levels do not correlate with severity or frequency of attacks.
- Elevated serum levels of IgA are observed in 80% of patients.

TREATMENT

- **Treatment is mainly supportive.** Colchicine, corticosteroids, and nonsteroidal antiinflammatory drugs (NSAIDs) fail to abort acute attacks.
- HMG-CoA reductase is an enzyme preceding MVK and, if the excess mevalonic acid is contributing to the pathogenesis of HIDS, **HMG-CoA reductase inhibitors might be beneficial.** A double-blinded randomized controlled trial of six patients with HIDS treated with simvastatin 80 mg/day demonstrated a decrease in urinary mevalonic acid in all the six patients along with significantly fewer febrile days in five of the six patients.[3]

TNF RECEPTOR–ASSOCIATED PERIODIC SYNDROME

GENERAL PRINCIPLES

Definition

TRAPS, previously known as familial Hibernian fever and benign autosomal-dominant familial periodic fever, is an **autosomal-dominant** disease characterized by recurrent episodes of fever, migratory rash, and ocular findings.

Epidemiology

- Prevalence is unknown but is thought to be the second most common hereditary periodic fever syndrome.
- Although TRAPS was initially described in people of Irish and Scottish descent, there is no ethnic predilection.

Pathophysiology

- TRAPS is caused by mutations in *TNFRSF1A,* a gene encoding the p55 receptor for TNF. Currently, over 50 disease causing mutations have been found.
- Initial studies suggested that pathogenesis occurred by sustained TNF stimulation of target cells by the **impaired shedding of the p55 component.** Recent data suggests that the **intracellular retention of misfolded p55** receptor may be contributing to the inflammatory response.[4]

DIAGNOSIS

Clinical Presentation
- The first clinical episode occurs during childhood or adolescence.
- **Febrile episodes with a distinctive migratory rash and myalgia, ocular involvement, and serositis** last anywhere from 1 to 6 weeks.
  - The migratory rash associated with TRAPS is distinctive. It is an erythematous macule associated with a significant amount of soft tissue swelling and myalgias of the muscles underlying the skin. The rash typically starts on the trunk or proximal limbs and migrates distally.
  - Ocular involvement seen in TRAPS consists of periorbital edema and conjunctivitis. Uveitis is not seen.
  - Serositis can involve pleura, peritoneum, and pericardium but is typically less severe than seen in FMF.
- **Amyloidosis** occurs in about 15% of TRAPS patients. It is unknown whether long-term treatment prevents amyloidosis.

Diagnostic Testing
Laboratories
- Acute phase reactants are elevated during attacks.
- Diagnosis is confirmed by the presence of a *TNFRSF1A* mutation known to cause disease.

Imaging
MRI of areas with the typical TRAPS rash demonstrates **panniculitis and fasciitis** of the underlying muscles; myositis is not seen.

TREATMENT

- **NSAIDs** can be used in mild episodes.
- **Corticosteroids** are used for more severe attacks. However, the dose of corticosteroids necessary to abort attacks escalates during the course of the illness.
- Small prospective trials have demonstrated partial efficacy of **etanercept** in both preventing attacks and aborting them.
- **IL-1 receptor antagonists** have been used successfully to both prevent and abort attacks in patients who have failed etanercept.[5]

CRYOPYRINOPATHIES

GENERAL PRINCIPLES

- Cryopyrinopathies (cryopyrin-associated periodic syndromes, CAPS) are rare diseases caused by **dominantly inherited** mutations in *CIAS1* (also known as *NLRP3*), a gene encoding **cryopyrin** (also known as NAPL3).
- Familial cold autoinflammatory syndrome (FCAS), Muckle–Wells syndrome, and neonatal onset multisystem inflammatory disease (NOMID; also known as chronic infantile neurologic cutaneous and articular syndrome [CINCA]) are a

spectrum of diseases caused by *CIAS1* mutations. NOMID/CINCA is the most severe and FCAS is the mildest.[6]

- Cryopyrin is part of a macromolecular complex called "**inflammasome**," which activates an enzyme that cleaves IL-1β to its active form.
- The mutations in *CIAS1* result in **elevated IL-1β level at baseline or in response to certain triggers.**

DIAGNOSIS

Clinical Presentation

Familial Cold Autoinflammatory Syndrome

- About 150 cases have been reported in the United States.
- Symptoms typically develop in childhood.
- Patients develop attacks of fever, pruritic, and painful rash, and limb pain which is sometimes accompanied by abdominal pain and conjunctivitis.
- Attacks occur reliably 1 to 2 hours after generalized cold exposure.

Muckle–Wells Syndrome

- Symptoms develop in childhood.
- Like FCAS, patients develop attacks of fever, rash (urticaria), abdominal pain, and conjunctivitis. Unlike FCAS, patients do not have attacks reliably after generalized cold exposure and avoidance of cold exposure does not prevent attacks.
- Patients with Muckle–Wells syndrome develop progressive sensorineural deafness that can be reversible with treatment.
- 25% of patients may develop systemic amyloidosis.

Neonatal Onset Multisystem Inflammatory Disease

- Febrile episodes start during infancy but then start to become more chronic than recurrent acute episodes.
- Along with fevers, rash, and sensorineural hearing loss, patients develop uveitis, disabling arthropathy due to overgrowth of the patella and epiphyses of long bones, and chronic aseptic meningitis with cerebral atrophy and mental retardation.
- 25% of patients may develop systemic amyloidosis.

TREATMENT

All the three cryopyrinopathies show a dramatic clinical and laboratory response (including the amyloidosis) to treatment with **IL-1 inhibitors** including anakinra (IL-1 receptor antagonist), rilonacept (IL-1 Trap, a fusion protein of the extracellular domain of the IL-1 receptor and the Fc region of IgG), and canakinumab (monoclonal antibody against IL-1β).[7]

REFERENCES

1. Masters SL, Simon A, Aksentijevich I, et al. Horror autoinflammaticus: The molecular pathophysiology of autoinflammatory disease. *Annu Rev Immunol.* 2009;27:621–668.
2. Goldfinger S. The inherited autoinflammatory syndrome: A decade of discovery. *Trans Am Clin Climatol Assoc.* 2009;120:413–418.

3. Simon A, Drewe E, van der Meer JW, et al. Simvastatin treatment for inflammatory attacks of the hyperimmunoglobulinemia D and periodic fever syndrome. *Clin Pharmacol Ther.* 2004;75:476–483.

4. Kimberley FC, Lobito AA, Siegel RM, et al. Falling into TRAPS-receptor misfolding in the TNF receptor 1-associated periodic fever syndrome. *Arthritis Res Ther.* 2007;9:217–225.

5. Jacobelli S, Andre M, Alexandra JF, et al. Failure of anti-TNF therapy in TNF receptor 1-associated periodic syndrome (TRAPS). *Rheumatology (Oxford).* 2007;46:1211–1212.

6. Hoffman HM, Wanderer AA. Inflammasome and IL-1 beta mediated disorders. *Curr Allergy Asthma Rep.* 2010;10:229–235.

7. Neven B, Marvillet I, Terrada C, et al. Long-term efficacy of the interleukin-1 receptor antagonist anakinra in ten patients with neonatal-onset multisystem inflammatory disease/chronic infantile neurologic cutaneous articular syndrome. *Arthritis Rheum.* 2010;62:258–267.

Index

Note: Page locators followed by f and t indicates figure and table respectively.